ABORTION AND THE STATUS OF THE FETUS

PHILOSOPHY AND MEDICINE

Editors:

H. TRISTRAM ENGELHARDT, JR.

Center for Ethics, Medicine, and Public Issues, Baylor College of Medicine, Houston, Texas, U.S.A.

STUART F. SPICKER

University of Connecticut Health Center, Farmington, Connecticut, and the National Science Foundation, Washington, D.C., U.S.A.

VOLUME 13

ABORTION AND THE STATUS OF THE FETUS

Edited by

WILLIAM B. BONDESON

University of Missouri-Columbia, School of Medicine, Columbia, Missouri

H. TRISTRAM ENGELHARDT, JR.

Center for Ethics, Medicine, and Public Issues, Baylor College of Medicine, Houston, Texas

STUART F. SPICKER

University of Connecticut Health Center, Farmington, Connecticut, and the National Science Foundation, Washington, D.C.

and

DANIEL H. WINSHIP

University of Missouri-Columbia, School of Medicine, Columbia, Missouri

D. REIDEL PUBLISHING COMPANY

A MEMBER OF THE KLUWER ACADEMIC PUBLISHERS GROUP

DORDRECHT / BOSTON / LANCASTER

Library of Congress Cataloging in Publication Data
Main entry under title:

Abortion and the status of the fetus.

   (Philosophy and medicine; v. 13)
   "This volume grew out of a symposium, 'The Concept of person and
its implications for the use of the fetus in biomedicine', held October 29,
30, and 31, 1980, at the Health Science Center of the University of
Missouri–Columbia under the sponsorship of the Departments of Medicine
and Philosophy, and the Program in Health Care and Human Values" –
Editorial pref.
   Includes bibliographies and index.
   1.   Abortion–Moral and ethical aspects–Congresses.   2.   Fetus–
Research–Moral and ethical aspects–Congresses.   I.   Bondeson, William
B., 1938–   .   II.   University of Missouri–Columbia. Dept. of Medicine.
III.   University of Missouri–Columbia. Dept. of Philosophy.   IV.   Series.
HQ767.3.A255   1983   179'76   83-9506
ISBN 90-277-1493-2

Published by D. Reidel Publishing Company,
P.O. Box 17, 3300 AA Dordrecht, Holland.

Sold and distributed in the U.S.A. and Canada
by Kluwer Boston Inc.,
190 Old Derby Street, Hingham, MA 02043, U.S.A.

In all other countries, sold and distributed
by Kluwer Academic Publishers Group,
P.O. Box 322, 3300 AH Dordrecht, Holland.

Printed in The Netherlands.

TABLE OF CONTENTS

EDITORIAL PREFACE

The topic of abortion is, in our culture, a troubling one. It excites strong passions, which have provided the impetus for political movements. This is undoubtedly the case in great proportion due to the interest of many of the Christian religions, as well as the interest of many Jews, in abortion as a sinful act. The tone of much of the concern regarding abortion and the proper use of the genitals might in fact suggest to the uninformed that Christianity was more interested in sexual truancy than in feeding the poor, the Gospels notwithstanding. However, abortion and contraception are no longer issues unconnected with feeding the poor. The ability in general to control population growth, and the ability of lower income families in particular to limit the number of children they will have, bear directly upon the amount of food available for the poor. The issue of abortion thus arises against the background of concerns to enable those in marginal economic situations to improve their positions when contraception fails or when adequate contraception or contraceptive information is not available.

Moreover, abortion has a special place as an element of women's taking possession of themselves. Humans generally have through technology been increasing their control over their own condition. Nature, which was before often alien and uncontrolled, has come ever more under the control of persons. One might think here of interventions from dams to vaccinations. However, abortion is of special moral interest as an element of rendering the body responsive to goals chosen by persons. Hence, it is in a special sense an element of the liberation of women, an emancipation from the other, blind, uncaring, biological forces of reproduction. Abortion allows individuals not only to control the number and spacing of children, but to ensure the quality of children through prenatal diagnosis. Abortion, then, is not just an issue of the status of the fetus, but of the status of persons and of women in particular. It is a part of increasing the capacity of persons to chart their own destinies without the unchosen intrusions of nature.

Given all the goods that flow from the availability of abortions, one might wonder whence the hesitations surrounding its use arise. Surely there are reasons for showing concern regarding any invasive surgical procedure. Further, there is disquietude aroused by a technology that allows greater control of reproduction and therefore brings greater responsibility to persons. The more human reproduction is in the control of persons, the more what could in the past be accepted as the will of God, must now be shouldered as an element of the responsibility of persons. Responsibility is always troublesome. If one continues with a pregnancy, defective or otherwise, it is now one's responsibility for having done so. One could have had it otherwise. As a consequence, we are forced to reflect on which pregnancies ought to go to term and which not, and under what circumstances. However, the central source of moral hesitation turns on the status of the fetus itself.

Exploring the status of the fetus is, as this volume indicates, of one fabric with the more general philosophical endeavor of assaying the significance of being a human or being a person. As we persons come to gain greater control over our human nature, that nature is rendered an object for our manipulation and therefore becomes the singular vehicle for our own self-creation. A line is presupposed between that life which is human and that which is also personal. As we declare brain-dead but otherwise alive humans dead, we draw a line between human biological and human personal life. Understanding the status of human fetal life will thus be a part of better understanding the distinctions we must discern among life in general, human biological life, and the life of persons. Analyses such as these will help to clarify language and concepts recruited for service in political and religious disputes. They may help as well to quell some unwarranted concerns. They will, however, surely contribute to the endeavor of better understanding the place and predicament of persons in the world. This volume is offered as a contribution to the better understanding of both abortion and the status of the fetus. As such, it is also meant as a contribution to the development of our understanding of what it means to be a person.

This volume grew out of a symposium, "The Concept of Person and Its Implications for the Use of the Fetus in Biomedicine", held October 29, 30, and 31, 1980, at the Health Science Center of the University of Missouri– Columbia under the sponsorship of the Departments of Medicine and Philosophy, and the Program in Health Care and Human Values. We are very grateful for the support of the National Endowment for the Humanities through grant number RD–20017–80–1305, the Education and Research Foundation of the American Medical Association, the Graduate School of the University of Missouri at Columbia, and D. Reidel Publishing Company. In addition, the Extension Division of the University of Missouri–Columbia gave important aid for which we are very thankful. Most, but not all, of the presentations made at that conference are found here. Those here have developed, some in major ways, since the conference was held. In addition, four essays have been added.

Much labor, from many individuals, has made this volume possible. Here we can mention only a few of those who contributed generously in time, effort, and insight: Guilio Barbero, M.D.; Jane Backlund; Gladys Courtney, R.N., Ph.D.; Sandra Davenport, M.D.; S.G.M. Engelhardt; Mary Ann Gardell; Charles Lobeck, M.D.; Allen E. Smith; J.D., and Lynn F. Thomas. We wish as well to thank those who attended this conference and whose ideas contributed in various ways to refashioning these essays into the present volume. We wish to thank them in addition for having demonstrated that these issues, which often incite unruly quarrels, can be the subject of serious investigation by individuals dedicated to the exploration of the concepts that frame our moral lives and our cultural expectations.

This volume appears after major legal changes in the area of reproductive liberties. It has only been a decade since the right to abortion on request was recognized in *Roe v. Wade* (410 U.S. 113 [1973]) and *Doe v. Bolton* (410 U.S. 179 [1973]), and not yet two decades since similar rights regarding contraception were protected by the Supreme Court in *Griswold v. Connecticut* (381 U.S. 479 [1965]). This is a very short period of time. Not yet a generation has passed since these rights to the control of one's own reproductive destinies were acknowledged. Yet in this time there has been a rather widespread use of these prerogatives. We are entering a period in which individuals take for granted their control over when and under what circumstances they will have children. A reproductive ethos is evolving based on the easy availability of contraception and abortion. Abortion and contraception will soon, if they do not already, frame our everyday understanding of ourselves as sexual beings. This volume offers a sketch of the conceptual presuppositions, shifts, and tensions that underlie this major development.

January 22, 1983
WILLIAM B. BONDESON
H. TRISTRAM ENGELHARDT, JR.
STUART F. SPICKER
DANIEL H. WINSHIP

H. TRISTRAM ENGELHARDT, JR.

INTRODUCTION

The issue of abortion is in part so intractable because it is not one issue, but many. It is many issues because it involves diverse goals and clusters of rights. It is complex also because it is problematic on various levels: religious, metaphysical, and what one might term a secular, ethical level. Considered only in terms of philosophical issues, it has evoked an immense and diverse literature, which can only be indicated via an arbitrary selection.[1] This volume addresses the issue of abortion by examining the status of the fetus with a secular, ethical framework. In so doing, it confronts many issues besides abortion: *in vitro* fertilization with and without embryo transfer, fetal experimentation, the rights of women, and the significance of sexuality. Abortion, here, serves as the titular focus for these other concerns with the fetus. They are problematic for many of the same reasons that abortion is. Abortion, as fetal research or *in vitro* fertilization, raises questions both ontological (e.g., concerning the nature of fetuses and of persons) and ethical (e.g., about the proper treatment of fetuses and persons). It forces us to clarify our views regarding what it means to be a person, in contrast to being a human. It forces us as well to clarify our views concerning the values at stake in human life and reproduction. Since the ontological theme (i.e., What does it mean to be human or a person?) is key to many of the issues raised by biomedical interventions involving the fetus, it is one of the central leitmotifs of this volume.

The debate concerning abortion in America and in Europe is occurring in pluralist, secular societies. As a consequence, the debate appears on two levels. On one level it involves discussions within particular communities sharing moral and metaphysical convictions. One might think here of debates regarding abortion within Roman Catholicism or within Judaism.[2] However, it is also sustained on the level of a public policy debate fashioned in secular terms. Because on this level many common ethical and metaphysical suggestions cannot be presupposed, the debate forces all who wish to participate to look for general grounds for agreement. As a consequence, much that one might hold with certainty within one's own community of faith cannot be presumed to hold as part of the general moral fabric of a pluralist society. This is disturbing for it condemns individuals who wish to live peaceably in a

xi

William B. Bondeson et al. *(eds.), Abortion and the Status of the Fetus*, xi–xxxii.
Copyright © 1983 *by D. Reidel Publishing Company, Dordrecht, Holland.*

secular, pluralist society to conduct their lives within two disparate contexts: that of their particular moral community and that of the general secular society. There will unavoidably be a tension between these levels. Moreover, if the state is not to take sides with one particular community against others, one will need to establish the extent to which common rational considerations can support one moral or ontological approach. In doing so one will be exploring and developing this secular level of moral discourse. This volume is a part of that endeavor. It is an attempt to see the extent to which moral and metaphysical convictions regarding abortion and the status of the fetus can be established in a secular, pluralist society. Where this volume does not support the moral views of a reader's particular ethical viewpoint, he or she is encouraged to see this not as a rejection of that viewpoint, but rather as an indication that such a viewpoint is not likely to be established as an element of the moral web of a peaceable, pluralist society.

This volume is offered as a step towards reassessing the significance of human life. Even theological reflections suggest the difference between being a human and being a person. Not all persons are humans. The persons of the Holy Trinity, as well as angels, are persons, too. The recognition of evolution and the possibility of life on other worlds suggests that, in addition, embodied moral agents may have developed on other worlds. For that matter, there is speculation that some linguistically competent chimpanzees should count as persons [25]. In any event, there is the possibility that a large proportion of the persons in this universe are not humans. On the other hand, recent definitions of death and the apparent status of the fetus have suggested that some humans may not be persons ([12], [13]).

This point can be seen by examining the force of the definition of death. The development of the brain-oriented definitions of death can be interpreted as the acquisition of a rather straightforward ontological conviction: when there is no longer the possibility of sapient action in the world, one is no longer in the world. This point can be extended to human ontogeny. It would appear that before one is sapient, one is not *yet* in the world. Or more simply, one is not yet in existence. The distinction between human biological and human personal life which these realizations presuppose can be put more graphically by way of an illustrative parable. Consider, for example, being confronted by a neurologist's diagnosis that one has a disease that will destroy one's entire brain, but that the powers of modern science will allow one to live a normal lifespan. A reasonable response would be that it would not just be senseless to continue living under such circumstances, but that one would not in fact be *there* as the supposed beneficiary. One would no longer exist.

This parable can lead further. The neurologist can revise the initial diagnosis and say that at least the lower parts of the brain, such as the medula, pons, and cerebellum (which are involved in reflexes, posturing, and complex motions), can be preserved. However, the higher brain associated with consciousness will be destroyed. If one still concluded that not only would it be senseless to preserve one's life under those circumstances, but that one would not in fact 'be' there, one has then taken firm possession of the notion of drawing a line between human biological and human personal life.

Such a set of considerations will, however, argue for a neocortically oriented, not simply a whole-brain oriented, definition of death. Since all tests have risks of both false positive and false negative determinations, one may still accept a whole-brain oriented definition of death. One may be willing to act as if certain dead individuals are alive in order to avoid the risks of false positive determinations, though conceptually one holds a neocortically oriented definition of death to be correct. Such concerns regarding false positive determinations of death may account in part, at least, for the reason why individuals such as Karen Quinlan are not declared dead [21]. Though it would be very difficult to hold that there is any person such as Karen Quinlan still existing in the world, one might still be reluctant to establish canons for a definition of death that would allow her to be declared dead, because one has an interest in avoiding criteria for the declaration of death with unproven risks of false positive determinations of death. Further, one would need to consider the emotional trauma involved in disposing of a living body, even though it is no longer the body of a person. We persons treat with respect many objects in the world that are not persons. For all these reasons one might then be willing to declare individuals dead only when easily determinable, necessary conditions for the possibility of persons being in the world are absent, even when it might be fairly certain that all of the sufficient conditions for being present in the world have not been fulfilled. This consideration should remind us why the presence of EEG activity in a fetus does not indicate the presence of a person, though the absence of these findings may indicate the absence (i.e., death) of a person. There is a difference between necessary and sufficient conditions for persons being present. It should also suggest why entities that are not persons strictly are treated as if they are persons strictly. Here one might think not only of the ways in which infants, but also the severely mentally retarded, and the senile, are treated with respect as if they were persons in the strict sense, though they can be the bearers only of rights, not of duties. In short, examining the distinction between human biological and human personal life will disclose further ontological complexities including the fact that we employ more than one concept of person in our moral practices.

In drawing a line between human biological and human personal life, one is presupposing a concept of person. The concept of person is, one should note, not simply biological. One can see this when one considers what would be involved, for example, in asking whether an intelligent being from another planet is a person. One would be asking how to identify beings who are morally equivalent to us: we who write books on philosophy or read them. Persons are important in moral discourse because they are the origin of moral questions and answers. They are in the end the moral judges of the significance of the universe. One might think here, for example, of John Rawls's characterization of persons:

Moral persons are distinguished by two features: first, they are capable of having (and are assumed to have) a conception of their good (as expressed by a rational plan of life); and second, they are capable of having (and are assumed to acquire) a sense of justice, a normally effective desire to apply and act upon the principles of justice, at least to a certain minimal degree. We use the characterization of the person in the original position to single out the kind of beings to whom the principles chosen apply ([29], p. 505).

This is a point that has been made clearly since Kant: persons are the sustainers of the world of moral concerns, and they are rational, self-determining entities ([23], p. 448). What we will count as persons will need to possess at least the capacity to reason, to choose freely, to have interest in goods, and to have the capacity to be concerned about the nature of proper conduct.

This sense of person stands out if one considers the minimum notion of ethics. Though it may be very difficult to establish by reason alone the correctness of one particular, concrete view of the good life, still, the very enterprise of resolving moral disputes by reasons and peaceably forwarded considerations, not force, presupposes mutual respect among the participants in such disputes. Only moral agents can be participants in such disputes. They must be respected as a condition for the possibility of ethics as an alternative to force, before and beyond any ability to discover or create a particular view of the good life. Killing, imprisoning or hurting innocent moral agents, as a result, count as paradigm evil acts, whether or not the beings are human. The relevant ontological concept of person is thus found through an inquiry as to the nature of the beings who would ground the very possibility of moral interests.

These considerations have application at the beginning of human life.

Though it is usually possible to speak of what one did at the age of six, it requires use of metaphor to speak of what one did at, say, the age of one month. We were not there, much less doing something. There was surely an organism present from which we would come. But we, as moral agents, as the person known to ourselves and others, did not yet exist. It is only later that we appeared and united in a stream of memories and actions the enterprises which are our lives. Early in human development, there is in fact less of 'someone' there, than in the case of adult non-human mammals. This would suggest that treating infants as persons is a conservative compromise, between restricting abortions and allowing infanticide — somewhat like employing whole brain oriented definitions of death rather than neo-cortically oriented definitions. Yet in the case of possible death, one can know for certain that there at least had been a person. One is concerned about mistakenly declaring that person dead. In the case of the one-month-old infant, however, there is no evidence that a person in a strict sense is present. The organism shows none of the mental capacities of a mature non-human primate.

Zygotes, embryos, and fetuses, like brain-dead but otherwise alive human beings, give no evidence of being persons. Nor will it help to say they are potential persons. Y's that are potential X's are *a fortiori* not X's. If fetuses are to be treated with respect greater than that accorded to non-human animals of similar development, it will be because of the value of such a practice, not because of the intrinsic value they possess (at least insofar as general, secular arguments are concerned). One will have to determine whether the competing moral issues at stake in abortion are in any fashion similar to those that would allow (or forbid) infanticide of children up to a week of age — one might think here of the issues that Richard Feen raises in his essay reporting the practice of infanticide employed by our antecedents in classical Greece and Rome.

The distinction between being a human and being a person, which these considerations presuppose, should not appear arbitrary. Being a human is a biological designation. It indicates membership in the genus *homo*, or perhaps more narrowly in the species *homo sapiens*. What is of prime moral interest is not species membership, as the above indicates, but whether an entity is in fact a person. (However, as one should note, some moral objects, which are not subjects, are of great significance — consider the moral regard of non-human animals.) The distinction between those stages in human development that involve the life of a person, and those that do not, is not unprecedented. St. Thomas Aquinas, and the Roman Catholic Church until recently, distinguished between the morality of early and late abortion on the grounds that early abortion did not involve taking the life of a person.[3] In this, the medieval church was influenced by Aristotle's view that the animal soul appears only after conception, forty days after for males and ninety days after for females (*Historia Animalium*, 7.3. 583b). The Old Testament, on the other hand, appears to presuppose that only at birth need killing a human be regarded with the same seriousness as killing an adult person.[4]

In the Middle Ages, these issues were as much discussed around concerns for setting the date for the Feast of the Immaculate Conception of the Virgin Mary as they were with regard to the question of abortion. Because the birthday of the Blessed Virgin had already been established as September 8, the controversy concerning the point at which the soul entered had direct relevance for the disputes regarding the proper date for celebrating the Immaculate Conception. St. Thomas Aquinas's reflections concerning the appearance of the soul after physical conception had implications as well for the significance of the doctrine of the Immaculate Conception. As one commentator notes, "The fetus, being not yet animated by a spiritual soul, could not be a subject of grace — or of sin either, for that matter . . . Before the creation of Mary's soul, that which was to become her body shared the common life; but before the creation of her soul, *Mary* did not yet exist" ([27], p. 333). That is, according to St. Thomas, there was a developing embryo that was to become the body of Mary. Because of these and other controversies, the date of the Immaculate Conception varied from December 8 to the first week in May ([2], pp. 125–126), until in 1708, Pope Clement IX set the date as December 8, as an observance for the whole church.[5] This decision was fateful because it suggested that Mary's conception as a person occurred nine months prior to her birth and presupposed the doctrine of immediate animation.[6] This decision undermined as well the distinction presumed by St. Thomas and the others between the pre-personal and personal life of the fetus. Finally, Pope Pius IX, who proclaimed the doctrine of the Immaculate Conception in 1854, in the Bull "Ineffabilis Deus" held that Mary was free from original sin "from the first instant of her conception" ("in primo instanti suae conceptionis") ([9], p. 562). It was Pope Pius IX who then in 1869 removed from Canon Law the distinction between the abortion of an ensouled versus an unensouled fetus.[7] It is ironic that these changes in canon law were made just as biology was establishing a developmental view of embryology which could have sympathetically construed St. Thomas Aquinas's stage-wise account of fetal development. Indeed, the evolutionary perspective fostered by Charles Darwin and Alfred Russel Wallace's publication of *The Origin of Species* in 1859 suggested that early stages of the fetus should be seen as more equivalent to prior evolutionary stages [19].

The 18th and 19th centuries were also marked by radical changes in the understanding of the authority of the state, which changes would in the 20th century have implications regarding the morality of proscribing abortion. Americans in 1776 and the French in 1789 attempted to fashion nations founded not on a particular religious authority, but on the rights of free individuals. Though the American government in its Declaration of Independence spoke of men being endowed by their Creator with certain inalienable rights, the First Amendment to the Constitution of 1787 both established the right to the free exercise of religion and prohibited the establishment of religion. In so doing, it anticipated the fact that Western governments would, save for a few residual ceremonies, conduct themselves in ways that did not require appeals to a divine authority. In the American experience, this understanding of government became explicit in the Texas Declaration of Independence of March 2, 1836, which spoke of inalienable rights, but did not appeal to a deity for their foundation ([41], pp. 98–99). In this, the Texans resembled the Virginians, who in their 1776 Declaration of Rights appealed to Nature, not to God.[8]

To ground rights, the Texians appealed to the notion of a peaceable community of persons. Thus, the Declaration of Rights of the Constitution of the Republic of Texas (17 March, 1836) states simply, "First. All men, when they form a social contract, have equal rights ... " and "Second. All political power is inherent in the people and all free governments are founded on their authority and instituted for their benefit; and they have at all times an inalienable right to alter their government in such manner as they think proper" ([41], p. 105). As a consequence of this shift, the Texas government retreated from many of the views of other Anglo-American jurisdictions, which saw themselves with an authority to enforce good public morals, even when these depended on a particular religious view of proper conduct. An example is found in the original Texas refusal, now reversed, not to hold aiding and abetting suicide to be a criminal act, despite what offense to morals such actions might cause.[9]

One sees, in short, the crumbling of what one might term the monotheistic presumption: that there is in fact *a* concrete view of the good life that can be rationally discovered, and that a government would therefore have the right to impose a particular view of the good moral life upon the private conduct of its citizens. As a result of the Enlightenment and its removal of the deity of any particular religion as authority-giver of the state, and the Enlightenment's subsequent failure to discover through reason a convincing view of the good life, the state was left only with the moral obligation of protecting the negative freedoms of individuals (e.g., not to be touched without their consent) and of creating refusable rights to welfare. Here one might think of the passage in Hegel's *Philosophy of Right* that speaks of civil servants as the universal class, individuals who will with equal reliability (or non-partisan unreliability) protect the civil rights of Christians and Jews alike (*Philosophy of Right,* # 197). With these developments the state is reconceived within a post-Enlightenment, post-Christian context in which justifiable intrusions into the private lives of citizens in order to enforce particular views of the good life are ever less plausible. Consider the example of the states of the United States which forbid oral intercourse, even between married partners. These are at best now seen as the vestiges of a time when the state could reasonably view itself as the custodian of a particular view of the good moral life of private citizens. Given these changes, the rights and duties to be enforced by the state become those that are integral to having a free, peaceable community, or which are created by common consent as entitlements to refuseable welfare rights.

Undoubtedly, we are still in the midst of coming to terms with these conceptual shifts. They are shifts, if rightly understood, that return to us what might be termed a polytheistic presumption, namely, that there are likely to be various competing views of the good life, many of which cannot be excluded as improper on the basis of reason alone. Thus, the nation-state ceases to be one moral community in the sense of being committed to one concrete view of the good moral life. It becomes instead a peaceable fabric embracing a wide range of communities: Catholics, Protestants, Hindus, Buddhists, atheists, heterosexuals, and homosexuals. It becomes like the Roman Empire, which tolerated the peaceable worship of a wide range of gods and goddesses. In this context, the decision in *Roe v. Wade* [30] is quite understandable: acknowledging a fetus to be a person in a strict sense would require a commitment to a particular metaphysical or religious viewpoint. The state may not choose one such viewpoint to enforce. It can at best create practices to protect some of the goods at stake in fetal life, as long as these do not collide with the rights of individuals who form the compacts that constitute free governments (e.g., competent women).

It is no secret that this state of affairs is found by many to be vexatious. They are far from accepting the notion that life in a pluralist secular society will require a two-tier morality: one tier in which one will be able to live out one's commitment to a particular community of beliefs (e.g., as a Roman Catholic, a Hassidic Jew, or a Southern Baptist), and a second tier in which public policy will be fashioned for a nation state, and in which one will need to find ethical principles that appeal generally to individuals apart from their commitment to a particular community of religious or meta-physical beliefs. If one fails to make this distinction, one will run the risk of the state's imposing a particular moral or metaphysical viewpoint to the prejudice of other viewpoints. Such a circumstance would return the state to a pre-Enlightenment position of wielding inquisitorial powers in the regulation of the private lives of citizens. It is no accident that attempts to proscribe abortion through constitutional amendment by removing cases involving the proscription of abortion from review by federal courts [33], or by defining fetal life as human life [32] should also be forwarded by individuals interested in allowing prayer in public school. One must realize that the purchase price of a government which is party to no *particular* religious or metaphysical viewpoint, and therefore able to embrace peaceably communities with widely divergent views of how citizens should live their private lives, requires forgoing the temptation to impose by state force one's own view of proper private morality. A peaceable pluralist society can be achieved only at the price of toleration. One will need to be content with converting others by witness rather than constraining conformity through force.

Fashioning public policy with regard to abortion will require assessing how much secular human reasoning can conclude regarding the morality of abortion and what limits exist upon the state's authority to forbid abortion. The essays in this volume are offered as helpful voices in such public policy discussions. To this end, this volume sketches the conceptual issues regarding abortion and the use of the fetus, especially as these turn on the status of the fetus. The volume opens with a review of ethical and public policy discussions concerning the status of the fetus. First, Thomas Shannon examines the range of attitudes regarding abortion, as well as difficulties involved in moving from private moral viewpoints to public policies. In doing so, he offers an overview of the evolution of abortion legislation from the 19th to 20th centuries in America. As LeRoy Walters indicates, attempts to forge public policy from private moral viewpoints regarding abortion have had, since *Roe v. Wade* [30], a peculiar character. On the one hand, it has been established at law that fetuses are not persons, while on the other hand policymakers controlling the use of federal funds for fetal experimentation or *in vitro* fertilization have proposed guidelines to protect and support a special moral regard for the fetus or early embryo in federally funded research.[10] As a point of public policy, this can be usefully rationalized as the difference between recognizing the proper limits on the law's prerogative to constrain the free choices of persons (e.g., here, pregnant women seeking abortions), and the right of the state to set special restrictions on the use of tax monies in areas where there is significant moral disagreement (i.e., where some groups in fact hold fetuses to be persons). After all, the recommendations of the National Commission and the Ethics Advisory Board of the Department of Health, Education, and Welfare, were not made in order to forbid either fetal research or *in vitro* fertilization and embryo transfer. They were developed simply as restrictions on those activities in institutions receiving federal funds.

John Biggers, in his article, offers a sketch of the history of views regarding the development of fetuses and an exploration of current scientific findings in the matter. Of most interest are the data he cites with regard to the high loss of early embryos in natural gestation, a point that he also raised in an earlier paper presented to the Ethics Advisory Board [1]; Nearly two-thirds of all zygotes never implant. It becomes difficult, then, as a public policy matter to treat such as persons. In fact, since the great proportion of the early embryos lost possess serious genetic abnormalities (e.g., trisomies), one may be tempted to see the practice of amniocentesis and selective abortion as simply the enterprise of completing a general project of nature to eliminate severely deformed fetuses. As George Agich suggests, in agreement with Walters and Biggers, one finds an intermixing of empirical, ethical, and public policy issues framing the development of the controversies regarding the fetus over the last decade.

In discussing current and possible future research involving human embryos, the late Pierre Soupart completes this volume's background sketch of the empirical issues underlying the debate concerning abortion and the use of *in vitro* fertilization. He also underscores the large amount of natural wastage of embryos in normal gestation in order to suggest that there is not a difference in kind between the risks to the embryo in normal gestation versus *in vitro* fertilization. By developing a sketch of the avenues that are currently open, or will in the future be open to exploration through *in vitro* fertilization, he places the moral issues raised by the use of the fetus within a larger framework. Where abortion in many cases involves only the interest of a particular woman, research with early embryos offers possible benefits, as Soupart indicates, to society generally, through the development of better contraception, the better understanding and treatment of infertility, and the better control of cancers such as choriocarcinomas. Besides these goals of a more immediate social nature, such research could as well give insight into man's evolutionary origin by comparing the compatibility of gametes from human and other higher primates. Finally, *in vitro* fertilization could be used for genetic screening and determining the sex of the human embryo.

In addition to his sketch of the techological promises of *in vitro* fertilization, Soupart offers material for a revealing thought experiment with respect to the extent to which being a human should count as a sufficient or necessary condition for being a person. In exploring the possibility of uniting gametes from humans and gorillas to form a hybrid, he raises the question of how the product of such a union should be regarded. If such were indeed self-conscious moral agents, they would likely plead their case before the law and the conscience of other persons to be recognized as "reasonable creatures in being, and under the King's peace", to take a line from Sir Edward Coke's *Institutes* (3 *Institutes* 47).

The three essays that follow outline the development of the concept of personhood in the law and its relationship to the standing of the fetus. As the essays by Leonard Glantz and Patricia White show, the law has developed notions of person to answer particular questions, and has avoided general, precise definitions. The history of the law suggests that one may bewitch oneself with the fact that there is only one word, person, though many concepts. Glantz outlines the vagaries of Anglo-American law in its determination of the point at which fetuses should be regarded as persons. As he shows, though courts have held that fetuses *in utero* are not persons, there has been much dispute about the extent to which a fetus needs to be totally separated from the mother in order to have standing as a person in criminal law. Defenses against manslaughter or homicide have turned on the extent to which a fetus has been totally expelled, drawn an independent breath, or had the umbilical cord severed. However, the courts did not examine in criminal, or for that matter in civil cases the notion of personhood itself, as a general philosophical idea. Concepts of personhood were, however, presupposed. In criminal law the question was the point at which prosecution for homicide could be initiated. Abortion was not considered an act of homicide. In civil cases the issue was under what circumstances a fetus could, should it survive, collect for damages done *in utero*. As Margery Shaw indicates in her commentary, these interests of the court have within the last few decades been joined to new grounds for suit, such as those on the basis of an alleged tort for wrongful life, in which individuals have held that others are civilly liable for their having been born. The moral force of these suits is that in circumstances in which a child is likely to be born severely deformed, there is an obligation to prevent conception, or in some cases to secure an abortion [20].

In her essay, Patricia White addresses the use of the concept of person in criminal and civil law through a detailed examination of its legal history in the United States. She finds in agreement with Glantz that no single coherent concept of person has developed in the law, but rather various notions of person have been elaborated in particular judicial findings or have been presupposed by particular statutes. She develops further the recognition that the fetus was not construed as a person in the law prior to birth,[11] though various sanctions were developed against abortion, some tied to the period of gestation at which the abortion was performed, and though the law evolved grounds for individuals to recover for injuries sustained *in utero* or in some jurisdictions for an estate to recover if the fetus is born dead. In the latter cases of recoveries for wrongful death, the acts under which recovery is possible have sought to compensate survivors for their losses, rather than to preserve a right of the dead fetus. In cases of recovery by the child for damages *in utero*, the fetus functioned as a place-holder for rights that could be achieved or actualized only if the fetus were born alive, thus gaining standing to sue. However, despite the wide range of interests that has moved the law in both criminal and civil cases, it becomes quite clear that legal personhood in American law is achieved only at birth. This posture, one should again note, has ancient lineage. It appears very similar to much of Jewish law, which treats the killing of the fetus as murder only when the fetus's head (or its greater part) had emerged from the vagina.[12]

The ways in which one appreciates the status of fetuses or of newborns depends on a rich web of cultural presuppositions, as Perkoff shows. In cultures where there are high neo-natal death rates, infants are often not named, or are not accorded the status of persons, until some period after birth. This was the posture, for example, of the Graeco-Roman West in classic times, as the article by Feen in this volume indicates. Indeed, the West has continued to puzzle concerning the points at which one ought to confer personhood, or full personhood. Perkoff notes, for example, that Roman Catholic canon law until 1869 drew a distinction between early and late abortions. This distinction, in fact, had been established in canon law from 1234 with a three-year exception between 1588 and 1591.[13] In any event, the lines of distinction can be multiple, suggesting degrees of conferral of personhood. Thus, for example, orthodox Judaism does not require mourning for the death of a child who dies within thirty days of birth.[14] Many social interests, as well as ontological concerns, have been balanced in the history of the West's attempt to assess the significance of human ontogeny. And, as Perkoff shows, the pre-reflective sentiment held by many in the West regarding fetuses is the result of various expectations sustained by Western culture. Westerners are more likely to feel that fetuses should be treated as persons than will individuals innocent of our particular religious and metaphysical concerns.

The volume then turns to the examination of what it is to be a person and the extent to which fetuses could be such. As Puccetti suggests, it will be very difficult to talk of later gestation fetuses or newborn children as persons in the sense that we are, and surely impossible to regard early fetuses as such. He thus suggests a distinction between beginning persons, which he would have include late gestation fetuses, and actual persons, conscious entities who build a personal life from their own agency and experience. To draw from an image in Puccetti's essay, before the development of a conscious life and after its cessation, there is no one home in the body. There is no one there, even if complex reflex activity is in place. As I have indicated, puzzles regarding the ontological significance of the development of human life and its cessation push us to draw a line between human personal and human biological life. I develop these points further in my essay through exploring the concept of viability. I argue that secularly defensible understandings of the status of the fetus will not secure it rights against women seeking abortion. As a result, in a peaceable pluralist society, one will need to develop a criterion of viability, *not* based on the capacity of medical technology to render fetuses viable, but rather one based on the need to allow sufficient latitude for women to make their own decisions with regard to the abortion of the fetuses they carry. Neither arguments for potentiality nor interests in human life as such can give sufficient support for the status of the fetus as a moral object, much less as a moral subject, to justify restricting the free choice of women in such matters. Potential persons have only potential rights, and simply being human does not confer sufficient moral standing to constrain the freedom of women seeking abortions. A candid examination of the status of the fetus leads one in fact to recognize that there cannot be only one sense of person. One is led, as I have argued above, to distinguish between not only human biological life and human personal life, but between those entities who are persons in the sense of moral agents (i.e., self-conscious, free, rational agents with moral interests) and those entities on whom many of the rights of persons in this first sense are conferred (e.g., infants). Thus, though fetuses are best treated as only human biological life, infants are given the status of persons out of a complex set of considerations and moral practices. Both birth and viability are lines upon which moral significance is conferred. However, these lines do not possess intrinsic moral significance. It is only persons in the strict sense of moral agents who have moral standing in and of themselves.

Robert Solomon is less optimistic than I with respect to the possibility of producing general secular arguments to secure the intrinsic dignity of persons, much less fetuses. In holding that such arguments for the status of persons fail, he is left with examining only the extrinsic values that fetuses or adult humans have, that is, the values they have for others in the particular communities in which they live. However, as he indicates, secular pluralist nations such as the United States are constituted out of numerous communities, which in many areas have widely divergent views of what ought to have value. The issue of abortion, as he argues, is such a point of divergence par excellence. The proscription of abortions would not find support in a general moral consensus, and would in fact be subversive of the very peaceable character of a secular, pluralist society.

However, even if one had grounds to hold that fetuses were persons, it would not follow from that alone that women would lose the right to abortion. The question would rather be under what circumstances women would have a responsibility to fetuses that would constrain them not to evict them from their bodies. This point, which has in part been explored by individuals such as Judith Jarvis Thomson [36] and Susan Nicholson [28], is elaborated in this volume in an analysis by Holly Smith of the extent to which a woman, by having sexual intercourse, waives the right to her body in favor of a fetus. As she shows, it is implausible to hold that most women, by intercourse, do in fact waive that right. As a result, it would not be proper to constrain women's choices on the supposition that they had waived that right, as would occur in anti-abortion laws. In short, Smith offers a re-examination of the bond between sexual intercourse as a social or recreational act, and sexual intercourse as a commitment to reproduction, showing that it is not plausible to view the obligation to carry a fetus to term as the just deserts of a women engaging in intercourse.

In her essay, Caroline Whitbeck takes this point further by exploring attitudes towards women, pregnancy, and the ways in which abortion is appreciated. As she shows, abortion is not pursued for its own sake, or as a goal in itself, but because of inadequate contraception, inadequate financial means to raise a child, fetal defects, the stigma of bearing an illegitimate child, rape, or other undesirable or constraining circumstances. Indeed, the language of the discussion of abortion has in great measure been the language of constraint. The discussions of the desirability of forbidding abortions are often tied to concerns with population dynamics and interests in having more citizens, in particular, more workers or soldiers. These considerations have not only led Communist countries at particular points in history to forbid abortion [11], but have also been forwarded as considerations in debates concerning abortion policy in Western countries. To conceive of the issues in these terms is to understand women as an extension of state breeding policies, rather than to acknowledge them as free individuals with the right to choose their own reproductive destinies. The abortion debate must therefore be appreciated not only in terms of the rights of women and the putative rights of fetuses, but also in terms of the ways in which women are viewed as extensions of social policy, the ways in which women understand themselves, and in terms of the evils avoided through the lesser evil of abortion.

These analyses of the relation of intercourse to the obligation of women to their fetuses and of the significance of pregnancy, indicate reasons for reassessing the ways in which sexuality and pregnancy are to be understood. Such a reassessment will lead to new appreciations of reproductive responsibility. As Margery Shaw argues, the capacity to control the quality of one's reproductive outcomes imposes moral obligations due to the availability of safe and effective abortion techniques. There could be moral grounds for holding, as *Curlender v. Bio-Science Laboratories* [7] [15] illustrates, that a woman should be held responsible for conceiving a high-risk pregnancy when she knew of such a risk, and when she could reasonably have avoided it. Further, once pregnant, if fetuses are not persons, she would be responsible for not having aborted a fetus which she should have known was defective. Such an omission would involve not simply a breach of responsibility to others (e.g., society) who will have to share in the costs of the care of the defective infant, but could be considered an injury to the child itself. In short, Shaw employs a case from the law to illustrate the moral implications of the issues raised by tort for wrongful life suits (i.e., suits by children for having been born under compromised circumstances). Reproduction is not an enterprise involving only a male and a female. Further, rights to reproduction are restricted not only by obligations to avoid injuring society, but also by obligations to avoid injuring the future actual persons such reproduction could produce.

Such a concern with social responsibility, since it stresses the obligation not to injure others who have not consented to the injury, is fully compatible with the rejection of the notion that a state may properly impose upon its citizens a duty to reproduce. In both recognizing the obligations of responsible reproduction (i.e., avoiding the birth of defective children), and recognizing the propriety of rejecting the purported right of the state to require reproduction, one is respecting the freedom of persons. This reappraisal of reproductive obligations suggests as well, to put it somewhat provocatively, that arguments for fornication as a basic human right are much stronger than secular moral arguments for the right to reproduce. Fornication is, after all, an act between consenting individuals, which will, as such, not cause unconsented injury (i.e., presuming that the general canons of civility in trysting are observed; indeed, in the general course of things one would expect the cost-benefit ratio to be quite positive for the individuals involved; but in any event, *volenti non fit injuria*). In contrast, sexual activities for the purpose of reproduction involve possible costs to unconsenting individuals, including the individual who is to be born from the act. The right to reproduction is therefore likely to be much more severely limited by moral considerations (e.g., obligations of the parents to ascertain that they will not be passing to their children any serious genetic or infectious diseases; hence, the obligations of physicians and would-be mothers to test for syphilis during pregnancy), than is the right to make love with consenting partners.

One finds discussions about the morality of abortion and the status of the fetus set, thus, within general concerns about the nature of sexuality and the obligation of individuals to take control of their own destinies, while respecting the freedom of their associates. Such understandings of human sexuality and of responsibility in reproduction are new in the sense of being for the first time widespread and enabled by modern technology. They contrast with traditional views that have construed the fetus to be a person, the goal of sexual intercourse to be reproduction, and children to be the gifts of God, not the chosen outcomes of human actions.

In the final section of the volume the reader is offered essays that sketch the roots of the traditional views concerning the status of the fetus and the obligations associated with reproduction and sexuality. In the first of these essays, Richard Feen provides an account of the ancient Greek view of the status of the fetus and the nature of reproductive responsibility. As he indicates, both abortion and infanticide immediately following birth were allowed. Contrary sentiments were to be found for the most part in the mystery cults and later in Christian sources. His essay shows the attempt of the ancient world to erect a line in human development that allowed interventions to control population and to avoid the burden of defective

children. He shows as well the development of the concern addressed by the
second contributor to this section: the determination of the point at which
an immortal soul enters the body of an embryo or fetus. Father Moraczewski
provides what has come to be understood as a traditional Roman Catholic
account, though it has been only recently that the Catholic Church has come
somewhat uniformly to hold that human life should be treated as the life of
a person from the moment, or from close to the moment, of conception.
Moraczewski attempts to place the moral arguments regarding the fetus
within a frame of general metaphysical presuppositions concerning the
infusion of an immortal soul, and within a doctrine of potentiality that holds
that potential entities should be treated as if they were the actual things
they could, potentially, become. Father James McCartney outlines the
recent background of such views in order to indicate the actual diversity of
Catholic moral positions and the fact that Roman Catholicism is by no means
committed to the notion that a fetus is a person from the moment of conception. Rather, as he shows, Catholic doctrine reflects an attitude towards
the significance of sexuality which militates against persons directing reproductive outcomes (i.e., through either contraception or abortion). These
three articles thus provide an overview of a number of the roots of traditional
concerns regarding abortion. They show that these concerns in part involve
interests in the control of reproductive outcomes, and in part interests
of a metaphysical or religious nature. Finally, Mary Ann Gardell closes
this section with a comparison of a number of the essays in the volume as
attempts to fashion a public policy regarding abortion in the absence of
general rational arguments (i.e., arguments outside *particular* religious,
metaphysical or ethical traditions) against abortion. As she indicates, *Roe v.
Wade* [30] is best understood as a compromise between the Greek allowance
of infanticide and the Christian proscription of abortion. It allows control
of reproduction, including the avoidance of the birth of defective children,
while allowing reverence for human life in a very singular way from the
moment of birth.

This attitude towards abortion and the control of reproduction is tied
to major changes in modern moral viewpoints (e.g., seeing reproduction as
a biological process to be controlled; seeing human biological life as material
for persons to refashion). As this volume has indicated, some of these changes
will not be fully accepted without considerable struggle, including conceptual
struggle. It is here that the general importance of these changes lies. We are,
through these conceptual struggles, coming to understand ourselves anew and
to appreciate our position in nature as persons in control of, and therefore

able to shape, our human nature. We are the result of blind evolutionary forces that have adapted us to environments in which we no longer live. However, we are as well persons who can decide which of the deliverances of nature we wish to accept, and which we wish to change. Abortion is but one of the ways in which we have learned to control our reproductive capacities and focus them to serve the capacities of persons. This volume thus gestures beyond the issue of abortion, and towards general concerns in philosophy regarding the significance of persons, and the ways in which persons through science and technology are fashioning themselves anew.

January 1983

NOTES

[1] There is a wide range of philosophical, theological, and legal issues raised by contemporary authors writing on the status of the fetus and the morality of abortion. See, for examples, [34], [44], [26], [15], [17], [3], [42], [37], and [36].

[2] Compare the views expressed by Grisez [18] and Curren [8] within the Roman Catholic tradition or the discussions held by Feldman [16] and Rosner [31] on the question of fetal status within the Jewish tradition.

[3] Following Aristotle, St. Thomas held that there was a sequence of three souls, only the last being rational and immortal, which are acquired in a process involving substantial change and development (*Summa Theologica*, Part I, Question 118, Art. 2). He relied on this distinction to argue that abortion before animation, that is, before "sense and motion", was less of an evil than abortion thereafter (*Opera Omnia*, XXVI, *In Aristotelis Stagiritae: Politicorum seu de Rebus Civilibus*, Book VII, Lectio XII, p. 484). Abortion was not a homicide before animation (*Summa Theologica*, II–II, Question 64, Article 8). Although it was a moral sin, it was "however less [of a sin] than homicide, for to that point conception could be prevented by another method" (*Opera Omnia, XI, Commentum in Quartum Librum Sententiarium Magistri Petri Lombardi*, Distinctio XXXI, Exposito Textus, p. 127, my translation).

[4] Consider the passage from *Exodus*:

"If men strive, and hurt a woman with child, so that her fruit depart from here, and yet no mischief follow: he shall be surely punished, according as the woman's husband will lay upon him; and he shall pay as the judges determine. And if any mischief follow, then thou shalt give life for life . . . " (*Exodus* 20: 22–23).

In the Septuagint version of the Old Testament, this distinction is drawn between whether the fetus was formed or unformed, that is ensouled or unensouled (*Exodus* 21: 22).

[5] See the Commentary on Section 1400 in [9]. The fact of this decision is explicitly mentioned, for example, in a daily missal widely used until the establishment of the vernacular mass [24].

6 The dispute regarding whether the soul enters at this moment of conception or later has been styled in Roman Catholic theology as the dispute between those who advocate immediate versus mediate animation. For literature on this, see [10].

7 No distinction is made in the present canon of the Roman Catholic Church between abortion in the early stages vis-à-vis later stages of gestation. It treats all abortions as if they were homicide ([4], Canons 985, Note 4, and 2350, Section 1).

8 Consider this passage from the Virginia Declaration of Rights (1776):

"That all men are by Nature equally free and independent, and have certain inherent Rights, of which, when they enter into a State of Society, they cannot, by a Compact, deprive or divest their Posterity; namely, the Enjoyment of Life and Liberty, with the Means of acquiring and possessing Property and pursuing and obtaining Happiness and Safety" ([43], p. 3).

9 The precedent setting cases were: *Grace v. State*, 69 S. W. 529, 530 (Tex. Crim. App. 1902), and *Sanders v. State.*, 112 S. W. 68, 70 (Tex. Crim. App., 1908). The State of Texas criminalized aiding and abetting suicide in 1973. See Tex. Penal Code Annotated 22.08 (1974).

10 One finds, for example, in 1975, Theodore Cooper, Assistant Secretary of Health, stating that "It is expected that no procedures will be undertaken which fail to treat the fetus with due care and dignity, or which affront community sensitivity" ([5], p. 33527). This language is found as well in the recommendation of the National Commission for the Protection of Human Subjects of Biomedical and Behavioral Research:

"Although the Commission has not addressed directly the issues of the personhood and the civil status of the fetus, the members of the Commission are convinced that moral concern should extend to all who share human genetic heritage, and that the fetus, regardless of life prospects, should be treated respectfully and with dignity" ([40], p. 62).

Finally, this language is employed as well in the report of the Ethics Advisory Board of the Department of Health, Education, and Welfare regarding *HEW Support of Research Involving Human IN VITRO Fertilization and Embryo Transfer*: " ... the human embryo is entitled to profound respect; but this respect does not necessarily encompass the full legal and moral rights attributed to persons" ([39], p. 101). In short, there is an interest in treating human embryos and fetuses with dignity, but not a commitment to regard them as persons. For current regulations concerning the use of embryos and fetuses, see: *Code of Federal Regulations*, 45 CFR 46. 201–46.211.

11 Even the California law that makes killing a fetus outside of abortion murder does not thereby recognize the fetus as a person "in the whole sense" (*Cal. Penal Code*, Section 187).

12 For a treatment of the fetus's life as not equal to that of the mother, see from the Mishna, *Oholot* 7: 6. The Jewish viewpoint with regard to the morality of abortion and the status of the fetus is a complex one. For more information, see [22].

13 See [14]. For an example of the distinction in canon law between murder and the destruction of an early embryo, see [6].

14 See *Kitzur Shulhan Arukh*, by Rabbi Solomon Ganzfried (the standard condensed

version of the Code of Jewish religious law, entitled *Shulhan Arukh*, compiled by Joseph Karo (1488–1575), Section 203, Paragraph 3: " . . . if an infant dies within the first 30 days of its life, or even on the 30th day of its life, and even if there has been growth of its hair and nails, you do not follow any of the observances of mourning, because it is as if there had been a miscarriage" [adapted and translated by Professor Isaac Franck]).

[15] One might note that legislation in California has since been passed which precludes offspring from suing parents for "wrongful life" (Cal. Civ. Code, Section 43.6 (1982); added to Assembly Bill 627, Chapter 331). Further, there have been contrary rulings [38]. We use Curlender [7] in this volume as a case involving important moral issues, not as forwarding a legal precedent.

BIBLIOGRAPHY

1. Biggers, J. D.: 1979, '*In Vitro* Fertilization, Embryo Culture, and Embryo Transfer in the Human', in U.S. Department of Health, Education, and Welfare, Ethics Advisory Board, *HEW Support of Research Involving Human IN VITRO Fertilization and Embryo Transfer: Appendix*, Department of Health, Education, and Welfare, Washington, D.C., Essay 8.
2. Bouman, C. A.: 1958, 'The Meaning of the Immaculate Conception in the Perspective of St. Thomas', in E. D. O'Connor (ed.), *The Dogma of the Immaculate Conception*, University of Notre Dame Press, Notre Dame, Indiana.
3. Brody, B. A.: 1975, *Abortion and the Sanctity of Human Life: A Philosophical View*, The MIT Press, Cambridge, Massachusetts.
4. *Codex Juris Canonici*, Typis Polyglottis Vaticanis, Vatican, 1965.
5. Cooper, T.: 1975, 'Protection of Human Subjects: Fetuses, Pregnant Women, and IN VITRO Fertilization', *Federal Register* 40, 33526–33551.
6. *Corpus Juris Canonici Emendatum et Notis Illustratum, cum Glossae: Decretalium d. Gregorii Papae Noni Compilatio*, Rome 1585, *Glossae ordinaria* at Book 5, title 12, Chapter 20, p. 1713.
7. *Curlender v. Bio-Science Laboratories*, 106 Cal. App. 3d 811 (1980).
8. Curren, D. E.: 1974, 'Abortion: Its Legal and Moral Aspects in Catholic Theology', *New Perspectives in Moral Theology*, Fides Publishers, Notre Dame, Indiana.
9. Denziner, H. (ed.): 1965, *Enchiridion Symbolorum Definitionum et Declarationum de Rebus Fidei et Morum*, rev. A. Shön-Metzer, 33rd ed., Herder, Barcelona.
10. Donceel, J. F.: 1970, 'Immediate Animation and Delayed Hominization', *Theological Studies* 31, 76–105.
11. Endres, R. J.: 1971, 'Abortion in Perspective', *American Journal of Obstetrics and Gynecology* 3, 436–439.
12. Engelhardt, H. T., Jr.: 1975, 'Defining Death: A Philosophical Problem for Medicine and Law', *American Review of Respiratory Disease* 112, 587–590.
13. Engelhardt, H. T., Jr.: 1978, 'Definitions of Death: Where to Draw the Line and Why', in E. McMullin (ed.), *Death and Decision*, Westwood Press, Boulder, Colorado, for the American Association for the Advancement of Science, Selected Symposia Series 18, 15–34.
14. Engelhardt, H. T., Jr.: 1974, 'The Ontology of Abortion', *Ethics*, 84, 217–234.

15. English, J.: 1975, 'Abortion and the Concept of a Person', *Canadian Journal of Philosophy* 5, 233–243.
16. Feldman, D. M. (ed.): 1974, *Marital Relations, Birth Control, and Abortion in Jewish Law*, Schocken Books, New York.
17. Green, R.: 1974, 'Conferred Rights and the Fetus', *Journal of Religious Ethics* 2, 55–75.
18. Grisez, G. G.: 1970, *Abortion: The Myths, The Realities, and The Arguments*, Corpus Books, New York.
19. Haeckel, E.: 1866, *Generelle Morphologie der Organismen*, Georg Reimer, Berlin.
20. Holder, A. R.: 1981, 'Is Existence Ever an Injury?', in S. F. Spicker, J. M. Healey, Jr., and H. T. Engelhardt, Jr. (eds.), *The Law–Medicine Relation: A Philosophical Exploration*, D. Reidel Publ. Co., Dordrecht, Holland pp. 225–240.
21. *In the Matter of Karen Quinlan*, D. N. Robinson (intro.), University Publications of America, Inc., Arlington, Virginia, 1976, Vols. I and II.
22. Jakobovits, I.: 1975, *Jewish Medical Ethics: A Comparative and Historical Study of the Jewish Religious Attitude to Medicine and its Practice*, Bloch Publ. Co., New York.
23. Kant, I.: 1968, *Grundlegung zur Metaphysik der Sitten*, Vol. IV, Königliche Preussische Akademie Edition, Berlin.
24. Lefebvre, G.: 1953, St. Andrew Daily Missal, E. M. Lohmann, Saint Paul, Minnesota.
25. Marx, J. L.: 1980, 'Ape-Language Controversy Flares Up', *Science* 207, 1330–1333.
26. Nelson, J. A.: 1980, *Abortion and the Causal Theory of Names*, State University of New York, Buffalo, Ph. D. Dissertation.
27. Nicholas, M. J.: 1958, 'The Meaning of the Immaculate Conception in the Perspective of St. Thomas', in E. D. O'Connor (ed.), *The Dogma of the Immaculate Conception*, University of Notre Dame Press, Notre Dame, Indiana.
28. Nicholson, S. T.: 1978, *Abortion and the Catholic Church*, Religious Ethics, Inc., Knoxville, Tennessee (Journal of Religious Ethics, Studies in Religious Ethics, II).
29. Rawls, J.: 1971, *A Theory of Justice*, Harvard University Press, Cambridge, Massachusetts.
30. *Roe v. Wade*, 410 U.S. 113 (1973).
31. Rosner, F.: 1972, *Modern Medicine and Jewish Law*, Yeshiva University, New York.
32. S. 158, 97th Cong., 1st Sess. (1981).
33. S. J. Res. 110, 97th Cong., 1st Sess. (1981).
34. Saponpzis, S. F.: 1981, 'A Critique of Personhood', *Ethics* 91, 607–618.
35. Sumner, L. W.: 1981, *Abortion and Moral Theory*, Princeton University Press, Princeton, New Jersey.
36. Thomson, J. J.: 1971, 'A Defense of Abortion', *Philosophy and Public Affairs* 1, 47–66.
37. Tooley, M.: 1972, 'Abortion and Infanticide', *Philosophy and Public Affairs* 10, 607–618.
38. *Turpin v. Sortini*, 119 Cal. App. 3rd 690 (1981).
39. U.S. Department of Health, Education, and Welfare, Ethics Advisory Board: 1979, *HEW Support of Research Involving Human* In Vitro *Fertilization and Embryo Transfer: Report and Conclusions*, Department of Health, Education, and Welfare, Washington, D.C.

H. TRISTRAM ENGELHARDT, JR.

40. U.S. Department of Health, Education, and Welfare, National Commission for the Protection of Human Subjects of Biomedical and Behavioral Research: 1975, *Research on the Fetus: Report and Conclusions*, Department of Health, Education, and Welfare, Washington, D. C.
41. Wallace, E. with D. M. Vigness (eds.), 1963, *Documents of Texas History*, Steck Co., Austin, Texas.
42. Warren, M. A.: 1973, 'On the Moral and Legal Status of Abortion', *Monist* 57, 43–61.
43. *We the States*, William Byrd Press, Richmond, Virginia, 1964.
44. Zaitchik, A.: 1981, 'Viability and the Morality of Abortion', *Philosophy and Public Affairs* 10, 18–26.

SECTION I

HUMAN DEVELOPMENT:
SCIENCE AND PUBLIC POLICY

THOMAS A. SHANNON

ABORTION: A CHALLENGE FOR ETHICS AND PUBLIC POLICY

The purpose of this paper is to review and analyze several issues related to the debate about public policy on abortion. It will review some of the ethical and political issues raised on abortion, describe some aspects of abortion policy in America, identify ethical problems raised by some of the policy questions, and then discuss some of the ethical issues involved in these policy debates. I hope, in this way, to indicate some of the fundamental problems and the more substantive issues behind the debate.

I. A REVIEW OF POLICIES ON ABORTION IN THE UNITED STATES

In his book, James Mohr [10] traces the history of why in 1800 there were virtually no abortion policies and in 1900 every state had an anti-abortion law. While not wanting to rehearse all of the salient elements in Mohr's book, there are a few issues with respect to public policy and abortion that I want to emphasize.

Mohr identifies several motives concerning why the early abortion legislation came into being. The first motive focused on preventing the mother's death through the use of an abortifacient ([10], pp. 20–45). These laws, as Mohr notes, were primarily poison control measures focusing not so much on the fetus as on the health status of the mother and the safety of the procedure that was used. These laws also had the effect of reinforcing the traditional norm of "quickening" as the dividing line between abortions which were not governed by statutes and those which were. The other two motives, which Mohr says contributed to the increase in abortion laws that came to a climax at the end of the nineteenth century, have to do with changes in the perception of who was receiving an abortion and who was providing them. There was a growing fear that since first generation American women were receiving abortions at high rates, the White Anglo-Saxon Protestant population might be outnumbered by the immigrants. This perception was related to the developing nativist movement; consequently, statutes were enacted to restrict abortion, intending not the protection of the fetus, but the protection of the status and power of the established classes. Parallel to this was the growing professionalization of medicine. Physicians were interested both in developing and tightening their own standards of practice

3

William B. Bondeson et al. *(eds.), Abortion and the Status of the Fetus*, 3–14.
Copyright © 1983 *by D. Reidel Publishing Company, Dordrecht, Holland.*

and in eliminating from medicine those described as quacks. Physicians lobbied against abortion in order to eliminate from the profession individuals who would not abide by its rules and to control the standards of the members of the profession itself. The medical profession was further able to control abortion by helping define medical conditions under which abortion might be appropriate and by providing competent individuals to perform the procedure. Thus, by the end of the nineteenth century, abortion legislation was present in all of the states and was contrary to the earlier experience of the country when abortion was possible for those who wanted it. Again, the primary intent of this legislation was the protection of the mother and the enhancement of the social status of two different groups within society: the establishment and the physicians.

Mohr also describes the pressures that led to the re-evaluation of these anti-abortion statutes in our own time and resulted in the *Roe v. Wade* [12] decision in 1973 ([10], pp. 250–255). These pressures are: (1) the fear of overpopulation; (2) a growing concern for the quality of life of the fetus as opposed to the mere preservation of life; (3) the development of the Women's Rights Movement with its emphasis on a woman's right to control her body; (4) the growing safety of abortion done under appropriate medical conditions; (5) the fact that women were getting abortions in spite of restrictive legislation. One could also add to this list the movement of several states to relax their own abortion legislation. Ultimately, this led to the testing of restrictive state statutes in the Supreme Court. The legal history is sketched in some detail in this volume by Leonard Glantz [2] and Patricia White [19].

What it is important to notice here is that abortion legislation was developed primarily out of a variety of social issues that were not directly or quite possibly even indirectly related to concern for the fetus. The older use of the term "quickening", and its contemporary analogue, "viability", served as a touchstone for the limits of abortion. That is, in the early nineteenth century, abortion was not considered greatly problematic morally or medically until the point of quickening. In the view of many individuals, a similar argument is being used today from at least a medical, if not a moral, point of view. And, in fact, as Mohr indicates, the *Roe* decision is based somewhat upon this older traditional view within American society: abortions before quickening or viability are not problematic. Moreover, abortion statutes — whether pro or con — were based upon neither the sanctity of life of the fetus nor a disregard of it, but rather upon other social issues and concerns.

Another important review of abortion policies comes from a recent article by Tatalovich and Daynes, entitled "The Trauma of Abortion Politics"

[16]. These authors indicate three significant periods in the history of the policy debate. First, in the early 1960s the basic issue was the building of a consensus toward abortion reform focusing primarily on the availability of therapeutic abortion. The authors note that the pro-abortion advocates shared similar assumptions, used similar arguments, and held common objectives with the abortion opponents. These proponents assumed, based on the American Law Institute's recommendations, that abortion should be permitted only to a limited number of women and that it should be performed for therapeutic reasons. This position defines abortion primarily in medical terms, not moral ones. The abortion reformers were not making any radical claims. All of the abortion statutes in effect permitted therapeutic abortions when the mother's life was in danger. Some states allowed abortion when the mother's health was threatened. What the reformers were arguing for was an incremental change in the abortion laws allowing this more expanded exception. And at that point in time, as Tatalovich and Daynes note, approximately 80% of the general population favored some abortion reform; while this support came from both Catholics and Protestants, Catholics did not support the reform at the same level that the Protestants did ([16], p. 645).

A second critical period that the authors identify is 1969 to 1973, which was marked by three interrelated developments. First, the pro-abortionists shifted towards repeal of all abortion laws as opposed to therapeutic reform. Second, opposition to abortion began to focus on opposition to *any* change, thereby opposing not only the new movement towards total repeal of abortion laws, but even the incremental changes that were desired earlier. Third, the proponents of abortion began to shift their strategy to the use of the judiciary to achieve reform rather than expend their limited resources on attempts to change legislation state by state. This strategy culminated in *Roe* which had the sense of being a "winner take all" case. This court decision made it difficult for any compromise posture to be taken and helped change the nature of the debate. Interestingly enough, the authors point out that there were ample court precedents on either side of the issue and that the court was not inherently locked into a pro-abortion decision. But had the court come out the other way, there still would have been a public policy debate, with the sides reversed. A major problem is not so much the court's decision, as the winner-take-all character of the decision which has in effect polarized the debate.

The third issue has to do with this polarization of perceptions on abortion, as well as with strategies to achieve the ends of the anti-abortion groups.

One of the by-products of this polarization has been the legislative maneuver-
ings of the anti-abortion group. Picking up their cues for strategies for reform
from the pro-abortion groups, the anti-abortion groups have escalated the
level of content of the debate, and have chosen to follow a route towards
change via neither state legislatures nor the judiciary, but rather are attempting
to circumvent the entire judicial system by having certain kinds of legislation
declared off limits from federal judicial review. The anti-abortion people
recognize that state-by-state campaigns will be costly and time consuming;
they realize that a constitutional amendment may be very difficult to achieve.
One effective strategy is to circumvent these processes by having Congress
declare certain forms of legislation off limits to judicial review. They are
also attempting to devise federal legislation to restrict public monies for
abortion to as few cases as possible, so that those who wish abortions must
pay for them themselves. Two important moves here have been legislation
introduced to define life as beginning at conception [14] — thus ensuring
a fetus constitutional rights, making abortion illegal, and raising constitutional
problems regarding certain forms of contraception — and the Hatch amendment [15] recently passed by the Senate Judiciary Subcommittee, which
states that the right to an abortion is not secured by the Constitution and
that the states and Congress shall have power to restrict and prohibit abortions. This amendment gives a state law precedence if it is more restrictive
than federal legislation.

Thus the third major phase of the debate that these authors identify
consists of a conflict at a very high and intense level among groups who
are violently pro or con abortion, while simultaneously denying to legislatures
the ability to make compromise moves. By focusing on an either/or position,
consensus is more difficult to achieve and consequently no policy is able
to gain legitimacy. Our current debate is characterized by polarization and
a move from a debate of the issues to personal confrontations in which
parties are perceived to be liberal or conservative with respect to how they
perceive this particular issue.

II. OPINIONS REGARDING ABORTION

It is important in developing a public policy to ensure some sense of legitimacy
by rooting it in the beliefs of the citizenry so that the policy at least to some
degree will be acceptable and workable. I am not arguing that the morality
of abortion will be settled or determined by poll-taking; I do think it is
important, with respect to proposing and implementing policy, to attend

to perceptions about abortion and to determine if there are possible connections between the pro and con abortion groups that might help facilitate some kind of compromise to enable a policy to be developed.

We need to examine first what reasons for abortion people find persuasive. One important finding is that there is an average approval of 67% for six specific reasons for abortion: a woman's health is seriously endangered by the pregnancy; the pregnancy is a result of rape; there is a strong chance of a serious defect in the baby; the family has a low income and cannot afford any more children; the woman is pregnant and does not want to marry the man; the woman is married and does not want any more children ([4], pp. 251–252). The last three reasons are known as the "soft" reasons for abortion and there is no solid social consensus on these three. The average consensus for the first three reasons, the "hard" reasons, averages about 85%, whereas it is about 50% for the soft reasons. There is clearly strong social consensus around the broadened concept of a therapeutic abortion. There is less, but slightly increasing, support for the more social or personal reasons for wanting an abortion. It is also important to note that the average approval has changed only four percentage points since 1972. There was a jump of twenty-two points between 1965 and 1972. But there has been a remarkable stability in the approval rate since 1972 ([4], p. 252).

With respect to the profiles of those engaged in the debate, there are some interesting correlations. First, two relevant differences between those who are pro and con abortion is that those who are anti-abortion tend to feel that obedience is more important and that curiosity during child development is less important than do those who are in favor of abortion. Second, a finding which should surprise no one, the higher a person's social status, the greater is their tendency to approve of abortion. In fact, one study indicated that a formal education is the best predictor of abortion attitudes. Third, the more one disapproves of activities such as premarital sex, extramarital sex, and homosexuality, the less one favors abortion. Fourth, differences between Protestants and Catholics with respect to favoring or not favoring abortion increase in proportion to degree of education. Finally, for both Protestants and Catholics, approval of abortion decreases as religiosity indexes increase, with the notable exception of Episcopalians who are more likely to approve of abortion the more religious they are ([4], pp. 257–258). What is significantly interesting and important in one study was the allegation that the Protestant–Catholic difference accounts for only about 1% of the variation in abortion attitudes over the years ([4], p. 257). This leads to the interesting hypothesis that the religious differences are not the critical differences in the abortion debate and that to cast the debate in terms of religious preference is both mistaken and particularly counter-productive for policy debates. These studies would indicate that the critical variables are those beyond religion and have to do with feelings about child rearing, social practices, education, and class ([4], p. 258).

A study of differences between members of the National Abortion Rights Action League (NARAL) and the National Right to Life Committee (NRLC) showed some interesting differences with respect to what the membership of each organization felt about abortion ([3], pp. 157–163). These findings are of particular importance for policy making. More than 95% of NARAL members and fewer than 5% of NRLC members approve of legal abortion when there is a strong chance of a serious defect in the baby, when the woman is married and wants no more children, when a woman's husband will not consent to an abortion, when the family is too poor to afford more children, when parents will not consent to a teenager's abortion and when an unmarried woman wants to have an abortion. These data are not surprising, especially insofar as they refer to the soft reasons for abortion. However, it's interesting that 73% of NRLC members favor making abortion available to women whose life is endangered by continuation of the pregnancy. Also 15% of NRLC members approve of abortion if the pregnant woman's physical health is seriously endangered by carrying the pregnancy to term and 7% to 8% favor legal abortion if pregnancy is the result of rape or incest. These data indicate that members of the NRLC do not present as monolithic and absolutistic a position on abortion as might be assumed. While the policy that could be based on such feelings may not be acceptable to all, nonetheless it does indicate that there are possibilities for some movement. Compromise, of course, will be called for.

Another relevant factor revealed by this survey indicates that NRLC activists are not only generally more conservative on moral issues but are also likely to describe themselves as conservatives, as Republicans, and to oppose government action to reduce income differences between rich and poor. As important as those differences are, the NRLC members are much more likely than NARAL members to give priority to their views on abortion over their views on social issues. Eighty-four percent of NRLC members as opposed to 47% of NARAL members say that abortion is so important that they would refuse to support a candidate whose position on abortion was unacceptable. This may mean that in elections or in debates of public policy, all other things being equal, there may be a strategic advantage to having a group which has the higher percentage of single issue voters on its side.

An interesting perspective is revealed on the single-mindedness of many of the right to life movement by another analysis of activists in the pro-life movement [6]. Kelley identified some general reasons why they were concerned for only one issue. First, abortion stops a human life and is, therefore, a unique issue. Second, a single issue focus protects the right to life movement from being absorbed or manipulated by any political party. Third, the passage of a human life amendment to the Constitution would require a political coalition of people with different ideologies and, therefore, strategically they wish to avoid being perceived as members of any other group. There seems to be a recognition that the alliance present in the pro-life movement is very tenuous and that it might not be able to stand the strain of having to deal with social problems that may not be perceived as having the same importance or solution, e.g., nuclear war or social welfare programs.

It would be interesting to know how the structure and impact of the pro-life movement will be affected by the interior tensions that are present, at least with respect to differences in the kinds of approvals of abortion that are tolerated by some members. The monolithic unity of the pro-life movement may be a perception, not a reality. One could assume that much of the energy of the pro-life movement needs to be spent in making sure that potentially disruptive issues do not enter into the dialogue and that no relationship between the ethical values surrounding the evaluation of abortion and other social issues be made, i.e., extending a pro-life stance to evaluate nuclear war. One could make a reasonable case that such a position will continue to become more and more difficult as time goes on and that members of pro-life groups will have to make more and more difficult choices with respect to the supporting of political candidates, especially when these candidates present viewpoints on a variety of issues that may, in fact, appeal to different populations within the pro-life movement.

III. VALUE AND ETHICAL DILEMMAS AND PROBLEMS IN THE PUBLIC POLICY DEBATE

The first problem is that there are few, if any, good alternatives to abortion. Adoption clearly is an alternative to abortion, but choosing adoption requires that the woman still carry the child to term and deal with the reality of separation from the newborn, a painful experience even if the woman is highly motivated. Even in the best of circumstances such a separation will not easily be made and when there is the suggestion of coercion or significant familial or other social pressure to carry the child to term rather than abort, the separation will be much more problematic. Even for women who choose to carry a child to term in the expectation of allowing the child to be adopted, there may be lack of good or even adequate social, physical, and economic support systems to make such a process easier to accomplish and to ensure the health of the mother and the newborn. Thus as much as a woman may desire to have the child adopted, she may not have either the physical or social support to do so.

Also we need to keep in mind the other alternative to abortion, carrying the child to term and keeping the child. There are a growing number of women who choose to keep their babies, especially among the teenage population [13]. Among the issues here are the ability and appropriateness of such young mothers' caring for their child, as well as problems related to adequate financial and psychological resources to provide an appropriate setting for the rearing of the child. Oftentimes teenage mothers need to interrupt their high school education; they frequently live at home with their parents. These individuals are often already on welfare or will need such assistance. In the light of economic policy initiated by the Reagan administration, it appears that reliance on that particular means of provision will be either not adequate or no longer available.

Thus, even though many individuals see adoption or the keeping of the child by the mother as preferable to abortion, there are many problems involved in doing this, especially in light of the unavailability of social programs to provide a context which would facilitate these kinds of decisions. Even though a variety of both counseling programs and economic assistance programs have been made available on a private basis, these programs are simply not adequate to deal with all of the needs presented by those individuals who might wish to carry a child to term and either have the child adopted or keep their child.

A second major problem has to do with the perception, if not the reality, of discriminatory treatment of women who choose abortion.[1] This relates first to the policy of the federal government which funds both pre- and post-natal services under Medicaid. The argument here is that if the government funds these types of services it should also fund services for abortion. This position has been argued before the Supreme Court and the decision was that the government does not discriminate by refusing to provide funds for abortion under Title 19 of the Social Security Program [5]. Such a requirement, however, means that such funds cannot come out of the federal budget. It is possible, and in fact many states have, continued to support such abortion programs out of state funds. Nonetheless, Medicaid-funded abortions dropped from 295 000 in FY 1977 to about 2000 in FY 1978 ([1], p. 13).

The other problem that raises the issue of discrimination has to do with the fact that those who will be affected most by cuts in programs will be the poor. Those individuals who are able to afford abortions will continue to be able to afford them, whereas individuals who either cannot afford to have an abortion or who live in states which do not provide funds for abortion may not be able to obtain them. However, one study suggested that the majority of women who wanted an abortion and who would previously have qualified for Medicaid assistance still obtained one ([18], p. 129). The fiscal, physical, and psychological costs of doing this are not known. Also, approximately one-fifth of Medicaid-eligible women were not able to receive abortions because of funding restrictions ([18], p. 130). Thus the issue is: will a particular group in our society have to bear a disproportionate share of the burden of such funding policies? The consequence of such a policy is that the government's position is not seen as neutral but rather as an aggressive policy designed to decrease the number of abortions. And since it can only do that in cases where it provides the funding, of necessity such restrictions have their most significant impact on the poor and the disadvantaged.

There are several subsidiary issues in this problem, among which are determining how abortion fits into the delivery of health care services and the perception that abortion may be a cost-effective method for solving many of the budgetary problems of welfare programs. It is more cost-effective to provide abortions than to provide continuing welfare payments. But such an observation does not begin to touch or even analyze the structural arrangements of our society that ensure that a certain number of individuals will always be disenfranchised both politically and economically. We can also ask what government neutrality with respect to abortion might mean. Does this mean that the government should provide nothing in the way of funds for abortion, that the government should not interfere with anyone who wishes to obtain an abortion, or that government should help fund any health-related service a person may want, including abortion?

A third major set of issues has to do with the religion—government relation. Here I will only mention one, the problem of how one translates one's religious beliefs or values into language which is appropriate for public debate. That is, is it possible to make insights and values that come from one's religious tradition or experiences accessible to people who do not share those experiences or traditions? The problem here is twofold: being able to make one's self understandable to other individuals, and making the depth of one's convictions accessible and intelligible to individuals who do not stand within that particular tradition. Another issue has to do with one's ecclesiology. How does one see the role of the church with respect to the larger society? Is the church to witness its values to society or is the church to analyze and evaluate, and occasionally reject social values? If one's ecclesiology leads one in the first direction, then it will not be as important to devise a means of translating one's insights so they can be understandable in a broader arena. If one chooses to use the second approach, it will be extremely important to develop a language that is widely accessible so that one can easily and helpfully engage in policy debates.

The fourth and most significant problem has to do with how the abortion debate can be conducted in the public arena. Alasdair MacIntyre, in his perceptive article, "How to Identify Ethical Principles" [9], and recent book, *After Virtue* [8], argues several theses, one of which is extremely important for the consideration of ethical issues in the public policy debate with respect to abortion. His primary claim is that morality is at war with itself because each moral agent reaches conclusions by valid forms of inference but that there is no agreement about the correctness or appropriateness of the premise with which the argument begins. MacIntyre then argues that moral philosophy in general, and I would argue our culture in particular, has no procedures for weighing rival value premises. MacIntyre relates this to our cultural and political background, which consists of fragments of a variety of social philosophies.

There are two major dimensions to this particular situation. First, we have not inherited a social or cultural context in which we can both understand and apply a philosophical theory. Second, we have inherited conflicting theories of ethics or social philosophy. Thus MacIntyre argues that what we perceive to be the social-philosophical context out of which our country developed its political philosophy comes from Aristotle, Cicero, Locke, and Sidney. Each of these presents conflicting claims with respect to what is good for humans and, even if one could resolve the epistemological problems with respect to adjudicating the truth of these different systems, one would still have the practical problem of evaluating the various goods which they claim are in the interests of human beings and the community.

Briefly stated, we have inherited two conflicting world views. First, we have the classical world view that asks the moral question: How might humans together realize the common good? This position assumes that community is natural and normative, there are goods that human beings can rationally identify and agree upon, and that the common pursuit of these will bring both personal and social development. The second claim focuses on the moral question: How may humans prevent each other from interfering with one another as each goes about his or her own concerns? This viewpoint assumes that being autonomous is the appropriate state from human existence, that individuals may not have interests or values in common, and that liberty and the pursuit of interests will maximize individual and social goods. With MacIntyre, we must wonder whether there will be common premises available for the resolution of the debate concerning abortion or regarding other uses of the fetus in biomedicine. We must wonder as well how we will acquire common conceptual commitments to the status of the fetus, the meaning of personhood, and the rights of society to impose a particular point of view of the common good, especially as this relates to the balancing of interests in autonomy and the maintenance of community standards of morality. Exploring these probabilities, as this volume does, will indicate the scope and power of ethics, and its implications for public policy.

Worcester Polytechnic Institute

NOTE

[1] The perception certainly approaches reality when one hears Senator Hyde, who sponsored legislation to restrict abortions paid for by Medicaid to those which threatened the life of the woman, say:

"I certainly would like to prevent, if I could legally, anyone having an abortion, a rich woman, a middle-class woman or a poor woman. Unfortunately, the only vehicle available is the HEW Medicaid bill. A life is a life" (*The Congressional Record*, 17 June, 1977, p. H. 6083; quoted in [18], p. 121).

BIBLIOGRAPHY

1. Alan Guttmacher Institute, 1979, *Abortion and the Poor: Private Morality, Public Responsibility*, Alan Guttmacher Institute, New York.
2. Glantz, L.: 1982, 'Is the Fetus a Person? A Lawyer's View', in this volume, pp. 107–117.
3. Granberg, D.: 1981, 'The Abortion Activists', *Family Planning Perspectives* 13, 157–163.
4. Granberg, D. and B. W. Granberg: 1980, 'Abortion Attitudes, 1965–80: Trends and Determinants', *Family Planning Perspectives* 12, 251–252.

14   THOMAS A. SHANNON

5. *Harris v. McRae*, 448 U.S. Reports 297 (1980).
6. Kelly, J.: 'Beyond the Stereotypes', *Commonweal* 107, 654–659.
7. Kelman, H. C. and D. P. Warwick: 1980, 'The Ethics of Social Intervention: Goals, Means, and Consequences', in B. H. Raven (ed.), *Policy Studies Review Annual*, Sage Publications, Beverly Hills, California, pp. 44–46.
8. MacIntyre, A.: 1981, *After Virtue*, University of Notre Dame Press, Indiana.
9. MacIntyre, A.: 1978, 'How to Identify Ethical Principles', in U.S. Department of Health, Education, and Welfare, National Commission for the Protection of Human Subjects of Biomedical and Behavioral Research, *The Belmont Report: Appendix*, Volume I, Department of Health, Education, and Welfare, Washington, D.C., Essay 10.
10. Mohr, J. C.: 1978, *Abortion in America*, Oxford University Press.
11. Perkins, B. H. *et al.*: 1978, 'Intensive Care in Adolescent Pregnancy', *Obstetrics and Gynecology* 52, 179–188.
12. *Roe v. Wade*, 410 U.S. 113 (1973).
13. Rosenthal, P. A.: 1981, 'Adolescence and Pregnancy', Department of Psychiatry, University of Massachusetts Medical Center, unpublished manuscript.
14. S. 158, 97th Cong., 1st Sess. (1981).
15. S. J. Res. 110, 96th Cong., 1st Sess. (1981).
16. Tatalovich, R. and B. W. Daynes: 1981, 'The Trauma of Abortion Politics', *Commonweal* 107, 644–649.
17. Tietze, C.: 1981, *Induced Abortion: A World Review, 1981*, The Population Council, New York.
18. Trussell, J. *et al.*: 1980, 'The Impact of Restricting Medicaid Financing for Abortion', *Family Planning Perspectives* 12, 121–130.
19. White, P.: 1983, 'The Concept of Person, the Law, and the Use of the Fetus in Biomedicine', in this volume, pp. 119–157.

LEROY WALTERS

THE FETUS IN ETHICAL AND PUBLIC POLICY DISCUSSION FROM 1973 TO THE PRESENT

This essay will focus on three public-policy documents published in the United States between 1973 and 1979. All three documents include discussions of the ontological and/or moral status of the human embryo of fetus.[1] The three documents are: (1) the *Roe v. Wade* decision of the U.S. Supreme Court in 1973 [17]; (2) the report on fetal research of the National Commission for the Protection of Human Subjects published in 1975 [15], [16]; and (3) the report on in vitro fertilization by the HEW Ethics Advisory Board, published in 1979 [13], [14]. In my view, these three documents are the most important public policy discussions of the human embryo and fetus to have emerged in the United States during the decade of the 1970s.

The three documents will be discussed in chronological order since each succeeding document clearly presupposes the content of the preceding document or documents. This chronological approach will result in a partial reversal of the ontogenetic sequence: the postimplantation human embryo and fetus are the primary foci of the first two documents, while the third document concentrates on the preimplantation embryo.

Two discrete settings are envisioned in the three public policy documents, the research setting and a second setting which might, for lack of a better term, be called "clinical". The clinical setting is the one in which *in vitro* fertilization and embryo transfer are employed to overcome involuntary infertility and in which abortions are performed to terminate unwanted pregnancies.

I. *ROE v. WADE*: THE POSTIMPLANTATION EMBRYO AND FETUS IN THE CLINICAL SETTING

In Parts IX and X of the *Roe v. Wade* decision, the majority opinion proceeded as follows. First, the Court declared that the fetus is not a person within the language and meaning of the Fourteenth Amendment ([17], pp. 156–159). Second, the Court noted the wide divergence of opinion on "the difficult question of when human life begins". Examples of these diverse views are the beliefs of the Stoics, most Jews, many Protestants, "physicians and their scientific colleagues", medieval Aristotelians, and Catholics, as well as the

15

William B. Bondeson et al. *(eds.), Abortion and the Status of the Fetus*, 15–30.
Copyright © 1983 *by D. Reidel Publishing Company, Dordrecht, Holland.*

viewpoint of the English common law ([17], pp. 160—161). Third, the Court argued that in most areas, the law has been

reluctant to endorse any theory that life, as we recognize it, begins before live birth or to accord legal rights to the unborn except in narrowly defined situations and except when the rights are contingent upon live birth ([17], p. 161).

Given this series of arguments and observations and the Court's expressed objection to the Texas legislature's "adopting one theory of life" and thereby overriding the pregnant woman's privacy right, one might have expected the U.S. Supreme Court to prohibit all state efforts to protect embryonic or fetal life at any stage of gestation. This exclusive emphasis on the woman's right to privacy and therefore to abortion would not, of course, have been incompatible with procedural safeguards designed to protect the health of the pregnant woman.

As is well known, the Court did not in fact advocate an unqualified right to privacy. The general structure of the Court's ruling was the contraposition of fundamental individual rights and compelling state interests. With respect to the developing embryo or fetus, the Court argued that the state could have a compelling interest in "potential life" from the point of viability on, "because the fetus then presumably has the capability of meaningful life outside the mother's womb" ([17], p. 163). According to the Court, the state may (but need not) express this compelling interest by proscribing the abortion of viable fetuses, "except when it is necessary to preserve the life or health of the mother" ([17], pp. 163—164).

Three points should be noted about the Court's conception of viability. First, the court did not require that a viable fetus be able to survive on its own outside the uterus: it implicitly accepted the notion that "artificial aid" might be provided to the delivered infant. Second, the Court did not attempt to clarify the notion of viability by indicating, for example, what percentage of fetuses must be able to survive at a general point of viability; rather, the Court seems either to have subscribed to an individually-oriented notion of viability (the likelihood that this particular fetus would be able to survive) or to have left the entire question to the judgment of the medical profession. Third, the Court implicitly accepted a dynamic concept of viability, noting that the point of viability is usually placed at about 28 weeks "but may occur earlier, even at 24 weeks" [2] ([17], p. 160).

The Court's decision, though vigorously resisted by numerous state legislatures, resolved most public policy issues regarding abortion for the decade of the 1970s. Several unresolved questions remained, however, most of them located near the viability-watershed. For example, how were pregnant women and their physicians to proceed when it was uncertain whether the point of viability had been reached in a particular pregnancy? More specifically, was potential viability sufficient to justify a compelling state interest? Further, in doubtful cases, could the state require that the abortion technique selected be calculated to maximize the chances of fetal survival following the abortion procedure? Finally, what obligations did physicians have to preserve fetal or neonatal life either during or after abortion in cases where some chance of survival seemed to exist? These unresolved questions were contested in the courts during the second half of the 1970. They were also addressed in part by the National Commission for the Protection of Human Subjects.

II. THE NATIONAL COMMISSION: THE POSTIMPLANTATION EMBRYO AND FETUS IN THE CLINICAL SETTING

In retrospect, it seems clear that the fetal-research issue was first raised in the United States as a conservative response to the Supreme Court's *Roe v. Wade* decision. (In Great Britain, a public debate on the same issue had begun in 1970 and had been, for the most part, terminated by the publication of the "Peel Committee Report" in 1972 [9].) In the United States, publicity about the fetal-research issue during April of 1973 [3] led in May to proposed legislation which would have banned the use of federal funds for live-fetus research [12]. In November of the same year the National Institutes of Health issued a set of preliminary guidelines on fetal research, as well as on several other types of controversial research [8]. These guidelines would have permitted most types of fetal research to continue. In mid-1974 a compromise was reached in the fetal-research debate: fetal research would neither be banned, nor would it proceed in the manner desired by NIH; rather, the whole issue would be studied systematically by a National Commission which would, in turn, report its findings to the Secretary of Health, Education, and Welfare [11]. The Commission began its work in December of 1974, making the fetal-research issue its first item of business. Meanwhile, during the calendar years 1973 and 1974 no fewer than 15 states passed legislation which either prohibited or restricted research with human fetuses.

While the *Roe v. Wade* decision on abortion led directly to the fetal-research debate, one should not overlook the radically different public-policy contexts or the two discussions. The Supreme Court's abortion decision specified the limits of state interference within the sphere of privacy accorded to every citizen. In contrast, the National Commission was charged with formulating recommendations concerning the types of fetal research which the federal government should either conduct itself or support non-federal researchers to conduct. Thus, *Roe v. Wade* was concerned with a noninterference right, whereas the National Commission's deliberations had their primary impact on a welfare right.

Despite these different policy contexts, it may be instructive to reflect how the principles enunciated in the Supreme Court's *Roe v. Wade* decision might have been applied (by the Court or others) to the problem of fetal research. One can plausibly argue that the Court's principles would have allowed research on pre-viable fetuses without restriction. The one proviso which might have been added to this general permission is that the state does have an interest in preventing damage to pre-viable fetuses which will subsequently become viable fetuses and viable citizens. Thus, the *Roe v. Wade* principles seem most compatible with a policy on fetal research which allows both therapeutic and nontherapeutic research on pre-viable fetuses, whether *in utero* or outside the uterus and especially in cases where induced abortion has insured or will insure that the point of viability will not be reached. (I do not mean to say that innocuous types of research on pre-viable fetuses likely to be delivered later as infants would have been prohibited by *Roe v. Wade* principles; however, as noted above, a different state interest might have been considered to apply where live birth beyond the stage of viability was anticipated.)

The National Commission clearly subscribed to a "theory of life" different from the one implicitly accepted by the Supreme Court in its *Roe v. Wade* decision. Or, to phrase the point more cautiously, the Commission adopted, for the most part, a conservative position on the status of the pre-viable fetus in the research context, while the Court specifically prohibited the states from establishing any legal restrictions on the rights of women to abort pre-viable fetuses in the clinical context.[3] In addition to adopting a conservative theory of life, the Commission contributed several empirical and conceptual refinements to the Court's discussion of viability.

The Commission accorded significant moral status to the postimplantation human embryo and fetus. Indeed, with one possible exception, to be discussed below, it seems fair to assert that the Commission advocated that the human fetus be treated in exactly the same way that a newborn infant ought to be treated. Consider the following statements from the Commission's final report on fetal research:

Although the Commission has not addressed directly the issues of the personhood and the civil status of the fetus, the members of the Commission are convinced that moral concern should extend to all who share human genetic heritage, and that the fetus, regardless of life prospects, should be treated respectfully and with dignity.

. . . While questions of risk become less relevant [in cases involving the nonviable fetus outside the uterus], considerations of respect for the dignity of the fetus continue to be of paramount importance, and require that the fetus be treated with the respect due to dying subjects. While dying subjects may not be "harmed" in the sense of "injured for life", issues of violations of integrity are nonetheless central[4] ([16], pp. 62, 68).

As if to leave no doubt concerning its viewpoint on the respect due to the human embryo and fetus, the Commission explicitly adopted an equal-treatment principle: no research procedure should be performed on a fetus-to-be-aborted which would not also be performed on a fetus-going-to-term ([16], pp. 67, 74). Given the fact that parents-to-be often treat the developing fetus proleptically as if it were already a child, the equality principle set rather strict limits on the range of permissible fetal research.

At two points in the Commission's fetal research report an alternative perspective on the pre-viable (or nonviable) fetus was at least vestigially in evidence. According to this alternative view, a different notion of "risk" or "harm" can be applied to the fetus-going-to-term, on the one hand, and the fetus-to-be-aborted or the fetus-already-aborted, on the other. At least two versions of this alternative view were formulated by the Commissioners and their consultants. The more conservative version was that *specific procedures* – for example, the injection of a drug into the bloodstream of a pregnant woman – might not injure a fetus if it were aborted within the two weeks following the procedure but might injure a fetus allowed to go to full term. The more liberal version of the alternative view was that *in principle* one cannot do harm to a fetus destined to die within a few weeks or a few hours. In other words, since abortion results in fetal death, and since death is an infinite harm, no additional harm can be inflicted upon the fetus through the performance of experimental procedures upon it prior to its imminent death.

Critics of this alternative view pointed out that, in the case of the fetus-to-be-aborted, a pregnant woman might conceivably change her mind about abortion following the initiation of the research. In that case a fetus-to-be-aborted would make an unexpected transition to the category of fetus-going-to-term, and long-term damage to a future infant caused by the research procedures would become a possibility. Defenders of the alternative view responded by citing empirical evidence that such changes in decision by pregnant women occur only in 1–2% of cases following the initial contact with an abortion facility ([2], esp. pp. 16–17).

In its final recommendations the Commission explictly rejected the alternative view with respect to the fetus already aborted. The Commission noted that after abortion a pregnant woman can no longer change her mind and that any pre-viable fetus surviving abortion is, in effect, a dying subject. The Commission concluded: " ... Out of respect for dying subjects, no nontherapeutic interventions are permissible which would alter the duration of life of the nonviable fetus *ex utero*" ([16], p. 68). Concerning the fetus-to-be-aborted, the Commissioners remained divided to the end, with some Commissioners advocating an unmodified equal-treatment position, while others advocated the conservative version of the alternative view. The Commission's compromise was procedural: special problems in the application of the equal treatment criterion to the fetus-to-be-aborted are to be referred to a specially constituted national body for review [5] ([16], p. 68).

In addition to formulating guidelines for research on pre-viable fetuses, the Commission sought to refine the concept of viability. A study of available evidence covering survival of low-birth-weight infants, conducted by Drs. Richard Behrman and Tove Rosen of the College of Physicians and Surgeons at Columbia University, reached the following conclusions:

Despite differences in data base from various sources, two facts emerged clearly: probability of survival of infants weighing less than 750 grams was extremely small, and no cases were found from any documentable source of any infant surviving with a birth weight below 600 grams at a gestational age of 24 weeks or less. Some rare cases were documented of infants surviving with birth weights below 600 grams, but in each instance, the gestational age exceeded 24 weeks, and the cases thus represented more mature infants who for various reasons were small-for-dates. Other rare cases were documented of infants born before 25 weeks gestational age who survived, but in each instance birth weight exceeded 600 grams. Thus, on an empirical basis the current limits of viability are clear: there is no unambiguous documentation that an infant born weighing less than 601 grams at a gestational age of 24 weeks or less has ever survived ([16], p. 55).

In the light of these empirical findings, the Commission adopted 24 weeks' gestational age and a weight of 600 grams as its indices of viability, given the technological state of the art in 1975. The Commissioners then proposed three types of refinements to this rather clear numerical standard. First, with regard to the live "fetus" outside the uterus, the Commissioners created a twilight zone, a stage between nonviability and viability during which the fetus was considered to be "possibly viable". The numerical boundaries for this stage in the Commission report were 500 to 600 grams of weight and 20 to 24 weeks of gestational age ([16], p. 5). Second, with respect to the fetus *in utero*, the Commission allowed a margin for error in estimating fetal age or weight, stipulating that 20 weeks' gestational age was to be the upper limit for nontherapeutic research in anticipation of or during abortion ([16], pp. 68–69). Third, recognizing that advances in medical technology could reduce the .iumerical indices of viability still further in the future, the Commission called for periodic review and revision of its proposed viability standards ([16], pp. 5–6).

A backward glance at the Supreme Court's concept of viability reveals some striking differences between the views of the Court in 1973 and the Commission in 1975. In the abortion context the Court had set the lower limit of viability at 28 (usually) or 24 weeks. In the research context the Commission set the lower limit of viability at 24 weeks and 600 grams in cases where it could be measured accurately but placed the operational lower limit of viability for the fetus in utero at 20 weeks' gestational age. Unless fetuses mature more rapidly in the research context, one is hard pressed to explain the discrepancy between 20 and 24 or 28 weeks. Assuming that no major advances in neonatal care occurred between 1973 and 1975, the most plausible explanation is that the Court set the viability limit high to allow as much room as possible for the exercise of the pregnant woman's privacy rights, while the Commission set the viability limit low either because of its respect for the fetus or in order to minimize the probability that fetuses potentially damaged by research procedures would ever survive to become damaged (and possibly litigious) adults.

In our focus on the substantive standards proposed by the National Commission it is easy to lose sight of the context in which its recommendations were formulated. As we noted at the beginning of this section, the Commission was not determining what types of fetal research were ethically or legally permissible. Rather, it was recommending to the Secretary of Health, Education, and Welfare the types of fetal research which should be "conducted or supported" by DHEW[6]. Even the translation of the Commission's recommendations into federal regulations has had direct relevance only to the types of fetal research which are supported by public funds appropriated to the Department of Health, Education, and Welfare. Thus, a private sector remained where scientific investigators and private foundations could in principle reach different conclusions concerning the ethical permissibility of various types of fetal research — within the limits set by a fast-growing number of state statutes on this topic.

The Commission did not explicitly indicate what priority it assigned to the funding of fetal research by DHEW. The only hints of the Commission's position can be found in the fine print of its recommendations and in the dissenting statements contained in its final report. In only two cases did the Commission recommend that fetal research should be "encouraged" by the DHEW Secretary: these were the cases of *therapeutic* research directed toward the fetus or the pregnant woman ([16], p. 73). There was apparently less unanimous enthusiasm among the Commissioners regarding the various types of nontherapeutic fetal research.

III. THE ETHICS ADVISORY BOARD: THE PREIMPLANTATION EMBRYO IN THE RESEARCH AND CLINICAL SETTINGS

In May of 1978 the Ethics Advisory Board of the Department of Health, Education, and Welfare agreed to review a research proposal by Professor Pierre Soupart of Vanderbilt University. Professor Soupart proposed to perform laboratory studies on human embryos following *in vitro* fertilization of human ova. The studies were to be conducted within a few days of fertilization. Professor Soupart's research proposal had already been reviewed and approved for scientific merit by the appropriate review body at the National Institutes of Health. Coincidentally, during the summer of 1978 an infant was delivered in England following *in vitro* fertilization and embryo transfer. Thus, it seemed reasonable to the Ethics Advisory Board to consider the preimplantation embryo both in the setting of laboratory research and in the setting where embryo transfer and further development were envisioned. The Board's intensive study of *in vitro* fertilization, initiated in September 1978, culminated in a report to the HEW Secretary dated 4 May 1979.

While several of the Board's consultants discussed the moral status issue at considerable length [7], the Board itself included only a brief comment on the status of the embryo in its conclusions:

... The Board is in agreement that the human embryo is entitled to profound respect; but this respect does not necessarily encompass the full legal and moral rights attributed to persons ([14], p. 101).

In addition, the Board noted the high rate of embryo loss following *in vivo* fertilization, that is, following sexual intercourse. According to statistics presented to the Board by Professor John Biggers, only about 37% of all one-celled embryos survive to be delivered as live infants ([1], p. 10). However, the Board did not from this *factual* observation reach any conclusions regarding the *moral* status of the embryo. Rather, the Board noted that embryo loss following attempts at embryo transfer parallels such loss "in nature" and is therefore ethically acceptable ([14], p. 101).

There was relatively little debate among Board members concerning the status of the embryo in the clinical setting. The need for embryo transfer sets temporal limits on the duration of *in vitro* culture, and the mutual interest of prospective parents and clinicians in a healthy offspring provides strong incentives for the careful handling of embryos-to-be-transferred in the laboratory setting. What had once been thought to be a serious ethical problem — the fertilization of numerous ova following superovulation and the existence of a surplus following the selection of one embryo for transfer — had been solved by a purely technical change in procedure: no hormones are currently given to women prior to ovulation, and only one oocyte (ovum) is harvested during each menstrual cycle.

The Board did not comment on the fact that grossly abnormal early embryos will almost certainly be discarded, nor did it discuss the philosophically interesting question of the moral status of a frozen early embryo. In the breeding of certain types of domestic animals, embryos are routinely frozen prior to transfer; the reportedly successful effort at embryo transfer in India also seems to have involved the frozen storage of multiple human embryos from one menstrual cycle to the next [10]. Other potential developments which the Board probably considered too speculative to merit discussion are the sexing of embryos, the repair of genetic defects in the embryo, the replacement of embryonic nuclei (cloning), and the creation of human-human hybrid embryos following *in vitro* fertilization and prior to embryo transfer ([18], pp. 48–52).

The question of laboratory research with early human embryos gave some Board members pause for the following reason: such research involves the creation of early embryos by means of *in vitro* fertilization when one knows in advance that such embryos will either be killed or allowed to die within, at most, a few days of fertilization. In the end, the Board reached a compromise formula. The ethical questions concerning the clinical and the laboratory setting were considered together, in a single recommendation, and laboratory research with early embryos was adjudged by the Board to be ethically acceptable if its dominant thrust was to assess the risks of *in vitro* fertilization and embryo transfer in the clinical setting. The Board's precise wording of this stipulation was as follows:

The Ethics Advisory Board finds that it is acceptable from an ethical standpoint to undertake research involving human *in vitro* fertilization and embryo transfer provided that:

A. If the research involves human in vitro fertilization without embryo transfer, the following conditions are satisfied: . . .

2. The research is designed primarily:

(A) to establish the safety and efficacy of embryo transfer and (B) to obtain important scientific information toward that end not reasonably attainable by other means . . . ([14], p. 106).

To date there have been no test cases which would explore the boundaries of the Board's dominant-thrust criterion for laboratory *in vitro* fertilization research. Most if not all types of already-performed IVF research could be comfortably arrayed under this banner.

The Board did not exclude the performance of any type of research procedure on early human embryos. Nor did it explicitly comment on futuristic research possibilities discussed by some commentators on *in vitro* fertilization. Among the major categories of potential research with human embryos are research on parthenogenesis,[8] interspecies fertilization, nuclear transfer (cloning), human-human hybridization, and human-nonhuman hybridization ([18], pp. 43–48). The guidelines adopted by the Board did, however, implicitly rule out efforts to achieve ectogenesis, or extracorporeal gestation: one of the Board's conditions for the ethical acceptability of laboratory research was that "no embryos will be sustained *in vitro* beyond the stage normally associated with the completion of implantation (14 days after fertilization)" ([14], p. 107).

In developmental terms the Ethics Advisory Board's report neatly filled a lacuna which had been left by the earlier National Commission report. The Commission had defined the fetus as "the human from the time of implantation". The Board now developed a policy for the human from the time of fertilization until the time of implantation, either *in vivo* (following embryo transfer) or *in vitro* (the 14-day limit for nontransferred embryos).

As we have noted, the earlier report of the National Commission had been devoted primarily to a discussion of the types of fetal research which merited federal funding. In the Ethics Advisory Board's report an interesting reversal of emphasis occurred. Most of the Board's report and its explicit recommendation concerning research with human embryos were devoted to the *ethical acceptability* of such research. This emphasis can be traced in part to the Board's regulatory mandate, to render advice as to "the acceptability [of research] from an ethical standpoint" ([14], p. 15). An additional rationale for this ethical analysis was that the Board wished to provide guidance to local institutional review boards which might conceivably be called upon to review proposed research on human embryos which was funded by non-HEW sources ([14], p. 107).

The members of the Ethics Advisory Board were rather sharply divided on the question of HEW funding for *in vitro* fertilization research. Some Board members also argued that the Board lacked the kind of overview and expertise which would permit it to make prudent allocation decisions. Therefore, the Board deferred to the Department of Health, Education, and Welfare, suggesting ethical considerations which the Department should take into account in setting its priorities but rendering no independent judgment on funding ([14], p. 109). The Board noted that the Department would have to make funding decisions both about laboratory *in vitro* fertilization research and, more remotely, about clinical trials of *in vitro* fertilization and embryo transfer as techniques for overcoming infertility.

The Board's explicit distinction between ethical acceptability and federal fundability was reminiscent of an analogous distinction developed by the United States Supreme Court in a series of abortion decisions during the 1970s. As noted above, the *Roe v. Wade* decision in 1973 clearly affirmed the legal permissibility of induced abortion prior to the stage of viability. However, in its 1977 decision *Maher v. Roe* the Court held that even though states could not interfere with the right to abortion, they were not bound to include nontherapeutic abortions in their Medicaid plans ([4], p. 35). The Ethics Advisory Board appears to have transposed the Court's negative right/positive right dichotomy from the legal to the ethical sphere and from the issue of abortion to that of human *in vitro* fertilization.

IV. CONCLUDING COMMENTS

The ethical and public policy discussion concerning the human fetus during the 1970s was carried on by multiple groups with divergent goals. The discussion covered all stages of embryonic and fetal development — from the time of fertilization to the time of delivery, both in the womb and in the laboratory. In these concluding comments I will seek both to acknowledge the different policy contexts and purposes of the three documents analyzed above and to identify areas of substantive agreement and disagreement among them.

The Supreme Court, the nation's highest judicial body, is charged with determining whether state or federal laws are in accord with the United States Constitution. In *Roe v. Wade* the Court held that the human fetus is not a legal person enjoying constitutional rights and that prior to the stage of fetal viability there can be no state interest so compelling that it would justify a state's interfering with a pregnant woman's constitutional right of privacy.

The National Commission for the Protection of Human Subjects was established by the Congress to make recommendations on research policy to the Secretary of Health, Education, and Welfare. While the Commission was not a regulatory body, its recommendations were to provide the factual and theoretical basis for regulations to be promulgated by the DHEW Secretary. In its deliberations, the Commission adopted the principle that the human fetus in the research context should be accorded treatment equal to that of the fetus going to term. This principle, in turn, led the Commission to recommend rather conservative rules for fetal research conducted or supported by the federal government.

The Ethics Advisory Board was established by the Secretary of Health, Education, and Welfare both to fulfill a task mandated by federal regulation and to provide advice on controversial ethical and public policy questions. In its report on *in vitro* fertilization the Board rendered judgments concerning (1) the *general* ethical acceptability of certain types of research with early human embryos, as well as (2) the ethical acceptability of federal support for such research. While the Board did not make a specific recommendation concerning the funding priority to be given to research involving embryos, it did (3) outline ethical considerations to be taken into account by public officials in assigning a funding priority to *in vitro* fertilization research. The first of these judgments seems to have been strictly ethical, while the second and third were directed toward public policy.

In sum, the Supreme Court in *Roe v. Wade* specified a noninterference right, while the National Commission and the Ethics Advisory Board devoted primary attention to delimiting the scope of a positive right, namely, the right to federal research funds. In addition, the Commission implicitly and the Board explicitly rendered ethical judgments concerning the moral propriety of the federal government's funding certain types of fetal or embryonic research at all. Only the Board advanced a general ethical judgment concerning the ethical acceptability of performing certain types of research, even without federal funding.

Despite these differences in the scope and goals of their deliberations and decisions, there are significant areas of substantive consensus among the three policymaking bodies and the public policy documents they produced. At the later stages of the developmental spectrum, it seems clear that the moment of delivery is considered the most decisive watershed. The Supreme Court ascribed legal personhood to the newborn infant, and the National Commission erected a formidable hedge of protections around the viable and even the possibly viable infant in its guidelines for federal funding of research. According to the Commission, even the clearly nonviable delivered "fetus" is to be treated with the respect that is owed to dying subjects.

The viable fetus *in utero* was accorded a lower legal status by the Supreme Court: in the Court's view in *Roe v. Wade* the viable fetus is not a legal person. Yet the Court conceded that the interest of the state could become compelling beyond the point of viability and that the state could restrict the grounds for aborting a viable fetus, unless the fetus were directly impinging upon the pregnant woman's life or health. As the Court's holding has been applied, both in the laws of the various states and in the customary practice of health professionals, the viable fetus is accorded almost-personal status before the law. In the research sphere, the National Commission's guidelines for federal research funding allowed only no-risk or minimal-risk research involving the viable fetus *in utero*. Thus, the fetus *in utero* is less well protected than the newborn infant only in the senses that it is not a legal person and that it can legitimately be killed in cases of necessity involving the mother's life or health.

At the other end of the developmental spectrum is the human embryo during the first fourteen days following fertilization. While the Ethics Advisory Board argued that the early embryo should be treated with "profound respect", it conceded that "this respect does not necessarily encompass the full legal and moral rights attributed to persons". The Board then set loose limits on the range of ethically acceptable research goals and stipulated that the knowledge sought through research on early human embryos should be attainable in no other way. Beyond these caveats, however, the Board set no limits on the types of research procedures which may permissibly be employed in laboratory research with early human embryos. This relative silence by the Ethics Advisory Board stands in marked contrast to the National Commission's detailed discussion of research procedures involving the embryo and fetus at later stages of development. Indeed, the Board accepted the deliberate creation of human embryos for research purposes. Tacitly, at least, the Board seemed to be saying: "There is no problem of sentience in early human embryos and no problem of full personhood in the ethical or legal sense. Do not squander such embryos in unnecessary research, but do not hesitate to use early embryos in research which may be of significant benefit to present and future persons".

In the middle of the developmental spectrum is the most controversial stage of embryonic and fetal development — the stage between implantation and viability. The Supreme Court, in contradiction of existing laws in most states, accorded pregnant women the right to abortion during this entire

stage in its *Roe v. Wade* decision. Yet the Court also conceded in later decisions that the states and the federal government need not fund women in
the exercise of that right. The National Commission encouraged federal
conduct or support of therapeutic research involving the previable embryo
or fetus *in utero* and accepted federal conduct or support of carefully-
delimited types of nontherapeutic research. However, the Commissioners
disagreed on how the notion of "risk" should be applied to the pre-viable
fetus-to-be-aborted. Meanwhile, numerous state legislatures were passing laws
which either banned or sharply limited not merely the funding but also the
conduct of fetal research.

In sum, the three public policy documents discussed in this essay reached
a rough consensus on the status of the preimplantation embryo, the viable
fetus *in utero*, and the delivered "fetus" or infant. The major point of controversy remained, as it has for centuries, the appropriate treatment of the
implanted embryo and fetus prior to the stage of viability. Given the pluralism
of opinion reflected in these public policy documents and in polls of the
larger society, the prospects for an early resolution of this controversy
do not appear bright. Perhaps we shall have to learn to disagree on this
issue, within a legal framework which protects diversity of both opinion
and action.[9]

Kennedy Institute of Ethics,
Georgetown University, Washington, D.C.

NOTES

[1] In standard obstetrical and embryological parlance, the human conceptus is called
an embryo during the first eight weeks of development and a fetus for the remainder
of gestation. The title of this paper employs the term fetus in an extended sense to
refer to both the embryonic and fetal stages of development.

[2] For a penetrating critique of the viability concept in *Roe v. Wade* and a constructive
proposal for making viability the relevant legal standard, see [6].

[3] For an analysis of the contrasting views of the Supreme Court and the Commission
on the status of the fetus, see [7].

[4] Of the eight philosophers and theologians who served as consultants to the Commission on the ethics of fetal research, five espoused a relatively conservative position on
the moral status of the fetus, one a liberal position, and two a mediating position.

[5] One commentator has argued that the conservative position on fetal status adopted by
the Commission and reflected in later DHEW regulations based upon the Commission's
recommendations constitutes an establishment of religion [5].

[6] I am indebted for this insight to a comment by my colleague, H. Tristram Engelhardt, Jr.
[7] See especially the essays by Leon Kass, Charles Curran, and Samuel Gorovitz in [13], Essays 2, 3, and 4.
[8] Whether an ovum induced to develop without benefit of fertilization by a sperm is properly called an "embryo" is an interesting conceptual question.
[9] I am indebted to Professor George Agich and to my colleagues at the Kennedy Institute for their critical comments on an earlier draft of this essay.

BIBLIOGRAPHY

1. Biggers, J. D.: 1979, 'In Vitro Fertilization, Embryo Culture, and Embryo Transfer in the Human' ([13], Essay 8).
2. Bracken, M. B.: 1975, 'The Stability of the Decision to Seek Induced Abortion' ([15], Essay 16).
3. Cohn, V.: 1973, 'Live Fetus Research Debated', Washington Post, 10 April 1973, pp. A1 ff.
4. Flannery, D. M., et al.: 1979, 'Legal Issues Concerning In Vitro Fertilization' ([13], Essay 18).
5. Friedman, J. M.: 1977, 'The Federal Fetal Experimentation Regulations: An Establishment Clause Analysis', Minnesota Law Review 61, 961–1005.
6. King, P. A.: 1979, 'The Juridical Status of the Fetus: A Proposal for Legal Protection of the Unborn', Michigan Law Review 77, 1647–1687.
7. Menzel, P.: 1975, 'The Court and the Commission', Hastings Center Report 5, 14–16.
8. National Institutes of Health: 1973, 'Protection of Human Subjects: Policies and Procedures', Federal Register 38, 31738–31749.
9. Report of the Advisory Group: 1972, The Use of Fetuses and Fetal Material for Research, Her Majesty's Stationery Office, London.
10. 'Test Tube Baby, World's Second, Born in India', Washington Post, 6 October 1978, p. A16.
11. U.S.: 1974, 'An Act . . . to Establish a Program of National Research Service Awards . . . and to Provide for the Protection of Human Subjects . . . ', U.S. Statutes at Large 88, 342–354 (Public Law 93–348, approved 12 July, 1974).
12. U.S. Congress, House: 1973, 'A Bill to Prohibit the Use of Appointed Funds to Carry Out or Assist Research on Living Human Fetuses', H. R. 7850, 93rd Congress, 1st Session, 15 May, 1973 (Representative Angelo Roncallo).
13. U.S. Department of Health, Education, and Welfare, Ethics Advisory Board: 1979, HEW Support of Research Involving Human In Vitro Fertilization and Embryo Transfer: Appendix, Department of Health, Education, and Welfare, Washington, D.C.
14. U.S. Department of Health, Education, and Welfare, Ethics Advisory Board: 1979, HEW Support of Research Involving Human In Vitro Fertilization and Embryo Transfer: Report and Conclusions, Department of Health, Education, and Welfare, Washington, D.C.
15. U.S. Department of Health, Education, and Welfare, National Commission for the

Protection of Human Subjects of Biomedical and Behavioral Research: 1975, *Research on the Fetus: Appendix*, Department of Health, Education, and Welfare, Washington, D.C.
16. U.S. Department of Health, Education, and Welfare, National Commission for the Protection of Human Subjects of Biomedical and Behavioral Research: 1975, *Research on the Fetus: Report and Recommendations*, Department of Health, Education, and Welfare, Washington, D.C.
17. U.S. Supreme Court: 1973, 'Roe *et al.* v. Wade, District Attorney of Dallas County', *U.S. Reports* **410**, 113–178 (decided 22 January, 1973).
18. Walters, L.: 1979, 'Ethical Issues in Human In Vitro Fertilization and Research Involving Human Embryos' ([13], Essay 1). Reprinted in *Hastings Center Report* **9**, 23–43.

JOHN D. BIGGERS

GENERATION OF THE HUMAN LIFE CYCLE

I. INTRODUCTION

Current arguments about fetal and maternal rights frequently invoke fertilization and birth as mutually exclusive events on which to base moral judgments. For example, the two following contrasting positions appeared in the British newspaper, *The Guardian* (October 29, 1973):

"To my mind life begins at the moment of conception, and to suggest otherwise seems to me just the sort of casuistry which an anti-Papist might describe as Jesuitical. (Incidentally, I am not myself a Roman Catholic.) Conception is the magic moment . . ." (John Grigg, quoted by Glover [21], p. 119).

"I do not believe a fertilized ovum is human life in the commonsense meaning of the term. I believe human life begins at birth. Or more technically, when a foetus is sufficiently developed to be capable of living if removed from the mother's womb. That human life begins at the moment of conception is a religious tenet that makes no claim whatsoever to scientific truth" (Dee Wells, quoted by Glover [21], p. 119).

Are such disparate views justified? I suggest not, since it is incorrect to assume that fertilization and birth are events that can be considered in isolation. Conception and birth should be recognized merely as phases of a more fundamental biological process – the life cycle (see [11], for a thorough discussion of the nature of the life cycle).

The essential features of the human life cycle are as follows. The process of fertilization renews the life cycle by initiating a period of development and growth called embryogenesis, in which organs arise from the fertilized egg. This method of reproduction occurs in the mother's genital tract by processes called internal fertilization and viviparity, respectively. A baby is finally delivered at birth and continues to develop and grow. Maturity is eventually reached, and this phase is followed by sensecence and death. During the period of maturity, the individual may participate in the process of reproduction that renews the life cycle. Thus life never stops, for if it did extinction would result. Life is passed on from one generation to another, and it is therefore incorrect to claim that life begins at arbitrarily chosen points of the life cycle.

31

William B. Bondeson et al. *(eds.), Abortion and the Status of the Fetus, 31–53.*
Copyright © 1983 by D. Reidel Publishing Company, Dordrecht, Holland.

The recognition that life is a continuum required may centuries of thought, observation, and experimentation. In the words of John Maynard Keynes, in another context:

The difficulty lies, not in the new ideas, but in escaping the old ones, which ramify, for those brought up as most of us have been, into every corner of our minds (quoted by Mackay [34]).

Thus in the first part of this paper I will trace briefly the origins of our modern ideas on generation. Next I discuss the central idea that reproductive processes have evolved which promote the flow of genetic information between generations. Then the bearing of live young, a very specialized form of reproduction in which new individuals spend part of development within the body of their mother, can be placed in proper biological perspective. Finally embryonic, fetal, and neonatal wastage will be described in terms of natural errors in the physiological mechanisms that subserve the flow of genetic information between generations and the bearing of live young, including some mention of recent medical advances that could save individuals suffering from these errors.

II. EARLY IDEAS ON GENERATION

We know from the earliest written records that human beings have speculated on the origin of babies. Likewise, the anthropological literature shows that primitive human beings are also interested in the same problem. The question people in these societies try to answer is, "Which sex generates babies?" The answers vary enormously (see [12], [42], for extensive discussions of these views). By way of illustration, we may compare the Greco-Egyptian doctrine that, in the words of Needham, denies physiological maternity, i.e., the father alone gives rise to the child, with the Melanesian doctrine, held by the Trobriand Islanders, that denies physiological paternity, i.e., the mother alone produces the child.

The denial of physiological maternity was taught by Aristotle and seems to be based on the following observations: a baby is born only after coitus between a man and woman, the initial development of a baby occurs within a woman's body, at coitus a fluid — the semen — is transferred from a man to a woman, once a baby is present in the woman, the menstrual flow ceases. *Ergo*, the semen provides the "form" to the embryo and the menstrual fluid gets used up to provide sustenance to the embryo. The Trobriand Islanders' denial of physiological paternity seems to be based on a different set of observations and beliefs: a baby develops within a woman's body, married women are often sterile despite having frequent intercourse, unmarried women, permitted by custom to have intercourse, invariably remained sterile until officially married (presumably a manifestation of adolescent sterility). Thus, sexual intercourse has nothing to do with producing a baby. To explain generation, they believe in Tuma, a mystical spirit-world of the unborn. The menstrual flow is again allotted a nutritive role which is dammed up during pregnancy to provide shelter for a soul from Tuma.

European thought on generation was dominated until the 17th century by the Greco-Egyptian doctrine, championed by Aristotle. Towards the end of this period the words *viviparous* and *oviparous* appeared in the English language (see the Oxford Dictionary). They were used frequently by the British physician and author Sir Thomas Browne in a book published in 1646, commonly known as *Browne's Vulgar Errors*. The words are derived by the conjugation of the Latin root *parere* — to bring forth, with the Latin roots *vivus* — alive, or *ovum* — egg. Thus viviparous means the bringing forth of young in a live state, and oviparous means the production of young from eggs. Browne explicitly regarded the two forms of generation as totally distinct, eggs being "unformed" and passively delivered by the mother, in contrast to live young that are "formed", and who participate jointly with the mother at least in the mechanism of delivery at birth. His views are illustrated by the following passage in which he rejects the popular belief that bears are born in a very immature state and are "unformed".

It is moreover injurious unto reason, and much impugneth the course and providence of nature, to conceive a birth should be ordained before there is formation; for the conformation of parts is necessarily required not only unto the prerequisites and previous conditions of birth, as motion and animation, but also unto the parturition or very birth it selfe; wherein not only the Dam, but the younglings play their parts, and the cause and act of exclusion proceedeth from them both: for the exclusion of animals is not merely passive like that of egges, nor the totall action of delivery to be imputed to the mother; but the first attempt beginneth from the Infant, which at the accomplished period attempteth to change his mansion, and strugling to come forth, dilacerates and breaks those parts which restrained him before ([10], p. 116).

These remarks were made when the Renaissance was already underway, and new concepts about the nature of generation were beginning to challenge the traditional teaching. An important individual at this time was the brilliant English physician, William Harvey, more famous for his discovery that blood circulates through the body. In a less well-known book, *De Generatione*, published in 1651, Harvey wrote:

In the dog, rabbit and several other animals, I have found nothing in the uterus after intercourse. I, therefore, regard it as demonstrated that after fertile intercourse among viviparous as well as oviparous animals, there are no remains in the uterus either of the semen of the male or female emitted in the act, nothing produced by any mixture of these two fluids, as the medical writers maintain, nothing of the menstrual blood present as 'matter' in the way Aristotle will have it; in a word, that there is not necessarily even a trace of conception to be seen immediately after a fruitful union of the sexes. It is not true, consequently, that in a prolific connexion there must be any prepared 'matter' in the uterus which the semen masculinum, acting as a coagulating agent, should congeal, concoct and fashion or bring into a positive generative act . . . (Quoted by [19], p. 24).

As an alternative explanation for generation, Harvey suggested that all animals develop from eggs. This view is immortalized in his dictum *Ex ovo omnia* inscribed on the egg illustrated in the frontispiece of his book. Eighteen years later, another explanation of generation was introduced by Swammerdam. This theory is known as the preformation theory which states that all individuals are perfectly formed from the beginning and merely have to enlarge and unfold much like a butterfly emerges from a chrysalis. The early embryologists who thought an individual is already preformed in an egg constitute a branch of preformationists known as *ovists*. The ovists believed:

that all living things there were to be had, in fact, had been organized by God at creation and that encapsulated within the first parent, all future generations were present . . . Each generation would in turn come to maturity, and when all created germs had reached the adult form, the species would become extinct ([19], p. 42).

Ten years after Swammerdam, in 1679, spermatozoa were first described by the Dutchman, Antony van Leeuwenhoek, the inventor of the compound microscope. He reported the work of his pupil, Ham, who examined human semen. Six years later, Leeuwenhoek recovered spermatozoa from the uterus of a bitch immediately after copulation. Scientists of the 17th and 18th centuries, however, were not unanimous about the biological significance of the spermatozoa. A common belief was that spermatozoa were parasitic. Linnaeus regarded spermatozoa as independent organisms and classified them with the following curious list under the name *Chaos infusoria*: (a) the moist virus of syphilis, (b) the contagion of eruptive fevers, (c) the cause of paroxysmal fevers, (d) the aery mist floating in the month of blossoming, (e) Münchhausen's septic agent of fermentation and putrefaction [15]. Others, however, saw spermatozoa as the exclusive source of new individuals. Thus, in 1694, Hartsoeker illustrated a spermatozoon containing a manikin within its head [42]. This view introduced the *animaliculist* version of the preformationist theory which soon acquired a following. Thus, the primitive notion that one or the other sex is responsible exclusively for the generation of new individuals persisted in the conflicting preformationist theories that were popular during the 17th and 18th centuries. No thought that eggs and sperm are both necessary participants in generation was entertained until the middle of the 19th century.

That both the ovum and spermatozoon participate in the generative process began to be recognized by a few naturalists around 1850. According to Cole, these naturalists

played a very minor part in the solution of the problem of fertilization, since the phenomenon of penetration by a *single* sperm, the fate of the sperm within the egg, and the participation of egg and sperm nuclei in fertilization were only completely demonstrated by the researches of O. Hertwig, Weismann and Fol, between the years 1875 and 1879 ([12], p. 195).

Thus the unravelling of the essential features of fertilization occurred only 103 years ago.

III. FLOW OF GENETIC INFORMATION BETWEEN GENERATIONS

1. *Biological Role of Fertilization*

One of the most important of all discoveries in biology is the cell theory, which was formulated during the first half of the 19th century (see [13], for a review). The theory arose from the work of several botanists and zoologists. The theory states that:

(a) all organisms are composed of cells or cells plus their products;
(b) all cells are basically alike in their chemical construction;
(c) new cells are formed from pre-existing cells by a process called cell division;
(d) the activity of an organism as a whole is the sum of the activities and interaction of the cell units.

The recognition that the sperm and ovum are single cells was very important for it showed that fertilization involved the fusion of two different types of cells to form a new cell. This cell is called the *zygote*.

One of the earliest consequences of fertilization to be noticed was that it stimulates the zygote to divide and begin the developmental process that leads to an adult. This function of fertilization is called *activation*. The other major function of fertilization is to mediate the flow of genetic information from one generation to another. Many years had to pass after the recognition of fertilization before this second function was fully appreciated. It required the discovery of several major biological phenomena. These include the recognition of the life cycle by Weissman, the quantal nature of inheritance by Mendel, the discovery of the chromosomes by Waldeyer, the formal probabilistic laws of inheritance independently by Fisher and Sewell Wright, and the molecular basis of the gene. The molecular basis of the gene is a relatively new discovery that resulted from the demonstration of the chemical structure of the DNA double helix by Watson and Crick [48] in 1953. Detailed introductions to these central concepts in biology can be gained from the following references: Dunn, [17]; Judson, [29]; Maynard Smith, [47]; and Kimura and Ohta [30].

2. *Genetic Variation and the Uniqueness of the Individual*

The primary function of the reproductive process in almost all organisms is the generation of genetic variability. This variability exists because of differences between the sets of genes present within individuals. It has been estimated that each human individual possesses about 100 000 different gene loci [32]. Each locus is occupied by one of a set of alternative genes called *alleles*. Thus a population of individuals that is capable of reproducing by its members sexually interacting with each other shares a large number of genes. Such a group forms a species, and each individual member possesses a sample of the total pool of genes shared by the species.

Human beings are members of a large group of organisms called *Eukaryotes* in which the genes are located on the chromosomes. Each eukaryotic species is associated with a particular number of paired chromosomes. Each pair is called an homologous pair. In humans the number of pairs is 23; 22 of them are called autosomes, and the remaining pair, the sex chromosomes. With the exception of the XY pair in males each pair of chromosomes appears to be morphologically identical. This morphological similarity, however, is illusory since the members of each pair of chromosomes carry genetically different information, because genes occupying the corresponding loci may be different alleles. There is thus a large number of different chromosome constitutions that may form a homologous pair in an individual. Consider four sets of alleles, α, β, γ, δ, consisting of 2, 6, 4, and 5 genes, respectively. The following sets are five of the many possible combinations (the subscript identifies a particular gene):

I	II	III	IV	V
α_1	α_2	α_2	α_1	α_2
β_6	β_4	β_6	β_1	β_2
γ_4	γ_2	γ_1	γ_3	γ_1
δ_3	δ_1	δ_5	δ_5	δ_4

An individual could contain a pair of any of these numerous combinations including a pair of identical chromosomes.

How is the variability in the genetic make-up of eukaryotic individuals generated? The variation arises at two levels of organization: in the assembly of the characteristic number of chromosome pairs from the chromosomes derived from the parents, and in the generation of new individual chromosomes. These mechanisms involve three basic processes — meiosis, fertilization, and mutation. During meiosis homologous pairs of chromosomes become separated into two sets each containing one member of each homologous pair. In humans each set will consist of 22 autosomes and one sex chromosome. These sets then pass to the gametes, the ovum or sperm. Since the two members of each homologous pair of chromosomes separate at random, various combinations of chromosomes can pass to the gametes. If n is the number of homologous pairs of chromosomes the number of possible combinations within an individual is 2^n. In humans this number is $2^{23} = 8\ 388\ 608$. This process that generates variation between gametes is called *chromosome recombination*. However, meiosis also involves another process called *crossing over* which generates further variability by altering the combinations of genes within chromosomes (see Figure 1). At the beginning of meiosis the members of each homologous pair come to lie side by side. Each chromosome splits longitudinally but the two halves, called chromatids, are held together at one point by the centromere. The chromosomes may lie across each other at one or more points. If DNA breakage and repair occurs at these points segments of homologous chromosomes may be exchanged. The cell then divides and one reconstituted chromosome then passes to each daughter cell. The two chromatids then separate by splitting of the centromere to give rise to two new homologous chromosomes that then participate in chromosome recombination in the second meiotic division. Crossing over occurs in all pairs of chromosomes except the sex chromosomes, and it has the potential of generating far more variation than the recombination of chromosomes. Variation can also be introduced into individual chromosomes by *point mutation*, a local change in the chemical structure of the DNA in a single

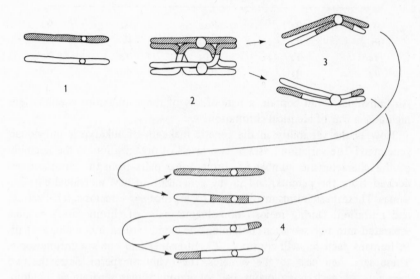

Fig. 1. Redistribution of the material of a pair of homologous chromosomes during the first and second meiotic divisions. In the first meiotic division the members of each pair of homologous chromosomes (1) divide with crossing-over (2) and separate to opposite poles (3). In the second meiotic division, the division of the centromeres gives rise to four genetically different chromosomes (4) each of which will form part of the haploid chromosome complement of a gamete. (From [25].)

gene. Mutations arise at a very low rate under natural conditions and only alter the composition of the gene pool very slowly [30].

The result of meiosis, and to a minor extent mutation, is to cause the production of sperm and ova containing different gene complements. The potential for variation is so large that almost all sperm and ova are genetically different and therefore capable of transmitting different genetic information. However, the potential for genetic variation between zygotes is increased even further by several orders of magnitude through the process of fertilization, in which an essentially unique sperm and an essentially unique ovum fuse. The potential number of types of pairs of alleles that constitute the genotype formed in a new zygote is astronomical, and for all practical purposes the zygote is genetically unique. Thus the genetic uniqueness of an eukaryotic individual depends on the combined processes of meiosis and fertilization. It is the continual production of new samples of the gene pool that allows a species, rather than its individual members, to adapt to the slow inexorable changes in the universe.

The modern epigenetic view of the life cycle holds that embryonic development proceeds from a set of coded instructions provided by the genes assembled at fertilization. This view is therefore very different from that held by the preformationists who thought that already formed manikins existed in ova or spermatozoa. Historically, there are signs that the idea of epigenesis was known by Aristotle, but it did not gain strong support and replace preformationist theories until the work of Von Baer in 1828 (see [23] for a review). Only in the last 20 years has epigenesis been formulated in chemical terms using the notion of informational molecules coded for by the DNA of individual genomes.

3. *Polyembryony*

The assembly of a new sample of the gene pool in a zygote does not necessarily determine the development of a single unique life cycle, since multiple genetically identical individuals can arise from a single zygote by a process called polyembryony. In mammals polyembryony can occur in three ways. One way is by the separation of the two blastomeres of a two-cell embryo. Each of these cells is totipotent, in that each has the capability of being able to develop into an independent individual, one of identical twins. Multiple birth ($\geqslant 2$) can also originate from a single blastocyst when multiple inner cell masses arise, or alternatively when multiple primitive streaks develop within a single inner mass. One obvious result of polyembryony is that all siblings will be the same sex.

Polyembryony has evolved as a normal reproductive pattern in a number of species and can result in the production of several offspring from a single zygote [41]. The phenomenon is a normal method of reproduction in the mammalian family *Dasypodidae* – the armadillos [43], which explains the observation of the early Spanish explorers of the New World that all members of litters of armadillos are of the same sex. For example, the nine-banded armadillo, the only armadillo that lives in the U.S.A., always has identical quadruplets, and the mulatta, an armadillo that lives in the Argentinian pampas, bears up to 12 identical young in each pregnancy (Fernandez, quoted in [3]). In human beings, polyembryony occurs in some pregnancies and is the cause of identical twins. It can arise by any of the three mechanisms described [14].

As the life cycles of these genetically identical individuals advance, they may acquire phenotypic variation among themselves as the result of exposure to unshared environmental influences during their development. Thus the uniqueness of individual siblings is not determined at fertilization but during the course of development. In a naturally reproducing eukaryotic species the zygotes that give rise to polyembryonic individuals will be heterozygotes, and the gametes each individual produces will show wide genetic diversity. However, the acquired characteristics that led to their uniqueness are unlikely to contribute to this diversity between their gametes [1].

4. *Extended Temporal Transitions Between Life Cycles*

In 1896 E. V. Wilson [51] coined the phrase "embryogenesis begins in oogenesis" to highlight the fact that some of the controls of development immediately after fertilization are laid down in the potential mother during the differentiation of the ovum. Nowadays developmental biologists distinguish between three types of gene products (informational molecules) necessary for development, based on whether they are synthesized during the development of the ovum or sperm prior to fertilization, or in the newly formed embryo after fertilization. They determine what are called maternal, paternal, and embryonic effects, respectively (see [38], for a review). The maternal contribution is likely to be much greater than the paternal contribution because of the large difference in size of the ovum and the spermatozoon.

Several studies on the mouse suggest that maternal gene products produced before fertilization control development entirely up to the 2-cell stage and partially up to the 8-cell stage. In the rabbit, α-amanitin does not inhibit development until after the 8-cell stage. Thus in this species the first three cleavage divisions do not require the synthesis of gene products after fertilization but are dependent on products synthesized during oogenesis. The activity of the embryonic genome in the mouse has been demonstrated by using genetic markers to show the activity of paternally derived genes. The earliest that has been demonstrated is β-glucuronidase [52] which appears at the 4-cell stage of development. Many proteins appear between the 2- and 8-cell stage in the mouse, and the 8-cell stage and early blastocyst in the rabbit. Whether these are the stages when the control of development becomes solely dependent on the embryonic genome has yet to be demonstrated [38].

Activation of mammalian ova can be induced experimentally without the participation of spermatozoa (see [24] and [49] for reviews). These embryos are called parthenogenones. They may possess the haploid number of chromosomes or the original haploid set may be replicated to give the diploid number. In the mouse both haploid and diploid parthenogenones develop to the blastocyst stage or early somite stage and initiate the decidual response in the uterus, but then they die. The reason these embryos die is far from understood, particularly in view of the work of Hoppe and Illmensee [27] on the effects of removal of a single pronucleus from a mouse zygote. In their experiments either the male or female pronucleus was removed, and the chromosomes in the remaining pronucleus caused to replicate by exposure of the eggs to cytochalasin, a procedure called *diploidization*. Such embryos are genetically equivalent to diploid parthenogenones; yet after transfer into the uterus of a surrogate mother they develop and rise to normal young. As pointed out by McLaren [38], it seems that some factor in the sperm other than its DNA is necessary to ensure later development. Presumably this unknown substance is synthesized by the father during spermatogenesis.

IV. VIVIPARITY

1. *Prenatal Development and Growth of a Baby*

Viviparity denotes the reproductive process in which embryogenesis and early growth of an individual occurs within the body of the mother. The process is initiated at fertilization and is completed at birth by the process of parturition. In women, this period of pregnancy lasts 270 days, with a standard deviation of 10 days. Viviparity is very widespread in the animal kingdom, but with varying degress of complexity.

Preimplantation development of human beings has been reviewed by Biggers [6]. Fertilization occurs in the upper part of the oviduct, called the ampulla. The zygote is activated and undergoes cell divisions until a ball of 16–32 cells is produced, called a morula. This process takes about three days. During this time the early embryo travels down the oviduct and enters the uterus. Throughout this period of embryonic life, each cell is essentially independent. Eventually a process called compaction occurs, in which the outer cells form the first tissue. This is an epithelium called the trophectoderm, which acts as an outer skin. The embryo can now control the chemical composition of its internal environment and begins to function as a multicellular individual [4], [9]. For three days it lies in the uterine secretions unattached to the mother's uterus. By the sixth day, most of the uterine fluid disappears, and the blastocyst becomes closely applied to the uterine epithelium. This event marks the beginning of implantation. The embryo then begins to invade the maternal tissue, and eventually it becomes completely embedded in the wall of the uterus. The process of implantation is now complete. The placenta then develops by the interaction of maternal and embryonic tissues, providing the organ through which the embryo receives nutrients and oxygen from its mother, and excretes its waste products. The net result at the end of pregnancy is a baby which normally weighs 3–4 kg. The magnitude of this process of growth can be appreciated by realizing that the zygote weighs only 1.25 μg, or that the newborn contains about $2^{42} \sim 4$ trillion cells which are all descendents of the original single-celled ovum.

The amounts of a few of the materials that are supplied by the mother through the placenta for the growth of the fetus are shown in Table I. Many other organic molecules are also supplied by the mother as well as the energy required for their transport, and the energy required for the biosynthetic processes in which these compounds are used to produce the fetus. An introductory account of fetal physiology has been written recently by Biggers [7].

TABLE I

Total amounts of water, N, Ca, Na, K and Cl in the human fetus at different stages of development (from [50], p. 91)

Body wt. (gm)	Approximate fetal age (weeks)	Water (gm)	N (gm)	Ca (gm)	Na (mM)	K (mM)	Cl (mM)
30	13	27	0.4	0.09	3.6	1.4	2.4
100	15	89	1.0	0.3	9	2.6	7
200	17	177	2.8	0.7	20	7.9	14
500	23	440	7.0	2.2	49	22	33
1000	26	860	14	6.0	90	44	66
1500	31	1270	25	10	125	60	96
2000	33	1620	37	15	160	84	120
2500	35	1940	49	20	200	110	130
3000	38	2180	55	25	240	130	150
3500	40	2400	62	30	280	150	160

The fetus also develops inside an embryonic sac called the amnion which is filled with amniotic fluid. The fetus, amniotic sac and its contents and the placenta which function jointly in pregnancy are called the conceptus. The relative weights of these components from 28–42 weeks of a human pregnancy are shown in Figure 2. The weight of the fetus becomes more and more predominant as the time of delivery is approached.

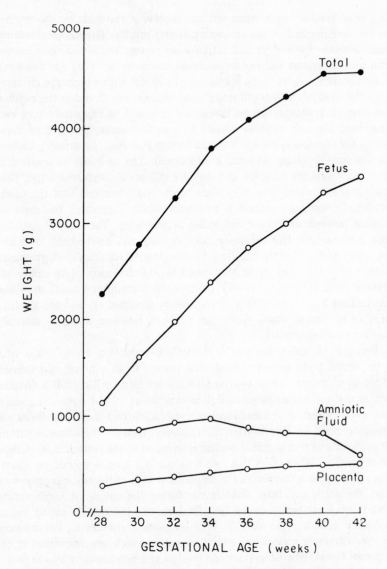

Fig. 2. Total weight of human conceptus and weights of fetus, amniotic fluid, and placenta from 28th to 44th week of conception. (From [7].)

2. *Embryonic-Maternal Interaction*

Pregnancy involves more than just the supply of materials by the mother
for the development of the conceptus. It also involves physiological interactions between the mother and intrauterine young. The interactions involve
both immunological and endocrinological functions (see [26] for a review).

Fertilization results in the formation of a zygote with a genotype different
from the mother, which will make some antigens not found in the mother.
The embryo is thus a foreign tissue, and it would be expected to provoke
a maternal immune response when it invades the uterus. The embryo, however, is not rejected as though it were a foreign skin graft, presumably because
the maternal immune response is suppressed. The mechanisms involved in
this suppression are complex and they are still poorly understood (see [20]
and [28] for recent reviews). Some recent work suggests that the newly
fertilized ovum may secrete a substance which suppresses the maternal
immune response at the very beginning of pregnancy. The name zygotin has
been proposed for this substance, and its assay may be the basis for a new
pregnancy test, called the rosette inhibition test, which can detect pregnancy
much earlier than can those tests based on the detection of an embryonic
hormone (see [45] for a review). If this work is confirmed it will show that
mechanisms have evolved that allow a newly fertilized egg and the resulting
embryo to protect itself from the mother's response which is naturally
hostile to a foreign tissue.

Fertilization occurs soon after the time of ovulation during the ovarian
cycle, which is the normal reproductive pattern in all non-pregnant women.
It occurs on average about 14 days after the last menstrual period. If fertilization is not successful, menstruation occurs about 12–14 days later, and a
new cycle begins. If fertilization is successful, further menstrual flows and
ovulation cease for the duration of pregnancy. Thus the reproductive pattern
characteristic of non-pregnant women is switched to the pattern characteristic
of pregnancy. When does this switch occur and how is it brought about?
The signal appears to arise in the trophoblast cells of the embryo on or soon
after the sixth day from fertilization during the course of implantation.
The trophoblast produces the first fetal hormone, a protein called human
chorionic gonadotropin (hCG). This hormone continues to be produced
in ever-increasing quantities, and soon reaches high concentrations in the
maternal blood. When this hormone reaches and is recognized by the ovary,
it causes the corpus luteum to persist and continue to secrete progesterone.
Thus the corpus luteum does not regress, as it would normally, shortly before

the next menstrual period is due. The persistent corpus luteum maintained by the action of hCG is called the corpus luteum of pregnancy, and its presence leads to the suppression of the menstrual cycle and the cessation of ovulation. It is only when this switch in endocrine function is achieved that pregnancy is physiologically established. Moreover, under natural conditions it is not until a menstrual period is missed that a woman becomes aware that she might be pregnant.

The process of parturition is also a complex series of interactions involving mother and fetus. However, a signal originating in the fetus is also necessary for the termination of pregnancy. This fact is supported by studies of the congenital defect called anencephaly, which is well known in human beings and as a genetic trait in cattle. In this condition the head regions of the fetus are grossly underdeveloped and a pituitary gland does not develop. Parturition can be severely delayed if this type of fetus is present with serious consequences caused by overgrowth of the fetus, so that it becomes too big to be delivered in the normal way. The fetal signal necessary to initiate the birth process is believed to be fetal adrenocortical hormone.

V. DISTURBANCES OF THE GENERATIVE PROCESS

1. *Imperfections in the Samples of the Gene Pool*

There is abundant evidence that the flow of genetic information between generations is far from perfect, so that zygotes arise with defective samples of the gene pool. Nevertheless, many of these zygotes are capable of partial development and give rise to abnormal individuals. Two main classes of error may arise in samples of the gene pool: (1) point mutations, and (2) cytogenetic aberrations (see [36] for an introduction to this field).

Point mutations arise through local chemical changes in the nucleotides which are the building blocks of DNA. The local changes occur at random in the cells of individual organisms. If they arise in the somatic cells they perish with the death of the individual. When they are produced in germ cells they may pass into the gene pool, and be transmitted to other individuals. These chemical changes in the genes may cause the production of abnormal proteins when DNA is transcribed and translated, and result in disease. Classical examples of diseases that are transmitted in this way are hemophilia and phenylketonuria. Two other such diseases, sickle cell anemia and Tay–Sachs disease, have become of social importance in recent years. Approximately 1000 genetic diseases of mutational origin are known to affect the human species [35], and at least 75 can be diagnosed using amnio-centesis [46], and fetoscopy [22]. Some mutations may lead to prenatal death and several are known in mice (see [37] for a review). The mutation t^{12}/t^{12} leads to death of the mouse embryo before implantation. Prenatal death in the human being can also occur, as in α-thalessemia.

Cytogenetic aberrations are caused by changes in the number or structure of the chromosomes, each of which carries many genes. These aberrations arise during the development of ova and spermatozoa, or during the process of fertilization itself. Many of the zygotes that result are incapable of completing embryogenesis and result in fetal death. Some, however, can complete embryogenesis and be born. Examples of cytogenetic disease are Turner's and Klinefelter's syndromes, which are caused by abnormal numbers of sex chromosomes, and Down's syndrome, which is due to an extra member of chromosome number 21.

2. *Embryonic and Fetal Wastage*

It has been known since 1914 that a considerable number of embryos in mammals die early in pregnancy. This phenomenon is a characteristic of normally fertile animals (see [5] for a review). There is now a considerable amount of evidence that embryonic loss is particularly high in women (see [8] for a review). Figure 3 shows the estimates of wastage in women. The results demonstrate that there is only about a one in three chance of a human fertilized egg developing into a viable baby. Two-thirds of the embryos are lost during the first six weeks after fertilization. The causes of this wastage fall into two classes. One class originates in the embryo and is a result of the genetic mutations and chromosome aberrations already described. The other class originates in the mother and is due to normal aging processes, overt disease of the female genital tract, or the transmission of exogenous agents such as viruses and drugs. The relative frequency of these causes of wastage is largely unknown. However, there is evidence which suggests that 40–50 percent of human embryos are lost in early pregnancy because of cytogenetic aberrations in the embryo [44]. The majority of these abnormal embryos cannot develop beyond the 10th week after fertilization and consequently die because of a deficient genome. These deaths may account for many of the early spontaneous miscarriages in women. Should the embryos die very early in pregnancy a woman may never know she had been pregnant, and if the process is repeated often she may conclude that she or her husband is sterile.

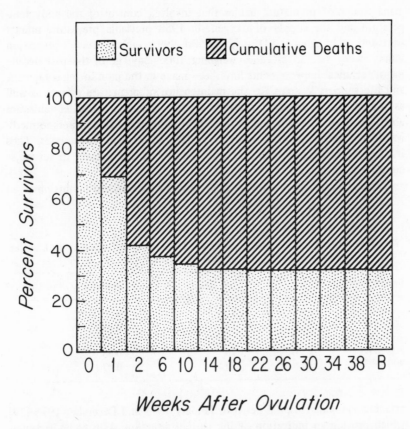

Fig. 3. Percentage of surviving and lost human embryos and fetuses at different stages of pregnancy. The figures are based on the life table of Leridon [31]. (From [8].)

3. *Neonatal Wastage – Viability*

Although pregnancy normally has a very fixed duration, babies can be born prematurely and survive. The ability to survive a premature birth is called *viability*. It is common to express viability in terms of birth weight rather than weeks of gestation, the former measure being more precise. The subject has been reviewed recently by Molteni and Jones [39].

Prior to 1940 perinatal mortality of human infants was high. In the 1940s, however, neonatal deaths were reduced by improvements in the management of premature babies that involved control of the body temperature and the supply of oxygen. In 1953 previable premature infants were defined by Arey and Dent [2] as 500–999 g, inclusive; viable premature infants were defined as those weighing 1000–2499 g. In the past decade major technical improvements have been made in the monitoring equipment and life support systems for the maintenance of premature infants as well as in diagnostic and nursing skills. As a result, smaller and smaller babies are able to survive. Fanaroff and Merkatz [18] pointed out that infants formerly considered previable now occupy 12–15% of neonatal care beds. Thus it must be recognized that the ability of premature infants to survive is continually changing.

Table II shows the survival rates of very low birth weight infants observed

TABLE II

The survival of very low birth weight infants at Johns Hopkins Hospital by birth weight from January 1977 through December 1978 (from [39], p. 167)

Body weight (g)	No. infants	Probability of survival
> 600	11	0
600–699	18	0.05
700–799	9	0.33
800–899	26	0.65
900–999	24	0.83

at Johns Hopkins Hospital between January 1977 and December 1978 [39] which provide an indication of the current situation. As is to be expected, the ability to survive varies between individual babies. The results suggest that the probability of infants weighing 750, 800, and 900 g of surviving is 0.25, 0.5, and 0.75, respectively.

Ethical discussions of viability frequently focus on the lower end of the distribution of survival rates. The subject was extensively reviewed in 1977 by the National Commission for the Protection of Human Rights. Of 276 531 births in the Province of Quebec, no premature infants weighing less than 600 g survived. This result agrees with the data in Table II, and data available from other centers in the United States. The Commission also examined eight cases frequently quoted of infants surviving with a body weight less than 600 g. They found the evidence for all of these cases questionable. For those who like to discuss viability in terms of gestational age, the evidence shows that no infant less than 24 weeks of age has survived, and that the probability of an infant 25 weeks old surviving is very small.

A major concern is whether such premature babies can develop normally or whether they will suffer severe handicaps or mental retardation as they develop. Advances in medical techniques during the past 25 years have changed the prognosis of conditions that formerly caused concern, and replaced them with new ones ([16], [33], and [39]). Drillien expressed the fear that as younger and younger infants are able to survive so there will be an increasing number of damaged children. Lubchenco and his colleagues reported that all infants weighing less than 1000 g have major defects, one of the most serious being spastic diplegia. Molteni and Jones's recent work [39], however, has shown a large reduction in survivors with major handicaps, spastic diplegia and low IQs, and they suggest that the former concerns may no longer be relevant. Instead, the pediatrician nowadays is more concerned with preventing death of these infants due to diseases such as hyaline membrane disease, bronchopulmonary dysplasia, sepsis and necrotizing enterocolitis.

VI. CONCLUSIONS

Physicians and biomedical scientists have always had to face very difficult ethical problems concerned with human life. The many questions are embraced by the title and rhetorical subtitle of Jonathan Glover's book, *Causing Death and Saving Lives*: Thou shalt not kill; but needst not strive officiously to keep alive? The problems have particularly intensified in the field of reproductive medicine in recent years for several reasons. Among these are concerns about population control and contraception, the emergence of prenatal diagnosis and fetal medicine, the treatment of a frequent cause of infertility by *in vitro* fertilization and embryo transfer, and the rights of people to reproduce outside traditional conjugal practices. Furthermore, there is much concern about the ethical aspects of scientific research on the human reproductive process. The many questions that arise require both scientific and non-scientific inputs so that they can be adequately answered. Although a biomedical scientist may be capable of participating totally in all aspects of the arguments involved, he or she has the important tasks of contributing the latest scientific views relevant to the questions under discussion, and of making sure that the scientific views are not misunderstood or misused.

In this paper I have summarized current views on generative processes in general terms, and described the specialized function of viviparity as applied to our species. I believe there are two major features of human generation which are relevant to moral discussions.

The first is that human life has never stopped since its appearance on this planet, for if it had stopped our species would have disappeared. The probability of the reappearance of a species on earth is miniscule. Thus it is wrong, or at best loose thinking, for theologians and others to insist that life begins at an arbitrary stage of the life cycle such as the completion of a process we call fertilization. What fertilization accomplishes is the final assembly of a new sample of genes which determine a unique individual who has the potential of living a life cycle that may generate new unique life cycles which will maximize the probability of life continuing in a slowly changing universe. The transition between generations is a complex process that begins in gametogenesis and ends sometime in preimplantation development.

To associate a particular stage of the life cycle with the conditions of becoming a person is entirely arbitrary and cannot be justified on scientific grounds. The association may be justified by some in terms of revelation, or as an axiom with which to begin a logical argument. In both situations the statement cannot be refuted, but this does not ensure the proposition has universal truth. The word *person* is also unsatisfactory in a scientific analysis because of its multiple vague meanings (see Webster's Dictionary). To many people, the word implies the ability to respond in a communicative way. In this sense an unborn child is not a person but a potential person. A sperm and an ovum are not potential persons since neither carries sufficient genetic information to code for development beyond birth. A zygote formed by the fusion of a sperm and ovum at fertilization is a potential person only if it contains sufficient genetic information to allow development beyond birth. It is not a potential person, however, if it carries incorrect genetic information so that it dies for example by the 10th week of gestation and is spontaneously aborted.

The second feature of human generation concerns viviparity. This involves the development of a highly integrated physiological relation between the fetus and mother. It is therefore biologically incorrect to regard the mother and fetus as independent physiological organisms. Pregnancy becomes established during implantation when a signal from the early embryo causes a switch in ovarian function. Moreover, a woman does not become conscious of becoming pregnant until menstrual cycles cease. It thus seems a very artificial idea to suggest that a sexually active woman could violate the rights of an early embryo when she has no idea of its presence. Her only choice would be to assume she were always pregnant and adopt a pattern of behavior which is unlikely to violate an embryo's rights. What this behavior should be is obscure.

Solutions to moral questions concerning human generation have been approached by imposing artificial constraints, such as equating the beginning of life with arbitrary stages of the life cycle, or separating the physiologically integrated components of pregnancy to discuss rights and duties of the fetus and mother. It would seem more acceptable scientifically to address the question: Do all phases of the life cycle have equal moral status?

Harvard Medical School,
Boston, Massachusetts

BIBLIOGRAPHY

1. Anonymous: 1981, 'Too Soon for the Rehabilitation of Lamarck', *Nature Lond.* 289, 631–632.
2. Arey, J. B. and J. Dent: 1953, 'Causes of Fetal and Neonatal Death with Special Reference to Pulmonary and Inflammatory Lesions', *J. Pediatr.* 42, 1–25.
3. Asdell, S. A.: 1964, *Patterns of Mammalian Reproduction*, 2nd ed., Cornell University Press, Ithaca, N.Y.
4. Benos, D. J. and J. D. Biggers: 1981, 'Blastocyst Fluid Formation', in L. Mastroianni, *et al.* (eds.), *Fertilization and Embryonic Development, in Vitro*, Plenum Press, pp. 283–297.
5. Biggers, J. D.: 1969, 'Problems Concerning the Uterine Causes of Embryonic Death, with Special Reference to the Effects of Aging of the Uterus', *J. Reprod. Fertil.* (Suppl.) 8, 27–43.
6. Biggers, J. D.: 1979, 'Fertilization and Blastocyst Formation', in N. J. Alexander (ed.), *Animal Models for Research on Contraception and Fertility*, Harper and Row, Hagerstown, Md., pp. 223–237.
7. Biggers, J. D.: 1980, 'Fetal and Neonatal Physiology', in V. B. Mountcastle (ed.), *Medical Physiology*, 14th ed., The C. V. Mosby Co., St. Louis, pp. 1947–1985.
8. Biggers, J. D.: 1981, '*In Vitro* Fertilization and Embryo Transfer in Human Beings', *New Engl. J. Med.* 304, 336–342.
9. Biggers, J. D. and R. D. Powers: 1979, 'Na$^+$ Transport and Swelling of the Mammalian Blastocyst: Effect of Amiloride', in A. W. Cuthbert *et al.* (eds.), *Amiloride and Epithelial Sodium Transport*, Urban and Schwarzenberg, Baltimore, pp. 167–179.
10. Browne, Sir Thomas: 1646, *Pseudodoxia Epidemica*, Book III, London, p. 116.
11. Calow, P.: 1978, *Life Cycles*, Chapman and Hall, London.
12. Cole, F. J.: 1930, *Early Theories of Sexual Generation*, Clarendon Press, Oxford, pp. 1–230.

13. Coleman, W.: 1971, *Biology in the Nineteenth Century*, Wiley, New York.
14. Corner, G. W.: 1955, 'The Observed Embryology of Human Single-Ovum Twins and Other Multiple Births', *Amer. J. Obstet. Gynec.* **70**, 933–951.
15. Dobell, C.: 1932, *Antony van Leeuwenhoek and His "Little Animals"*, Constable, London.
16. Drillien, C. M.: 1958, 'A Longitudinal Study of the Growth and Development of Prematurely and Maturely Born Children', *Arch. Dis. Child.* **33**, 417–431.
17. Dunn, L. D.: 1965, *A Short History of Genetics*, McGraw-Hill, New York.
18. Fanaroff, A. A. and I. R. Merkatz: 1977, 'Modern Obstetrical Management of the Low Birth Weight Infant', *Clin. Perinatol.* **4**, 217–237.
19. Gasking, E.: 1967, *Investigations into Generation, 1651–1828*, Hutchison, London.
20. Gill, T. J. and C. F. Repetti: 1979, 'Immunologic and Genetic Factors Influencing Reproduction', *Amer. J. Path.* **95**, 465–570.
21. Glover, J.: 1977, *Causing Death and Saving Lives*, Penguin Books, Harmondsworth, England.
22. Gohari, P. and A. Spinelli: 1979, 'Fetoscropy in the Practice of Perinatology and Obstetrics', *Obstet. Gynec. Ann.* **8**, 179–202.
23. Gould, S. J.: 1977, *Ontogeny and Physlogeny*, Harvard University Press, Cambridge.
24. Graham, C. F.: 1974, 'The Production of Parthenogenetic Mammalian Embryos and Their Use in Biological Research', *Biol. Rev.* **49**, 399–422.
25. Haggis, C. H., D. Michie, A. R. Muir, K. B. Roberts and P. M. B.: Walker: 1964, *Introduction to Molecular Biology*, Longmans and Green, London.
26. Heap, R. B., A. P. Flint and J. E. Gadsby: 1979, 'Role of Embryonic Signals in the Establishment of Pregnancy', *Brit. Med. Bull.* **35**, 129–135.
27. Hoppe, P. C. and K. Illmensee: 1977, 'Microsurgically Produced Homozygous-diploid Uniparental Mice', *Proc. Nat. Acad. Sci., U.S.A.* **74**, 5657–5661.
28. Johnson, P. M., P. J. Brown and W. P. Faulk: 1980, 'Immunological Aspects of the Human Placenta', *Oxford Rev. Reprod. Biol.* **2**, 1–40.
29. Judsoh, H. F.: 1979, *The Eighth Day of Creation*, Simon and Schuster, New York.
30. Kimura, M. and T. Ohta: 1971, *Theoretical Aspects of Population Genetics*, Princeton University Press, Princeton, N.J.
31. Leridon, H.: 1977, *Human Fertility* (translated by J. F. Helzner), Chicago University Press, Chicago.
32. Lewin, B.: 1974, *Gene Expression*, Vol. 1, Wiley, New York.
33. Lubchenco, L. O., F. A. Horner, L. H. Reed, I. E. Hix, D. Metcalf, R. Cohig, H. C. Elliott, and M. Bourg: 1963, 'Sequelae of Premature Birth', *Am. J. Dis. Child.* **106**, 101–115.
34. MacKay, A. L.: 1977, *The Harvest of a Quiet Eye*, The Institute of Physics, London.
35. McKusick, V. A.: 1971, *Mendelian Inheritance in Man*, 3rd ed., Heineman, London.
36. McKusick, V. A.: 1969, *Human Genetics*, 2nd ed., Prentice-Hall, Englewood Cliffs, New Jersey.
37. McLaren, A.: 1976, 'Genetics of the Early Mouse Embryo', *Ann. Rev. Genet.* **10**, 361–188.
38. McLaren, A.: 1979, 'The Impact of Pre-fertilization Events on Post-fertilization Development in Mammals', in D. R. Newth *et al.* (eds.), *Maternal Effects in Development*, Cambridge University Press, Cambridge, pp. 287–320.

39. Molteni, R. A. and M. D. Jones: 1980, 'Neonatal Management', *Clin. Obstet. Gynec.* **23**, 165–179.
40. National Commission for the Protection of Human Subjects of Biomedical and Behavioral Research: 1975, *Appendix: Research on the Fetus*, U.S. Department of Health, Education and Welfare, Washington, D.C.
41. Needham, J.: 1942, *Biochemistry and Morphogenesis*, Cambridge University Press, Cambridge.
42. Needham, J.: 1959, *A History of Embryology*, Cambridge University Press, Cambridge.
43. Newman, H. H. and J. T. Patterson: 1909, 'A Case of Normal Identical Quadruplets in the Armadillo and its Bearing on the Problem of Identical Twins and Sex Determination', *Biol. Bull.* **17**, 181–187.
44. Schlesselman, J. J.: 1979, 'How Does One Assess the Risk of Abnormalities from Human *In Vitro* Fertilization?', *Am. J. Obstet. Gynec.* **135**, 135–148.
45. Shaw, F. D. and Morton, H.: 1980, 'The Immunological Approach to Pregnancy Diagnosis: A Review', *Vet. Rec.* **106**, 268–269.
46. Simpson, J. L.: 1979, 'Antenatal Monitoring of Genetic Disorders', *Clin. Obstet. Gynec.* **6**, 259–293.
47. Smith, J. M.: 1978, *The Evolution of Sex*, Cambridge University Press, Cambridge.
48. Watson, J. D. and F. H. C. Crick: 1953, 'A Structure for Deoxyribose Nucleic Acid', *Nature* **171**, 737–738.
49. Whittingham, D. G.: 1980, 'Parthenogenesis in Mammals', *Oxford Rev. Reprod. Biol.* **2**, 205–231.
50. Widdowson, E. M.: 1968, 'Growth and Composition of the Fetus and Newborn', in N. S. Assali (ed.), *The Biology of Gestation*, Vol. 2, Academic Press, New York, pp. 1–49.
51. Wilson, E. V.: 1896, 'On Cleavage and Mosaic-work', *Arch. Entwicklungsmech. Org.* **3**, 19–26.
52. Wudl, L. and V. M. Chapman: 1976, 'The Expression of β-Glucuronidase During Preimplantation Development of Mouse Embryos', *Devel. Biol.* **48**, 104–109.

GEORGE J. AGICH

SCIENCE, POLICY, AND THE FETUS: COMMENTS ON WALTERS AND BIGGERS

The question of the status of the fetus, like the question of the definition of death, involves more than matters of fact which can be clarified through scientific research programs. Rather, such questions involve basic philosophical issues which provide the occasion for individuals to make decisions and for society to establish policies. Hence, an important starting point for this volume is with those policy discussions which have assessed the place of the fetus in biomedicine. Similarly, since the context of discussion involves biomedicine and since many policy considerations of the fetus seem to turn on distinguishing stages in the development of the fetus, it is also important to have before us a discussion of biological thinking regarding the development of early human life.

I interpret both Professors Walters and Biggers as providing a background for the main discussion and analysis of the issues surrounding the use of the fetus which will occur in later sections. Accordingly, it is not surprising that the two papers contribute more to the setting of the problem of the fetus in biomedicine than to its solution. I regard these contributions highly, insofar as the first philosophical and critical task is to understand the context in which ethical problems arise. Such problems arise within specific historical and social contexts. In this regard, it is especially important to have an early opportunity to frame questions regarding the historical and social factors which determine our present situation rather than engaging in immediate discussion of what we *assume* to be the central issues.

In his paper, 'The Fetus in Ethical and Public Policy Discussion from 1973 to the Present', LeRoy Walters [9] considers three public decisions regarding the status of the fetus: *Roe v. Wade* [8], the National Commission for the Protection of Human Subjects [7], and the Ethics Advisory Board [6]. In Walters' view, there is a remarkable continuity in these decisions which can be attributed to the way each addresses various stages in the development of the fetus. In fact, Walters ([9], p. 15) suggests a substantive relationship "since each succeeding document clearly presupposes the content of the preceding documents". Accordingly, one way to address the issues which Professor Walters raises is to consider the sense of continuity and to ask whether we should credit it to the discussions themselves or to Walters' own synoptic vision.

55

William B. Bondeson et al. *(eds.), Abortion and the Status of the Fetus, 55–66.*

My commentary will take the form of roughing what his presentation has so nicely burnished for us. I take this image from his own conclusion that "the three public policy documents . . . reach a rough consensus on the status of the pre-implantation embryo, the viable fetus in utero, and the delivered 'fetus' or infant" ([9], p. 28). I will argue that the consensus is indeed rough not only because these discussions have not closed off arguments regarding the moral and legal status of the fetus, but because the three discussions are discontinuous in significant respects. This makes it difficult to speak clearly of a consensus, rough or otherwise, regarding the fetus.

Granting that the substantive issues concerning the fetus are solidly embedded in the three main policy discussions which Walters considers, we must still decide how best to approach those discussions. There are at least two approaches that might be taken. We might approach the discussions historically, stressing the continuities and allowing the disagreements and the arguments at stake in each discussion to emerge only implicitly; or, we might proceed philosophically, focusing on the normative assumptions and claims made in each discussion, and critically analyze their validity. Walters has chosen the former approach. In so doing, he attributes a sense of continuity and consistency to these discussions which tends not only to minimize controversy, but which confuses philosophical analysis and justification with policy decisions. However, I am concerned not so much to criticize Walters' approach, as to set the stage for philosophical analysis by introducing breaks into his account and by pointing to alternative interpretations of the main issues involved in *Roe v. Wade*, the National Commission for the Protection of Human Subjects, and the Ethics Advisory Board.

Whether one describes the historical development of policy statements or evaluates them, it is imperative to be clear about what is meant by 'policy'. Policy decisions, even when they overtly include ethical considerations, necessarily go beyond ethics to consider questions of feasibility. Feasibility is

that quality whereby a proposed course of action is [judged] not merely possible but practicable, adaptable, as depending on circumstances, cultural ways, attitudes, or traditions of a people . . . ([5], p. 294).

Feasibility thus includes questions such as: Will the policy be obeyed? Is it enforceable? Is it the prudent thing to do given the policy's possible effect on other sectors of social life? This makes the analysis of policy statements a tricky business indeed. It makes it all the more imperative to distinguish philosophical 'closure' on an issue from the 'closure' demanded by feasibility requirements, on the one hand, and the openness prerequisite for ethical discourse from an openness which meets feasibility requirements, on the other.

Minimally, a 'policy' serves as a guide to action or choice. To establish a guide to action or choice involves, first, connecting the present capacity to act of some specified actor (individually or collectively) to a set of future outcomes and, second, the policy (or guide to action or choice) must order those alternative outcomes or actions in terms of a transitively ordered set of preferences already available or created for the occasion ([4], p. 188). Carrying out these tasks, it should be noted, involves both empirical and normative considerations. As Eugene Meehan has observed:

Reasoned actions always involve both empirical and normative factors and the empirical component is prior — there can be no normative judgment until the options have been established ([4], p. 188).

So understood, a policy is simply the rules of action or guides by which a priority structure is applied to a particular choice or set of choices. So, in describing a discussion in which a policy is formulated, it is important to distinguish the considerations supporting particular rules of action from those which establish the priority structure which the rules apply. But since the policy discussions under consideration involve both feasibility and ethical requirements, it is very difficult, yet so very important, descriptively to distinguish valid ethical argument from political and social concerns, because what is ethically permissible, strictly speaking, may yet be controversial and impracticable.

These problems of interpretation can be illustrated by turning first to the work of the Ethics Advisory Board. In Walters' view ([9], p. 24), the Report of this Board nicely fills a lacuna regarding the early developmental stages of the fetus. Together with *Roe v. Wade* and the National Commission's work on the fetus, the Ethics Advisory Board brings a sense of completion to the policy discussion of the fetus. However, it is unclear precisely what this sense of completion amounts to.

In the first place, there was a good deal of disagreement regarding the ethics of *in vitro* fertilization and embryo transfer in presentations made to the Ethics Advisory Board and referenced in the Board's Report. Some, but not all, had to do with the ontological and ethical status of the fetus. Regarding the human embryo in the laboratory setting, at least three distinguishable positions emerge which are described in the Report.[1] The content of these positions is not germane at the moment; what is important is that the Board described these positions without critically analyzing them.

Accordingly, it is difficult to know how the Board's final recommendations are to be justified on the basis of this fundamental disagreement. Second, in addition to disagreement over the status of the fetus, concerns were expressed that potential adverse consequences of this research would outweigh potential benefits. Such concerns are usually central policy worries, so it is surprising that they are not explicitly addressed in the Board's recommendations. In fact, the Board's Report is notably silent on these matters. By failing to provide a clear priority structure in terms of which to judge the most problematic cases, it is difficult to reconstruct the main argument seen as decisive by the Board.

For example, the Board did not explicitly comment on futuristic research possibilities which were presented by some commentators, such as parthenogenesis, interspecies fertilization, nuclear transfer (cloning), human-human hybridization, and human-nonhuman hybridization. Nor did the Board make a concrete recommendation regarding the research proposal which prompted the activation of the Board itself. So, if one requirement for any policy is that it be inclusive rather than exclusive of troublesome cases, it is not at all clear that the work of the Ethics Advisory Board constitutes an adequate statement of policy at all. In this regard, it is important to attend to the Board's own cautious characterization of its recommendations:

The Board is required by HEW Regulations to review research proposals involving human *in vitro* fertilization and advise the Secretary as to their "acceptability from an ethical standpoint". This phrase is broad enough to include at least two interpretations: (1) "clearly ethically right" or (2) "ethically defensible but still legitimately controverted". In finding that research involving human *in vitro* fertilization is "acceptable from an ethical standpoint" the Board is using the phrase in the second sense; the Board wishes to emphasize that it is *not* finding that the ethical considerations against such research are insubstantial. Indeed, concerns regarding the moral status of the embryo and the potential long-range consequences of this research were among the most difficult that confronted the Board ([6], p. 100).

This lack of a clear sense of 'closure' possibly reflects less on the philosophical issues surrounding the fetus than on the complex feasibility demands which configured the Board's deliberation. However, by not distinguishing philosophical and feasibility requirements, Walters conveys a sense of agreement — a "rough consensus" — without materially advancing our understanding of the issues which the Board faced and its conclusions. We are left, in short, with a rather bland sense of what might be, from a critical and evaluative point of view, a rather spicy stew.

We can carry this interpretive disagreement further by considering *Roe v.*

Wade. That decision turned on the recognition of the fetus *in utero* as a non-person in legal terms. For the most part, any right that a fetus can be convincingly asserted to have, it has *contingent* upon being born. Therefore, the fetus as such does not qualify for protection under the Fourteenth Amendment. On the other hand, the fundamental right to privacy of a pregnant woman does require that any limitation placed on the exercise of this right — as by State laws prohibiting abortion — be justified in terms of clear and compelling State interest. The Supreme Court held in *Roe v. Wade* that prior to the point of viability the only compelling state interest has to do with establishing standards and procedures reasonably to preserve and protect maternal health. The alleged state interest in "potential life" can come into play only at that "compelling point" when the fetus "has the capability of meaningful life outside the mother's womb" ([8], p. 163). However, this still does not mean that the fetus gains, at that point, the status of legal personhood.

One can read *Roe v. Wade* as consistent with the legal tradition which views alleged rights of the unborn — to property or to recover damages and compensation for injuries inflicted before birth — as contingent upon their being born. The reasoning central in this tradition has to do with the enforceability of the attributed rights. The right of the unborn conferred by law functions as a place holder or reservation for the rights he shall actually inherit only when he becomes a full-fledged being [2]. The unborn acquire rights only upon being born, because only then can their claims be enforced.

On this reading, the Court is saying nothing very new about the rights of the fetus. The concern of law seems to be restricted pragmatically to the requisites of the adjudication process. The Court hardly needed to recognize any specific theory of life when it had an ample legal tradition with which to work. In fact, one reason given for rejecting the Texas abortion statute had to do with its arbitrarily adopting a "theory of life" ([8], p. 162). For the same reason, the Court's definition of viability is admittedly unrefined relative to medical knowledge, but it is adequate in the pragmatically useful sense of sorting out the Constitutional issue which was before the Court. If this is so, then it is unclear how one can see the National Commission as refining *Roe v. Wade* as Walters suggests. The Supreme Court in *Roe v. Wade* was not concerned with defining viability. In fact, viability was not central to the main question before the court since *Roe v. Wade* clearly recognizes the woman's right to abort even a viable fetus to protect herself against the "stressful life and future" and the psychological, social, and medical harm that "additional offspring" may impose ([8], p. 153). Hence, *Roe v. Wade* says little regarding the ethics of abortion or regarding the status of the fetus except that under our Constitution we shall permit possibly immoral private actions when there is no compelling State or public interest to prevent them. That is to say, there still may be other interests and senses of personhood which are not exactly "State interests" or the legal concept of personhood which would argue against abortion either in general or in particular cases, but those interests and concepts of the person are not pertinent to the Constitutional protection of freedom of the pregnant woman to decide for an abortion. This conclusion admittedly poses a central question for the philosophical analysis of policy, namely, how should we define ethics in the context of a public policy. But this question can emerge only from a critical reading of policy discussions.

Walters, however, describes *Roe v. Wade* in terms which imply that its issues are the same as those before the National Commission for the Protection of Human Subjects and the Ethical Advisory Board regarding research with the fetus. For example, he notes that "several unresolved questions remained" after *Roe v. Wade* " . . . most of them located near the viability-water-shed" ([9], p. 26). All of these questions concern the "possibly viable" fetus and whether potential viability was sufficient to justify compelling State interest. Walters sees these questions partly addressed by the National Commission. He notes that these questions have been contested in the courts in recent years, but he does not discuss the general answer which the courts have developed over the years. This omission permits the suggestion of continuity and consensus in public discussions of the fetus which is surely not borne out by the facts.

The work of the National Commission on fetal research further illustrates the importance of not only attending to the particular policy context before drawing conclusions regarding philosophical issues, but of distinguishing feasibility from ethical concerns. The National Commission had the primary task not of determining which types of fetal research were ethically or legally permissible, but rather to recommend to the Secretary of HEW which types of fetal research should be "supported or conducted" by DHEW. For this reason, the National Commission for the Protection of Human Subjects of Biomedical and Behavioral Research matter-of-factly viewed the fetus as the *subject* of research in need of protection without actually addressing the question of the personhood of the fetus at various stages of development. Although the National Commission wrestled with distinctions such as the difference between a pre-viable fetus *in utero* and a pre-viable fetus *ex utero* and between research with a fetus to be aborted and one being carried to term in the context of considerations of risk and whether the research was therapeutic or nontherapeutic, the policy context of protecting "subjects" of research seemed to influence heavily how the question concerning fetal research was framed.

Indeed, the Commission itself notes:

Throughout the deliberations of the Commission, the belief has been affirmed that the fetus as a human subject is deserving of care and respect. Although the Commission has not addressed directly the issue of the personhood and the civil status of the fetus, the members of the Commission are convinced that moral concerns should extend to all who share genetic heritage, and that the fetus, regardless of life prospects, should be treated respectfully and with dignity ([7], pp. 61–62).

As a matter of fact, the Commission proceeded on the assumption that the fetus was a subject deserving of respect not simply in general terms, but in accord with the respect owed to infants and children. It went so far as to regard the non-viable fetus *ex utero* as a dying subject and, accordingly, prohibited non-therapeutic interventions which would alter the duration of the life of these fetuses ([7], p. 68). Accordingly, it seems natural to ask how this position can be justified. Does the research context itself and the fabric of protections accorded subjects of research justify this position or were there other considerations which proved decisive? If other considerations proved decisive, what were they? For instance, was there a compelling argument for the ontological equality of pre-viable fetuses and children or was the Commission persuaded by other considerations? Were these considerations ethical or political? These kinds of questions are central to a critical understanding of the Commission's work and they point to the need for an explanatory and evaluative concern beyond the descriptive. However, it should be stressed that we can raise these (and our earlier questions) thanks to Walters' overview. They naturally arise *on the basis* of his overview. And although these questions suggest the need for further interpretation of the policy discussions of the fetus, they should not be construed as denying the help which Walters' paper affords us in this enterprise by so succinctly presenting what is, indeed, a very complicated story.

In a similar vein, we can approach Biggers' [1] discussion of 'Generation of the Human Life Cycle' as setting out our present biological knowledge regarding development of the human fetus. This effort is particularly apropos since the policy discussions considered above focus on different stages or phases in fetal development and, in some sense, turn on an understanding of the developing 'personhood' of the fetus. So, it is important to have before us a review of biological thinking regarding development of early human life. The issue posed by Biggers' presentation precisely concerns the relevance of scientific thought to ethical questions regarding the fetus.

Biggers intends to show that popular positions regarding the definition of when human life begins, e.g., at fertilization or at birth, are unjustified, primarily because the question "when does human life begin" is itself non-sensical. The question is nonsensical from a scientific, biological point of view. According to Biggers:

Conception and birth should be recognized merely as phases of a more fundamental biological process – the life cycle .... Life is passed on from one generation to another, and it is therefore incorrect to claim that life begins at arbitrarily chosen points of the life cycle ([1], p. 31).

Of course, one might strenuously object that the question of the definition of human life is not a question regarding human life in general, but individual human life, especially individual human persons. Hence, Biggers' insistence on a universal life cycle as the concept central to the question of the begin-ning of human life seems misplaced. This kind of objection, however, misses its mark since Biggers does not unambiguously purport to offer a universal definition of human life relevant to ethical and policy issues regarding the fetus. Rather, he aims to outline the current state of scientific knowledge of early human development and implicitly argues that any view regarding the status of the developing fetus must come to terms with this understanding.

Biggers indicates that the understanding of human generation is susceptible to 'cultural loading' or determination as evidenced by early ideas on generation (i.e., denials of both physiological maternity and paternity). Early under-standings of generation reflect beliefs and explanations which correlated commonsense observations regarding intercourse, menstruation, conception, and pregnancy. Biggers illustrates quite well that even scientific thought on generation from the seventeenth century involved alternative and competing explanations, such as Harvey's suggestion that all animals develop from eggs and alternative preformation theories. In effect, Biggers traces a very complex story in which our present understanding of human generation grew from many sources. It was not primarily *observation* of the processes surrounding conception, e.g., the action of spermatozoa (which Linnaeus curiously termed *Chaos infusoria*) or Harvey's *inspection* of the uterus after intercourse (in which he found "there are no remains in the uterus either of the semen of the male or female emitted in the act, nothing produced by any mixture of these two fluids"), but rather certain ideas, such as cell theory, which organized observation and opened avenues for research.

Although Biggers speaks of the cell theory as a discovery, it should rather be regarded as a theoretical framework or as what Thomas Kuhn [3] has termed a 'paradigm', because it organized and oriented research questions in basically different directions. It is in this sense that Biggers' focus on the life cycle should be interpreted.

The point to be learned from Biggers' paper is that the question of the meaning or definition of human life is not something to be *discovered* in empirical, scientific terms at all, but rather must be *decided* upon. Thus, the question of the definition of human life and the status of the fetus is seen fundamentally as a conceptual, rather than empirical, question. Deciding whether any particular developing entity is 'human life' or a 'human person' requires an antecedent judgment or decision about how we will use the concepts of 'human life' and 'human person'. The decision about the use of these concepts will, of course, involve considerations which Biggers does not discuss, namely, values and purposes beyond the biological facts. Biggers' contention, in this regard, is that biology has, for its own purposes, already satisfactorily answered this question in terms of a universal life cycle. It is not germane in the present setting to evaluate this view of the theoretical importance of the concept of the life cycle, but it is important to point out, as Biggers does not, that the idea of the life cycle is not itself an empirical matter of fact, a discovered and verifiable scientific truth, rather it is a regulative idea in terms of which scientific investigation into a multitude of seemingly disparate occurrences and processes can be systematically organized. Even if this reading of Biggers' paper is correct, his view of the life cycle can nonetheless be criticized, but the criticism must be directed toward the regulative character of the concept of the life cycle. The main line of attack would be that 'life cycle' is understood too restrictively.

In the human species, at least, growth and development cannot be understood exclusively or reductively in physiological terms. Rather, we must speak of bio-psycho-social development, rather than biological development or life cycle alone. It is well-recognized that at certain stages, particularly infancy, any attempt to understand physiological development requires a consideration of the psycho-social interactions involving the infant, especially the interaction or bonding between the infant and its mother. Here, environment is not only physiological or physical, but psycho-social as well. And so, to understand human development we must appeal to a *specific* concept of the life cycle rather than the more general concept with which Biggers works. This concept is broader than Biggers' in seeing human development in more than biological or physiological terms, but is narrower in that it focuses on *human* life rather than *life* generally. An objection to Biggers' view of the life cycle based on the concept of human growth and development would be on a firm foundation indeed. However, we must ask at this point: Does recognizing this criticism allow us to accept Biggers' main thesis regarding the relevance of the scientific understanding of the life cycle and generation in general to moral issues regarding the fetus? If we regard Biggers as offering not a full treatment of *human* growth and development, but a view of physiological development in general and human *physiological* development in particular, is his discussion relevant to the ethical issues regarding the 'personhood' of the developing embryo or fetus as he implies?

Biggers concludes that the process of genetic determination of the individual and the specialized function of viviparity in the human species are "two major features of human generation which are relevant to moral discussions" ([1], p. 50). He argues that "to associate a particular stage of the life cycle with the conditions of becoming a person is entirely arbitrary and cannot be justified on scientific grounds" ([1], p. 50). Of course, there may be other valid, non-scientific considerations germane to the personhood of the developing fetus. But we must not forget the empirical conditions under which human persons develop. Basically, the process of fetal development is biological or physiological, though not exclusively so. Hence, any account of developing personhood must come to terms with current physiological knowledge. As Biggers points out, the concept of a person is vague and its application to the fetus problematic. Minimally, the concept of personhood implies the ability to communicate or to act independently. For these reasons, an unborn child is not a person, strictly speaking, but is seen as a *potential* person. But what does it mean to be a 'potential' person?

Biggers can be interpreted as arguing that biology can help answer this question by providing us with knowledge of the limiting empirical conditions of developing personhood. For example, one cannot speak of potential personhood without reference to a complete set of genetic information that allows for development beyond birth:

A zygote formed by the fusion of a sperm and ovum at fertilization is a potential person only if it contains sufficient genetic information to allow development beyond birth. It is not a potential person, however, if it carries incorrect genetic information so that it dies for example by the 10th week of gestation and is spontaneously aborted ([1], p. 50).

In other words, the concept of a human person, potential or otherwise, must include a possible embodiment. The process of embodiment or development of human personhood is open to biological understanding. Any definition of personhood which would ignore this understanding would do so at its own risk. But beyond these facts, what else has biology to contribute to the issue of the personhood of the fetus?

Here, Biggers points to viviparity:

This involves the development of a highly integrated physiological relation between the fetus and mother. It is therefore biologically incorrect to regard the mother and fetus as independent organisms ([1], p. 50).

As a matter of fact, then, the mother and fetus are not biologically independent organisms. Dependence is a physiological concept referring to the highly complex interactions which occur between the pregnant woman and the developing embryo at least from the time of implantation. The presence of physiological dependence establishes that the fetus has no biological claim to existence not bound up with that of the mother.[2] This factual connection, however, does not of itself establish any particular value judgments regarding the fetus. But the question of the ethical status of the fetus is, after all, a question of values, of how we should regard the developing fetus. On Biggers' view, this question is *arbitrarily* answered if we assume that the fetus is an *independent* organism by "separating the physiologically integrated components of pregnancy to discuss rights and duties of the fetus and mother" ([1], p. 51). In other words, in Biggers' view, biological knowledge of early human development is a side-constraint for ethical discussion and analysis. An answer to the conceptual question of the personhood of the fetus or the definition of when human life begins must be anchored in the empirical, scientific understanding of actual early human life. And so, like Walters, Biggers challenges us to articulate the values and concerns which orient our views of the ethical status of the fetus by sketching the terrain in which this orientation must occur. We owe both Biggers and Walters our thanks for this lesson.

Southern Illinois University,
School of Medicine,
Springfield, Illinois

NOTES

[1] These positions were advocated in testimony before the Board by Leon Kass, Charles Curran and Clifford Grobstein, and Samuel Gorovitz. Briefly, Kass argued that laboratory research with human *in vitro* fertilization and embryo culture is incompatible with the

respect that is due to early human embryos and that the potential adverse consequences of the research outweigh the benefits. A main concern of Kass was that many human embryos which would be studied in the laboratory would have been created solely for research purposes. Kass was impressed by the continuities in embryonic and fetal development and by the potential viability of the early human embryo if it is transferred at the proper time. Charles Curran and Clifford Grobstein argue separately for a similar position. Curran argues that truly human life is present two to three weeks after conception or shortly after the implantation of the embryo; hence, any attempts to culture embryos *in vitro* beyond this stage raise clear ethical problems. Grobstein argues that human cells, tissues, and organs that have no reasonable prospect of possessing a developing sentience or awareness should be seen as human materials rather than human beings or persons. Finally, Samuel Gorovitz argues that sentience, rather than the potential for sentience, is the primary criterion for determining the moral status of the human embryo or fetus.

2 *Roe v. Wade* notes the following: "The pregnant woman cannot be isolated in her privacy. She carries an embryo and, later, a fetus, if one accepts the medical definitions of the developing young in the human uterus" ([8], p. 159).

BIBLIOGRAPHY

1. Biggers, J. D.: 1983, 'Generation of the Human Life Cycle', in this volume, pp. 31–53.
2. Feinberg, J.: 1980, 'Is There a Right to be Born', in J. Feinberg (ed.), *Rights, Justice, and the Bounds of Liberty*, Princeton University Press, Princeton, pp. 207–20.
3. Kuhn, T. S.: 1970, *The Structure of Scientific Revolutions*, The University of Chicago Press, Chicago.
4. Meehan, E. J.: 1975, 'Policy and Philosophy Studies', in S. Nagel (ed.), *Policy Studies and the Social Sciences*, Lexington Books, Lexington, Massachusetts, pp. 185–200.
5. Micallef, P. J.: 1972, 'Abortion and the Principles of Legislation', *Laval Theologique et Philosophique* 28, 267–303.
6. U.S. Department of Health, Education, and Welfare, Ethics Advisory Board: 1979, *HEW Support of Research Involving Human in Vitro Fertilization and Embryo Transfer: Report and Conclusions* and *Appendix*, Department of Health, Education, and Welfare, Washington, D.C.
7. U.S. Department of Health, Education, and Welfare, National Commission for the Protection of Human Subjects of Biomedical and Behavioral Research: 1976, *Research on the Fetus: Report and Recommendations* and *Appendix*, Department of Health, Education, and Welfare, Washington, D.C.
8. U.S. Supreme Court: 1973, 'Roe *et al*. v. Wade, District Attorney of Dallas County', *U.S. Reports* 410, 113–178 (decided 22 January, 1973).
9. Walters, L.: 1983, 'The Fetus in Ethical and Public Policy Discussion from 1973 to the Present', in this volume, pp. 15–30.

†PIERRE SOUPART

PRESENT AND POSSIBLE FUTURE RESEARCH IN THE USE OF HUMAN EMBRYOS

I. INTRODUCTION

On July 25, 1978, a baby girl was born in Oldham, Lancashire, England, as a result of a new reproductive technology: *in vitro* fertilization of the human egg (IVF) and transplantation of the resulting preimplantation embryo (ET) into the uterine cavity of the egg donor [49].

A second birth, resulting from a similar procedure, but allegedly involving an additional technologic step — the cryopreservation of the preimplantation embryo — occurred in Calcutta, India, on October 3, 1978 [50]. It was the birth of another baby girl. The third successful birth occurred on January 14, 1979, in Glasgow, Scotland, when a baby boy was born, as a result of an IVF-ET procedure performed by Drs. Steptoe and Edwards. Although less celebrated than the previous two births, this was a most significant event because, from a strictly academic viewpoint, the birth of a male offspring following IVF-ET rules out the possibility of accidental activation of the human ovum, possibly due to extracorporeal manipulations, whereas the birth of female offspring does not.

The fourth successful birth, that of another baby girl, occurred on June 23, 1980, in Melbourne, Australia. In the latter instance, there was a significant difference as compared to the previous three, in that this birth was announced in a scientific report, published in the February issue of *Fertility and Sterility* [25], the official Journal of the American Fertility Society. Despite the spectacular and world-wide reported success of the events described above, human IVF-ET is by no means a routine procedure nowadays.

Neither Steptoe and Edwards, nor the Indian team, have to date published detailed accounts of their work. Yet, enough information is available, through presentations at scientific meetings and media interviews ([25], [28], [39] and [42]), for an analysis of problems encountered in IVF-ET over the past decade now to be possible.[1]

In discussing present and possible future research in the use of human embryos, two approaches are conceivable. LeRoy Walters [53], in his analysis of 'Ethical Issues in Human *in Vitro* Fertilization and Research Involving Early Human Embryos', has chosen to categorize ethical issues raised by

67

William B. Bondeson et al. *(eds.), Abortion and the Status of the Fetus*, 67–104.

human *in vitro* fertilization and related research techniques. In doing so, Walters greatly contributed to the clarification of such issues and of their relative importance, both at short and longer range. Walters' analysis, although thoroughly exhaustive, does not necessarily reflect the pragmatic approach of the biomedical investigator to aspects of IVF-ET that have to be further researched with a view to improving the success rate of the procedure, and we hope adding to our current knowledge of human reproduction mechanisms. Thus, in this presentation, it was chosen to start with the exposition of available biological facts, i.e., the analysis of problems encountered over a decade of IVF-ET development, and from there on proceed to the description of realistically attainable research objectives.

From an ethical and didactic viewpoint as well, it would seem important to be able clearly to distribute issues between two main categories, i.e., IVF research not involving ET, versus IVF research definitely involving ET. Yet, this is not so easily done, because in many instances research involving IVF but apparently not involving ET is aimed at the immediate improvement of the ET success rate. On the other hand, there are several IVF research applications, which do not require ET to reach their ultimate significance.

In order to make the reading of this contribution easier, some background material must be provided in the form of definitions and description of mechanisms.

II. BACKGROUND: DEFINITIONS AND MECHANISMS

1. *Infertility*

Infertility is seen as the inability to initiate pregnancy over a period of one year of unprotected and regular sexual intercourse in a couple in their reproductive years. How much of a problem infertility represents in Western societies is difficult to quantify with any degree of accuracy. From the fact that infertility is nowadays among the chief complaints presented to the practicing gynecologist, and from rough estimates, it is now recognized that infertility, of either male or female origin, is a problem of sizable magnitude. There are about 65 million couples of reproductive age in the U.S. Among these, 15%, i.e., over 10 million, present an infertility problem. Since the cause of the infertility problem is in roughly equal proportion of male or female origin, about 5 million American women suffer from infertility. Among the causal factors of female infertility, Fallopian tube pathology, of various origins, is found to be the villain in about 50% of the cases. Thus,

2.5 million women could be eligible for alleviation of infertility by means of IVF-ET. Granted, IVF-ET is not the only means of alleviating infertility resulting from tubal pathology. Over recent years, the development of micro-surgical techniques has permitted the restoration of patency in many cases of tubal obstruction. Yet, patency restoration is no guarantee of functional restoration of the Fallopian tube, thus, there is no guarantee that successful pregnancy will ensue [14]. The major complication of tubal microsurgery is ectopic pregnancy, i.e., the implantation of an embryo in the oviduct rather than in the uterus. This is a life-threatening condition, which guarantees further infertility since the emergency surgical treatment involves the excision of the involved Fallopian tube. Dr. Victor Gomel, a pioneer of Fallopian tube microsurgery, is currently guest-editor for Clinical Obstetrics and Gynecology of an international Symposium on 'Microsurgical Techniques in Infertility' [14]. Dr. Gomel has commissioned this reviewer to prepare an analysis of the 'Current Status of *in Vitro* Fertilization and Embryo Transfer in Man' [45]. Obviously, microsurgeons, primarily committed to the alleviation of infertility, are realistically aware of the limitations of their own technology and, therefore, are most interested in a back-up technique, i.e., IVF-ET.

Failures of reconstructing a functional oviduct are not all recorded in the treatment of tubal diseases of inflammatory origins. An increasingly large number of such failures is recorded in attempts at reversal of voluntary tubal sterilization. Available statistics over the period 1970–1978 indicate that the frequency of tubal sterilizations performed in the U.S., after steadily increasing during the first 3 years, has stabilized around half a million per year. Thus, today, there may be as many as five million women in the U.S. that underwent tubal sterilization. Owing to familial tragedy, the loss of one or several children, or remarriage to a man with no children of his own, it is not surprising that a significant number of these women are seeking reversal of their tubal sterilization. Considering the present modest success rate of tubal reconstruction, many women are looking at the IVF-ET procedure as a valid alternative for restoring their fertility.

But other factors also have favored the interest in the development of methods for the alleviation of infertility. Adoption, for instance, a traditional palliative to infertility, has become increasingly difficult if not impossible to achieve in many cases over the years, owing to the widespread use of effective contraception methods, the liberalization of abortion laws, the tolerant attitude of society toward the single parent, and the incredibly complex regulations governing adoption in the U.S. With regard to adoption, for instance, a typical example of the ineptitude of current regulations is that of a family in military service, otherwise satisfying all criteria of eligibility for adoption, which never meets the requirements for residence, simply because the man is constantly moved around, from one military installation to another, in the country or abroad. On the other hand, the advent and progressive acceptance of technological intervention in human reproduction, such as artificial insemination using the semen of the husband (AIH) or that of a donor (AID), has prompted many infertile couples to demand they be at least half if not full biological parents of their progeny. For many interviewed couples, adoption is no longer an acceptable solution to their problems. The spectacular success of IVF-ET, with the birth of Baby Louise Brown in England on July 25, 1978, and the attending ill-advised publicity, have convinced many infertile couples that the procedure is simple and bound to be successful in most of the cases. Consequently, in the U.S., clinics in the private and academic sectors of reproductive medicine, which have either announced their intent to offer this service or are known to have expertise in the techniques required by the IVF-ET procedure, have been flooded with requests for treatment of infertility resulting from tubal diseases. The volume of the demand is such that, considering the complexity of the IVF-ET procedure, clinics that conceivably could provide this service would be fully booked for the next five to ten years.

2. Fertilization

Our current knowledge of human fertilization mechanisms is derived from electron microscrope studies of oocytes fertilized *in vitro* [46], [47], and of a single fertilized ovum recovered from a surgical specimen [56]. From these studies, one may list the essential components of human fertilization in chronologic order, as follows: (1) Oocyte maturation, characterized by three different aspects: nuclear and cytoplasmic maturation, and functional stimulation of satellite cells (cumulus oophorus and corona radiata cells), which are all critical to successful fertilization. Owing to our current limited understanding of factors regulating oocyte maturation, ova suitable for fertilization are best obtained when they have completed most of their maturation *in vivo*. A detailed discussion of biological considerations regarding fertilization of mammalian (including human) oocytes can be found in a recent review [42]. (2) Sperm capacitation is the second prerequisite for successful fertilization. It consists of an as yet ill-defined physiological modification of sperm plasma membrane and outer acrosomal membrane, affecting the anterior two-thirds of the sperm head. This physiological change occurs in the female genital tract and leads to a further modification of the morphology of the sperm head, known as: (3) the acrosome reaction. This is a regulated vesiculation process by which sperm plasma membrane and outer acrosomal membrane are eliminated together. By this process, hydrolytic enzymes contained in the acrosome, a cap-like structure sitting on the tip of the sperm head, diffuse outside the sperm and contribute to the digestion of the outer egg investments, the viscous matrix of the cumulus oophorus and loosening of the corona radiata. In a spermatozoon with a reacted acrosome, the outermost structure of the anterior part of the sperm head is the inner acrosomal membrane. This inner membrane appears to be the site of a proteolytic enzyme, the acrosomal proteinase or 'acrosin', which allows for completion of the next step. (4) Sperm passage through the zona pellucida: the zona pellucida is a thick glycoprotein shell which completely surrounds the mammalian egg. With the help of the inner acrosomal membrane-bound acrosin, the sperm is able to digest its way through the zona pellucida and gain access to the perivitelline space, i.e., the space separating the inner aspect of the zona pellucida from the oocyte proper, leading to the next step in fertilization mechanisms. (5) Fusion of the fertilizing sperm plasma membrane to the oocyte membrane: having gained access to the perivitelline space, the fertilizing sperm always establishes contact with the egg membrane in a specific region of its head: the post-acrosomal cap. The very first contact between sperm membrane and egg membrane triggers three events of developmental significance. First, the initial contact triggers the so-called 'cortical reaction' in the egg. The unfertilized egg contains, just underneath its membrane, a layer of (electron-dense) granules, limited by a single membrane. The cortical reaction is achieved by fusion of the cortical granule membrane to the egg membrane, resulting in the extrusion of cortical granule contents into the perivitelline space, in a true exocytosis phenomenon. In some way, not yet understood, the extrusion of cortical granule contents is instrumental in the establishment of the block to polyspermy, a mechanism by which any sperm other than the fertilizing one is prevented from fusing itself to the egg. This is a most important safety device, because the addition to the fertilized egg of one or more chromosome sets would result in di- or polyspermy, a condition sooner or later lethal to the embryo. Second, the initial contact between sperm and egg membranes, in some way, sends a message which triggers resumption of meiosis in the egg. Just prior to ovulation, the mammalian oocyte had been maturing under the influence of the luteinizing hormone (LH) surge, but had its maturation physiologically arrested at metaphase of the second maturation division. The activating effect of the fertilizing sperm on the egg promotes the resumption of meiosis in the egg and its completion by the extension of a mini cell, known as the second polar body and containing egg chromosomes. Now, the fully mature egg contains only 23 chromosomes (in man) of maternal origin. Third, the fertilizing sperm, which during its transit in the female genital tract has developed the ability to fuse its own membrane to that of the egg [48], establishes a cytoplasmic bridge between itself and the egg. This cytoplasmic bridge, initially very small, goes on enlarging. This is the mode of delivery to the egg of the sperm payload of genetic material, 23 chromosomes of paternal origin in a highly condensed form. The sperm plasma membrane becomes incorporated into that of the fertilized egg and the sperm contents, nucleus and flagellum elements sink into the cytoplasm of the egg. At the beginning of membrane fusion between the two gametes, sperm motility which was essential to insure passage through the egg investments, has become irrelevant and has completely stopped. (6) The egg is now activated. It contains 23 chromosomes of maternal origin, and has just recieved 23 chromosomes of paternal origin in the form of a highly condensed sperm nucleus. Independently but synchronously, the sperm chromosomes and maternal chromsomes will rehydrate their respective chromatin. The rehydrating chromatin of each chromosome set will be wrapped in a nuclear envelope, resulting in the appearance of two distinct and separate structures, the male and female pronuclei. The activity going on in each of these pronuclei is the duplication of DNA, in preparation for the first division of the fertilized egg. The fertilized egg initially contains 46 chromosomes: 23 of paternal origin and 23 of maternal origin. Since, from the first division of the fertilized egg on toward each subsequent cell division in the developing embryo, each cell (blastomere) must contain 46 chromosomes, the initial duplication of DNA in both male and female pronuclei is of crucial importance. Duplication of DNA in both male and female pronuclei leads to the formation of 92 chromosomes: two sets of paternal origin, and two sets of maternal origin. When DNA duplication is completed in both pronuclei, chromosomes recondense (in the typical shipping form of chromosomes), pronuclear membranes break down, and microtubules appear which form the first cleavage spindle. The condensed chromosomes pair themselves on the equatorial plate of the first cleavage spindle and this is the culminating point of fertilization. The first cleavage of the fertilized egg, which is now imminent, represents the initial step of embryonic development. All morphological steps described above are documented at the electron microscopic level in previously published studies ([46], [47]).

At this point in time, it must be clearly realized that the most healthy human beings, both male and female, manufacture a small but significant proportion of faulty germ cells. Accidents of meiosis occur all the time; also, accidents of fertilization may occur, such as failure of the block to polyspermy and failure of completion of meiosis in the egg. To be aware of such failures is crucial for the understanding of the underlying causes of human natural embryonic losses, which will be discussed later on.

Much of the public concern about human *in vitro* fertilization undoubtedly relates to the ethical issue of initiating life outside the body. Therefore it seems important to ask at the outset what scientific evidence there is to support the view that fertilization represents the beginning of life. Here are some considerations taken from R. V. Short [40] and from our own contribution to the understanding of the significance of fertilization mechanisms [45].

Although there can be no doubt that fertilization of an oocyte by a spermatozoon is an important event in the development of a new individual, we also know that fertilization is not an essential step in this process. Parthenogenesis, or the development of an egg cell into a new individual in the absence of fertilization by a spermatozoon, is the normal method of reproduction in a number of insects. In birds, parthenogenetically derived fertile male cockerels and turkeys are known to exist, and in mammals such as rats, mice, rabbits, and guinea pigs, parthenogenones have been identified during the early stages of embryonic and fetal development, although they do not seem to survive until birth [29]. A laboratory simulation of membrane fusion events occurring between gametes at fertilization, namely the fusion of two oocytes to each other, also initiates embryonic development, which currently has progressed to the blastocyst stage in the mouse [45]. Although it is not yet known whether such a mode of initiating embryonic development will lead to live birth, there is no a priori reason to believe that it will not do so. Therefore, the argument that fertilization represents the beginning of life cannot be supported on scientific grounds. It seems better to regard life as a continuum of gradually increasing probability of reaching adulthood. There may be a quantum increase in this probability at the time of fertilization in mammals, but there are still many hazards ahead of the fertilized egg if it is to implant and undergo normal embryonic development; even the unfertilized mammalian egg has some limited expectation of normal embryonic development.

3. *Preimplantation Development: The Mammalian Embryo*

The reason why IVF and embryo culture are at all possible is that, from fertilization to the blastocyst stage of development, the mammalian embryo is unattached, floating in the fluid filling the oviduct lumen for the first 3 days, then in the fluid of the uterine cavity for another 3 days, before implanting itself into the endometrium. In all mammalian species, regardless of the size of the animal and the duration of pregnancy, preimplantation development takes approximately six days. Environmental conditions which support fertilization and preimplantation development in culture, as demonstrated by the birth of young after embryo transfer, have only been found thus far for 4 mammalian species: mouse, rat, rabbit, and man [2].

After fertilization of the human egg *in vitro* is completed, the first cleavage occurs resulting in a 2-cell embryo. Subsequent cell divisions will lead to 4-cell, 8-cell, 16-cell embryos, and so on. Upon the seventh cell division, the blastocyst stage of development has been reached. Presently, the only available guideline for judging whether human embryonic development is proceeding on schedule in culture is the exponential growth curve described by Edwards and Steptoe (in [39]). According to this curve the estimated midpoints of cleavage stages (in hrs ± SE) are as follows: 2-cell: 24.9 ± 1.9; 4-cell: 51.9 ± 1.9; 8-cell: 67.9 ± 2.5; 16-cell: 84.6 ± 3.4; morula: 100.2 ± 3.0; early blastocyst: 112.7 ± 3.8. Any significant departure from this curve would make a preimplantation embryo unfit for transplantation because, to insure successful implantation, strict synchrony between embryonic development and endometrium development is of the essence. A simple rule of thumb of mammalian embryo implantation is that "the embryo can wait for the endometrium, but the endometrium will not wait for the embryo".

At the 8- to 16-cell stage of development a dramatic change in the aspect of the embryo occurs, which is known as 'compaction'. Up to now, the blastomeres were still individualized, with a minimal cell-to-cell contact. At late 8-cell to early 16-cell stage, however, cell-to-cell contacts have been maximized and the cell shape has changed. The shape of the cells has been altered at their lateral border so that they now spread on each other. Various types of cell junctions appear between these cells and end up as a permeability seal, limiting the passage of molecules across an epithelium via the intercellular space. From now on, exchanges with the outside milieu will be tightly controlled, which later on will permit the accumulation of fluid leading to the formation of the blastocoele. Compaction can also be regarded as the initial step of morphogenesis, since the 'inside-outside' or cell position theory of development proposes that the determination of cells of the inner cell mass of the morula is due to their position inside the embryo, where an internal micro-environment is created by surrounding (trophoblastic) cells. Thus, at the morula stage cavitation occurs due to fluid accumulation inside the embryo. The blastocoele so formed enlarges progressively. The cells of the outer layer are flattening and form the one-cell-thick mural trophoblast, and the inner cells are pushed against the inner aspect of the mural trophoblast to become a crescent-like cluster of cells when seen in profile, occupying no more than about one-sixth of the mural trophoblast inner aspect, no more than 2-cell-thick in its center and one-cell-thick at its periphery. The blastocyst is now composed of four distinct components: (1) the zona pellucida, which is beginning to stretch and thin out; (2) the one-cell-thick layer of flattened cells constituting the trophoblast and entirely lining up the inner aspect of the zona pellucida; (3) the inner cell mass; and (4) the fluid-filled blastocoele. The next phenomenon is the 'hatching' of the blastocyst: the zona pellucida cracks open and the blastocyst literally crawls out of the zona pellucida. This is a most dramatic event when viewed in microcinematographic rendition. The trophoblast part of the embryo will be involved in the implantation into the endometrium and will contribute the embryonic component of the placenta, while the inner cell mass will evolve to become later on the fetus proper.

4. *Embryo Transfer*

The embryo transfer technique is non-surgical. The embryo is loaded in the tip of a fine nylon catheter filled with culture medium at body temperature. The catheter is threaded through the cervical canal and the embryo is delivered to the uterine fundus by the slow injection of 0.05 ml from the tip of the catheter in which the embryo has been sitting. After embryo delivery, the catheter is immediately checked under the microscope to insure that the embryo has not remained attached to its wall.

As simple as it may appear, embryo transfer remains a delicate operation. Bleeding, ever so slight, resulting from threading the catheter in the cervical canal and uterine cavity, may prevent implantation since a layer of fibrin deposited on the outer aspect of the zona pellucida would make blastocyst hatching impossible.

The preimplantation embryo enters the uterus approximately 72 hours after ovulation (and fertilization), when the embryo is at the very early morula stage, consisting of 8–16 cells. Literature survey shows that only 15 human preimplantation embryos have been recovered from the genital tract: 9 from the oviduct, 6 from the uterus. The most advanced developmental stage recovered from the oviduct was a 7-cell embryo [32] and the earliest developmental stage recovered from the uterus was a 12-cell embryo [16]; the age of both specimens was estimated at about 72 hours. The most advanced stage of development ever recovered from the uterus was a blastocyst expanded in the zona pellucida, consisting of 186 cells, and of an age estimated at more than 120 hours [6]. Thus, it would seem that preimplantation embryos could be transferred to the uterine cavity from the 8-cell stage up to the blastocyst stage, i.e., from 72 hours up to about 120 hours of development. Quite obviously, implantation cannot take place until blastocyst hatching is completed. The reason why the human preimplantation embryo does not migrate to the uterine cavity earlier than 72 hours of development, is most likely due to the fact that the uterine environment has not yet been suitably modified to support embryonic development. From laboratory animal work it is well known that the mammalian egg can be fertilized in the uterine cavity but that it will not survive there. Thus, reported attempts at transferring embryos 36–42 hours after insemination [33] represent wishful thinking, at best.

Edwards and Steptoe (in [39]) reported having transferred embryos at the 6–8 cell, 8-cell, and morula stages. They also reported successful implantation only when transferred embryos were at the 8–16 cell stage, and when the transfer was performed late at night. There is no physiological evidence in support of the latter statement, except perhaps the patient being soon asleep in bed. In the recent Australian experience [25], the embryo was transferred at the 8-cell stage, at 10:45 p.m., 74 hours after fertilization. The obvious advantage of transferring an 8-cell embryo is that it cuts down on the need for further culture in the laboratory.

Until now all embryo transfers have been carried out in the luteal phase of the cycle in which oocyte recovery was performed. In a soon-to-be-tested new approach to implantation (see below), embryo transfer will be deferred to a subsequent and completely unmanipulated natural cycle. Synchronous transfer (i.e., transfer of an embryo the developmental stage of which is in synchrony with that of the endometrium) timing will be decided by the interplay of three factors: (1) prospective determination of the LH (luteinizing hormone) surge by rapid radioimmunoassay or radioreceptor assay to predict the time interval when ovulation can be expected to occur; (2) time-lapse videorecording of real-time sonar scan during the time period when ovulation is expected to occur, in order to pinpoint exactly the moment of ovulation (sonar scan measurements of the follicle at ovulation show a reduction in volume due to the loss of egg, cumulus oophorus and follicular fluid, immediately followed by a gain in volume due to the formation of the corpus hemorrhagicum); (3) precise data on the timing of cleavage of the preimplantation embryo in culture, indicating that such development is proceeding on schedule.

5. Embryo Cryopreservation: State of the Art

The technology of mammalian embryo cryopreservation was first introduced by Whittingham, Leibo and Mazur [55]. In the ensuing years, numerous laboratories (ours included) have successfully used the procedure to freeze embryos of mice, rats, rabbits, sheep, goats, and cattle. The freezing of embryos has been the subject of one international course (sponsored by UNESCO-ICLA-ICRO), and of two international conferences ([10], [31]). 'Successful' freezing means not only that high percentages of frozen-thawed embryos are able to develop in culture (where culture techniques are available), but that they are able to develop into normal offspring when the thawed embryos are transferred into the oviducts or uteri (depending on development stage) of suitably prepared foster mothers. The state of the art of mammalian embryo cryopreservation can be summarized as follows: (1) the embryos of seven species (man included) have been successfully cryopreserved; (2) in one species (mouse) all stages of preimplantation development, from unfertilized egg to blastocyst, have been successfully cryopreserved; (3) the survival rate (as evidenced by live birth following ET) is greater than 90% in most cases; (4) the survival rate after 60 months of cryopreservation is equal to that after 24 hours.

A detailed description of the principles of embryo preservation can be found in a recent review by Whittingham [54]. The procedure for mammalian embryocryopreservation is currently well standardized. It involves: (1) addition of a cryoprotectant at $0°C$ (dimethyl-sulfoxide, glycerol, or ethylene-glycol) at a final concentration of 1.5 M; (2) cooling to $-6°C$ and induction of ice formation (seeding) in the extracellular solution; (3) slow cooling at -0.1 to $-0.5°C/min$, down to $-80°C$; (4) storage in liquid nitrogen at $-196°C$; (5) warming up at 4 to $20°C/min$ up to $0°C$; (6) careful, stepwise diluting out of the cryoprotectant at $0°C$. All these steps are designed to allow the embryos to remain in osmotic equilibrium with the suspending medium at all temperatures. During slow cooling the cells shrink due to loss of intracellular water to the hypertonic extracellular medium. This loss of water prevents the massive formation of intracellular ice, which has been shown to be the primary factor for cell death during freezing.

The prediction of optimal cooling rate for a given cell type can be deducted from a quantitative physicochemical model, derived to describe the kinetic response of cells when exposed to sub-zero temperature [26]. Very recent development, i.e., the injection into the mathematical model of variables such as the temperature coefficient of water permeability of a given cell type, which can be determined experimentally [22], lends a high degree of accuracy to the prediction of optimal cooling rate. It has been calculated that 3 determinations of the temperature coefficient of water permeability of the human oocyte would yield a good approximation of such a variable, while 15 such determinations would provide all desirable precision in the determination of this variable ([22], personal communication). This development is of utmost practical significance, in that the optimal cooling rate for cryopreservation of human embryos can be determined using an extremely small (15) sample of human preovulatory oocytes or fertilized ova. The clinical significance of human embryo cryopreservation will become evident when the current status of human IVF-ET is analyzed.

There is already some experimental support for the use of cryopreservation in clinical IVF-ET. Allegedly, the Indian team used such a technological step to produce the live birth which occurred in Calcutta on October 3, 1978. According to some reports [28], three preovulatory ova were obtained following a superovulation procedure and follicular aspiration. The 3 ova were fertilized, allowed to develop for 3 days in culture, then freeze-preserved for 53 days. Thus the transfer was performed 56 days after egg recovery, i.e., two menstrual cycles (of 28 days) later, in a totally unmanipulated natural cycle. Allegedly, the 3 embryos were transferred together in a single operation. One led to a live birth. Whether the other two embryos were damaged in the freezing process or suffered from later demise from other causes is not known. Data on the monitoring of that pregnancy are not available, except for the fact that no amniocentesis was performed [28].

6. Abortions: Definitions and Classification

(1) Abortion is the termination of a pregnancy, i.e., the state in which the uterine implantation of an embryo has been recognized by the maternal organism, before the embryo (so designated up to the end of the 8th week)

or the fetus (so designated from the beginning of the 9th week) is capable of extrauterine life (24 to 26 weeks in some cases). The chronology used here is standard chronology, to be found in any standard textbook of human embryology (e.g., see [30], pp. 2–4).

(2) Spontaneous abortion: all abortions not induced are spontaneous even if an external cause such as trauma or disease is involved.

(3) Preclinical abortion: a spontaneous abortion occurring so early after implantation that it is never brought to medical attention and no organic material is available for investigation.

(4) Clinical abortion: a spontaneous or induced abortion in which organic material (gestational sac and/or fetus) is brought to medical attention and is amenable to anatomical and chromosomal analysis.

(5) Iatrogenic abortion: an induced but unintended abortion, resulting from a complication of amniocentesis.

7. Natural Embryonic Loss in Man

Contrary to popular belief, the establishment of a pregnancy in man is a hazardous (for the embryo) and difficult business. Although suspected as early as 1949 [16], it was not until recent years that the magnitude of natural embryonic loss in man could be quantified with some degree of precision.

Leridon [23] used data on the incidence of blighted human ova together with data on fetal mortality to construct a "life-table of intrauterine mortality".

The results of his calculations show that 69% of human ova exposed to spermatozoa are lost by the expected time of birth. The results also show a large incidence of fertilization failure (16%) and a large incidence of embryo loss during the first 2 weeks following fertilization. Thus, by the time the woman would expect to miss her menstrual period, 58% of all potential conceptions have already been lost. Other series of independent evidence support the conclusion that high embryonic loss occurs spontaneously in man [34]. An estimate of between 69% and 78% embryonic loss, however, is reasonably consistent with data showing that it takes an average of 4 months to achieve pregnancy by artificial insemination. Thus, it may take an average of 4 months of continual sexual activity to establish a pregnancy capable of producing a normal offspring [27]. Embryonic loss also increases significantly with the age of the mother, particularly after the age of 35. Unfortunately, this is a circumstance much too frequent among patients eligible for IVF-ET. The death of embryos may arise from 2 primary causes: intrinsic abnormalities in the embryo that are lethal (such as unmasked recessive genes and chromosomal aberrations) and lethal environmental effects mediated via the female genital tract. The effects may be due to the normal aging process in the female tract, disease of the genital tract, or transmission of exogenous teratogenic agents. Studies on incidence of cytogenetic aberrations in spontaneous abortions show that a major factor in embryonic loss is chromosomal imbalance that arises during the maturation (meiosis) of both types of germ cells and during fertilization. It has been argued that chromosomal aberrations that arise during gametogenesis and fertilization account for a loss of 50% in human embryos that are potentially existent at the time of fertilization [5]. The cause of the 25% deficit between the estimate of 69% [23] and of 78% [34] and that of 50% [5], is presumably due to unmasked recessive genes and environmental factors of nongenetic origin. The true contribution of these factors is presently unknown. Much more is known, however, about cytogenetic factors involved in the loss of human embryos.

During meiosis, several accidents may occur, resulting in sperm and ova with abnormal numbers of chromosomes. Sex chromosomes may not separate, resulting in sperm that contain both X and Y chromosomes or no sex chromosomes at all, or in ova containing 2 X chromosomes or no X chromosomes at all. In the same way, any of the 22 pairs of autosomes may fail to separate. This type of aberration is called "nondisjunction". Fertilization, involving any of these abnormal sperm or ova, results in abnormal embryos. For example, if a normal ovum is fertilized by a sperm without a sex chromosome, an XO embryo is produced, which is affected by Turner's syndrome. Such an individual has only 45 chromosomes (45, XO) and is an example of a general class of aberration called *monosomy*. If an ovum with 2 X chromosomes is fertilized by a normal Y-bearing sperm, an XXY individual is produced, who has Klinefelter's syndrome. Such an individual has 47 chromosomes (47, XXY) and is an example of another general class of aberration called *trisomy*. Nondisjunction of the G class of chromosomes, i.e., chromosomes 21 or 22, can result in trisomy G, which causes Down's syndrome.

Other types of accidents can happen. Failure to complete meiosis may occur, so that an ovum or a sperm is produced that has the full set of chromosomes. Thus, if a diploid ovum is fertilized by a normal sperm, a triploid embryo is produced (69, XXY or 69, XXX).

Normally, only one sperm enters the ovum at fertilization. Then, entry of more than one sperm is prevented by the *block to polyspermy*. If this safety mechanism fails, one or more sperm may enter the ovum at fertilization, giving triploids, tetraploids, and so on. Fortunately, much abnormal fertilization does not result in viable embryos in man. Recent studies ([3] and [19]) suggest that most human triploid embryos are formed naturally by dispermic fertilization as the result of failure of the block to polyspermy. There is a significant absence of autosomal monosomies in spontaneous human abortions [5]. Boué and Boué [5] argue that these aberrations must be produced in numbers equivalent to the trisomies, but that they cause embryonic death so early that they cannot be detected. Their elimination may in fact occur before the first missed menstrual period (preclinical spontaneous abortions). My strong personal contention is that when we are able to analyze systematically the cytogenetics of human preimplantation embryos, we shall find that such aberrations actually occur and we shall be able to determine their frequency. Moreover, this will not be an artifact of IVF and preimplantation development in culture, but will reflect the true natural incidence of these aberrations.

What is the fate of cytogenetic aberrations? The presence of an abnormal number of chromosomes may or may not be lethal. For example, the XXY trisomy is compatible with postnatal life, the XO monosomy, as well as trisomy G, is predominantly lethal in fetal life, but some are born. Triploidy, however, is nearly always lethal in embryonic life and those that are born only survive for a short time. Studies on the chromosome complements in spontaneous abortions in women have provided information on when embryos die [5]. Some types, such as tetraploidy (karyotype: 92), trisomy C, and trisomy E, are, on average, lethal a few weeks earlier than other types, such as monosomy X, triploidy, trisomy D, and trisomy G. Nevertheless, nearly all of them become developmentally arrested by the 8th week of pregnancy.

Thus, there is strong evidence that there is a high incidence of embryonic death in the normal human reproductive process. A large component of this arises from errors in meiosis in the male and female and in errors of fertilization, such as failure of the block to polyspermy. Normally, most of the abnormal embryos die and are eliminated early in pregnancy. Nevertheless, a few do not die and are eventually born with congenital abnormalities. The incidence of these abnormalities at birth increases with maternal age.

Obviously, there are irreducible factors, the effect of which cannot reasonably be expected to be overcome by human IVF and ET. One has to be prepared to repeat embryo transfer in order to establish a pregnancy since the natural implantation success rate is only 69%. In this respect, freeze preservation of preimplantation embryos, following superovulation, would certainly improve the efficiency of the procedure, in that it would permit serial transfer without a need for repeated laparoscopies and would allow for delaying transfer to completely unmanipulated natural cycles. It can also reasonably be expected that advances in quality control procedures, such as the monitoring of failure of the block to polyspermy, digyny, karyo-typing the blastocyst, and perhaps, in the not-too-distant future, provided that genes are expressed this early in development, quantitative enzyme activity assays on single cells [18] will definitely help to avoid the transfer of intrinsically defective embryos, especially when it is already known that a projected pregnancy will have a high genetic risk associated with it.

8. *Note*

The research objectives described in this review concern only *in vitro* fertiliza-tion and the first six days of embryonic development. There is, however, one exception to the above statement: *in vitro* research on the biological origin of the hyatidiform mole and choriocarcinoma may culture extending beyond the first six days of embryonic development.

III. CURRENT STATUS OF IVF-ET IN MAN

1. *The World Record of IVF-ET*

If one looks critically at the current world record of IVF-ET, the success rate is not high, abnormal pregnancies have been produced, and abortions, both spontaneous and iatrogenic, have been recorded. Table I shows the distribution, as of October 1, 1980, of these cases, listed by country of origin.

The total number of pregnancies detected by sustained elevated titer of urinary gonadotropin amounts thus far to 11. Of these 11 pregnancies, 4 resulted in at term, live birth (36.4%). The 7 recorded abortions amount to 63.6% of all pregnancies. The 3 preclinical abortions are those in which the elevated titer of urinary gonadotropin suddenly faded away. Among the clinical abortions two categories must be distinguished. The clinical abortion recorded in Australia was not a spontaneous one but resulted from an accident of amniocentesis. The karyotype was that of a normal male. Thus, this is a clear case of iatrogenic abortion, without detectable genetic component.

TABLE I
World record of pregnancies established by IVF-ET

COUNTRY	PREGNANCIES	LIVE BIRTHS	SEX [a]	ABORTIONS	
				Clinical	Preclinical
Australia	3	1	F	1 [b]	1
India	1 [c]	1	F	– [c]	– [c]
U.K.	7	2	M + F	3 [d]	2
TOTAL	11	4	1M/3F	7	
%	100	36.4 [e]	25/75	63.6 [e]	

[a] Determined either at birth only or by karyotyping amniocentesis material and at birth.
[b] Resulted from an accident of amniocentesis. The karyotype was that of a normal male.
[c] No information available on previous attempts and on possible incidence of abortion.
[d] Includes one ectopic pregnancy.
[e] Probability of obtaining a live baby from an implanted embryo in IVF-ET: 36.4/63.6 = 0.57.

Among the 3 clinical abortions recorded in U.K. some distinction must also be established. The first one [49] resulted from an ectopic pregnancy, presumably due to the migration of a transferred embryo from the uterine cavity to a remaining oviduct stump. Hence, the recommendation that the cornua be cauterized at the time of preliminary laparoscopic evaluation. The second abortion occurred spontaneously 10 weeks after embryo transfer. The karyotype was 69, XXX. It was not possible from banding studies to determine whether the additional autosomal set was maternally or paternally derived. The third one occurred 20.5 weeks after embryo transfer. A karyotype, established on amniocentesis material obtained at 16 weeks, exhibited a large Y chromosome together with an additional fragment of one chromosome 15. Both of these anomalies were found to be present in the father. The infant was born alive, but died after 2 hours. It weighed 200 g and measured 18 cm in crown-rump length. No abnormality could be detected at autopsy in either the baby or its placenta.

Among the live births, all babies are free from congenital defects and, for the time being, seem to be normally developing.

Using data from Leridon [23], one can calculate that the probability of obtaining a live baby from an implanted embryo in human spontaneous pregnancy is: 31/69 = 0.45 [4] . Similarly, one can calculate (Table I) that the probability of obtaining a live baby from an implanted embryo in IVF-ET is: 36.4/63.6 = 0.57. Although these figures may seem close to each other, they are not quite comparable. The probability derived from Leridon's data takes into account only the effects of spontaneous abortions, while the probability derived from current IVF-ET results takes one iatrogenic abortion into account. Had this iatrogenic abortion been avoided, the current status of IVF-ET would read: 5 live births out of 11 implantations, i.e., 45% successes and 55% failures. The corresponding probability of obtaining a live baby from an implanted embryo would then be raised to: 45/55 = 0.82. The probability figures of 0.57 and 0.82 are most likely too high, owing to the small size of the sample currently available. What those figures strongly suggest, however, is that pregnancy resulting from IVF-ET is probably no more hazardous than spontaneous pregnancy in man.

Another clear indication given by current results of IVF-ET is that one has to be prepared to proceed with multiple embryo transfer in order to achieve one implantation. Biggers [4], using data from Leridon [23], has made some interesting statistical calculations regarding the efficiency of *in vitro* fertilization and embryo transfer. If it is assumed that the production of blastocysts and transfer of embryos is fully efficient, the probability of obtaining live babies after the transfer of 1, 2, or 3 blastocysts can be calculated using the binomial distribution (Table II).

TABLE II
Probabilities of failure and the birth of singletons, twins, and triplets
following human blastocyst transfer [a]

NO. BLASTOCYSTS TRANSFERRED	REQUIRED NO. OF OOCYTES	PROBABILITY			
		Failure	Singleton	Twins	Triplets
1	2	0.55	0.45	–	–
2	3	0.30	0.50	0.20	–
3	5	0.17	0.41	0.33	0.09

[a] Assumes full efficiency of oocyte *in vitro* fertilization, embryo culture and transfer techniques.
Source: Biggers [4], calculated from the life-table of Leridon [23].

The number of oocytes that need to be collected from the ovary to give 1, 2, or 3 blastocysts can also be calculated (Table II).

Since it is unrealistic to suppose the transfer technique is 100% efficient, similar calculations have been done assuming 25, 50, and 70% efficiency (Table III).

TABLE III

Probability of having a child (singleton, twin, or triplet) following human blastocyst transfer assuming different efficiencies of transfer

NO. BLASTOCYSTS TRANSFERRED	TRANSFER EFFICIENCY (%)			
	25	50	75	100
1	0.11	0.23	0.34	0.45
2	0.21	0.40	0.56	0.70
3	0.30	0.53	0.71	0.83

Source: Biggers [4].

From experience with embryo transfer in animals, it is more realistic (and conservative) to assume an efficiency of about 50%. Thus, if one blastocyst is transferred, the chances of obtaining a live baby are about 1 in 4. If 3 blastocysts are transferred in a single procedure, the chance of producing a live baby is raised to about 1 in 2, but this involves a 1 in 100 chance of triplets. Please note that the terminology of 'live baby' has been used and keep in mind that the 31 live babies that can be born out of 100 fertilizable ova will still contain a percentage of birth defects, unless advanced technology is applied for selecting out abnormal embryos prior to implantation and unless the pregnancies are carefully mentored afterward. The problem with increasing efficiency of the technique by transferring more than one blastocyst at a time would arise from the added difficulty of monitoring the normality of more than one fetus and then deciding what to do if abnormal and normal fetuses are developing together. Thus, it would seem simpler, and perhaps as efficient, although it may require more time to initiate pregnancy, to proceed with serial transfer of a single blastocyst, following superovulation, IVF, embryo development in culture and freeze storage of several embryos.

Finally, as modest as the IVF-ET world record is thus far, there is no evidence that such procedures add to the natural risk of chromosomal abnormalities at birth. To quote Dr. J. J. Schlesselman [36] from the Biometry Branch, NICHD: "Unless *in vitro* fertilization in man strongly contradicts the experience in domestic animal reproduction, which suggests no increased risk of abnormalities at birth, a large number of births would be required to provide a definitive assessment of risk" ([36], p. 135).

Such a statement, from an objective and independent biostatistician, is most encouraging.

2. IVF-ET's Main Problem: The Low Implantation Success Rate

The practical problems that have dominated human oocyte recovery in the early days as well as today are timing of recovery and an overall low yield. These problems were overcome, but it was found that their solution generated other problems. Hence, over the past 10 years, two different strategies were used for oocyte recovery.

(a) Egg recovery following hormonal induction of multiple follicle growth. The first approach was based on an adaptation to normally cycling women of the method designed to induce ovulation in anovulatory women, i.e., administration of gonadotropins. Such a treatment induces multiple follicle growth and ovulation following hCG (administered so as just to precede the natural LH surge) is expected 30–40 hours later. Thus, laparoscopy is timed to take place 32–34 hours post hCG, at a time when follicles should be ripe but not yet ruptured. Alternatively, clomid can be used instead of menotropins. Using such approaches, one preovulatory oocyte can on the average be recovered per patient, with a range of from 0 to 3 preovulatory ova.

After several years of using this approach, Steptoe and Edwards (in [39]) reported that 77 embryo transfers led to only 3 implantations, 2 of which faded away, and the third of which ended up in an ectopic pregnancy. On retrospective analysis, it was found that the principal difficulty lay in abnormalities of the luteal phase following induction of follicular development with gonadotropins in cycling women. It seemed that the higher the estrogen concentration, the shorter the luteal phase; many patients had only 9-day luteal phases [39].

A similar experience is reported by the Australian team of Monash University, Melbourne [25]. Over the period 1973–78 the results of IVF-ET following egg recovery in hormonally stimulated cycles were as follows: (1) No. of patients treated: 146; (2) No. of eggs inseminated: 322; (3) No. of eggs failing to become fertilized: 143 (43.5%); (4) No. of eggs fertilized: 179; (5) No. of eggs failing to cleave: 91; (6) No. of eggs cleaving: 88; (7) No. of embryos transferred: 34; (8) No. of transient implantations: 1; (9) No. of live births: 0.

However, the inadequate luteal phase following multiple follicle growth induction in normally cycling women may not have been the only source of the problem. A recent study by Soules *et al.* [41] strongly suggests that direct inhibition of ovarian steroidogenesis may result from (1) toxic effects of anesthetic agents; and (2) stress-induced changes in other hormone levels, e.g., hyperprolactinemia.

(b) Egg recovery in the course of a natural cycle. Thus, multiple follicle growth induction was abandoned in favor of egg recovery in the course of a natural cycle. A compromise was established between the increased difficulty of recovering one single preovulatory oocyte and the benefit of a presumably balanced luteal phase, thought most conducive to successful implantation. Yet, in this approach, one is confronted with several difficulties: (1) there is currently no practical method for the prediction of the LH surge, critical for the timing of egg recovery; (2) the possible inhibitory effect of general anesthesia was unknown at the time; (3) trauma of unknown magnitude may result from contents aspiration from a single leading follicle, thus possibly interfering with luteinization.

The results of this approach in England (Steptoe and Edwards, in [39]) were as follows: of 28 implantation attempts, only 4 (14%) succeeded which led to 2 live births. The Australian team, using the same approach, reported almost identical results [25]. From 14 embryo transfers, 2 resulted in successful implantation (14%), from which an iatrogenic abortion and one live birth resulted.

The success rate of implantation of 14%, reported by two independent groups, does not compare favorably with the natural implantation rate of 69% [23]. It is therefore quite clear that the major problem that IVF-ET researchers are facing is to improve the implantation success rate, if the IVF-ET procedure is to gain clinical acceptability.

IV. IMMEDIATE RESEARCH OBJECTIVES INVOLVING HUMAN EMBRYOS

The chief objective of what this reviewer considers to be the top priority research item involving human embryos is to improve the implantation success rate.

This major objective can realistically be attained by: (1) avoiding conditions adverse to implantation; and (2) screening out chromosomally defective embryos which would be demised before the end of the second week following fertilization.

The analysis of the current status of IVF-ET emphasizes that: (1) there is at present no evidence that the IVF-ET procedure adds to the natural risk of chromosomal or other abnormalities at birth; (2) ironically, almost all measures that were taken to improve on egg recovery and its timing turned out to be self-defeating. When a seemingly more physiological approach was adopted, adverse factors were still at play, limiting the implantation success rate, although, now, the procedure has led to the birth of normal offspring.

1. Adverse Factors and How to Avoid Them

To clarify the proposed method of procedure, it is useful to list the various factors adverse to implantation and to indicate the appropriate solution for each of them. (1) The induction of multiple follicle growth by hormonal pretreatment improves preovulatory oocyte yield and solves the problem of properly timing their recovery. However, this treatment, applied to normally cycling women, disrupts the endocrine equilibrium of the luteal phase, which is most often short, and therefore compromises implantation in the cycle of egg recovery. Since it is most advantageous to obtain several fertilizable eggs in a single recovery procedure, thus cutting down on the need for repeated laparoscopies and their attendant risks, the induction of multiple follicle growth remains a method of choice for the procurement of fertilizable ova. Logically, the solution to the problem of an ensuing hostile luteal phase is to defer embryo transfer to a totally unmanipulated natural cycle. (2) Until very recently [41], it has not been suspected that all general anesthetic agents could have an inhibitory effect on ovarian steroidogenesis, and there was only a slight hint that stress-induced changes in other hormone levels (e.g., hyperprolactinemia) may occur, therefore interfering most of the time with successful implantation. Once again, the logical solution to this problem is to defer embryo transfer to a totally unmanipulated natural cycle. (3) Aspirating follicular contents in a natural cycle, where there is only one leading follicle, may result in a trauma of unknown magnitude, which is bound to interfere with luteinization. The recently introduced technological development of repeatedly flushing the follicle with culture medium, after the initial contents aspiration, has certainly contributed to the improvement of preovulatory oocyte recovery from a single follicle. Yet, this procedure is bound to increase the trauma to the single leading follicle, thus further compromising luteinization. Here again, the logical solution to the problem seems to be the deferment of embryo transfer to a totally unmanipulated natural cycle. (4) In spontaneous human pregnancy there is a 16% incidence of fertilization failure. IVF is not expected to be more immune to failure than physiological fertilization. Next, there is a 15% cleavage failure in physiologically fertilized ova. Fertilization failure and cleavage failure of *in vitro* fertilized ova are easily recognized and therefore pose no practical problem. But, physiologically, 27% of implanting embryos will die before the end of the week required to complete implantation. In unassisted pregnancy, this loss, although considerable, goes unnoticed. Not so in IVF-ET. The cause of such failures rests with accidents of meiosis (monosomies and trisomies), of fertilization (polyspermy or digyny), and perhaps also of early cleavages. It would therefore seem to be self-defeating to transfer every single embryo developing in culture without thoroughly checking its chromosome make-up. The risk of implantation failure that would be taken on the basis of a defective chromosome complement, would be equal to 27 out of 69 implanting embryos according to Leridon [23], i.e., a 0.39 probability of not achieving implantation. Thus, if one wants to improve the implantation success rate of IVF-ET, one has to develop accurate procedures to screen out embryos which are intrinsically doomed.

The above analysis clearly defines what the two fundamental research efforts should be in the immediate future: (1) work out an effective method for the cryopreservation of human preimplantation embryos; (2) work out practical methods for the screening out of chromosomally defective preimplantation embryos.

2. *Embryo Cryopreservation*

As a top priority research item, the experimental approach to optimal cryopreservation of human preimplantation embryos will now be described. (1) Determination of the temperature coefficient of water permeability of preovulatory oocytes and of 1-cell fertilized ova (since these may be different), using the method of Leibo [22]. (2) Having determined the value of the temperature coefficient with sufficient precision (15 determinations should provide this degree of precision, according to Leibo), use this value in the computerized mathematical model of Mazur [25] to predict the optimal cooling rate for human preimplantation embryos. (3) Using a standard method for mammalian embryo cryopreservation [54], and the optimal cooling rate determined above, conduct an electron microscope study to determine any fine morphological alterations which may result from the cryopreservation procedure. Controls in this study should be unfrozen specimens, developing synchronously with the frozen ones, both types being obtained from the same egg donor. (4) Using the same cryo-preservation methodology, determine the ability of cryopreserved embryos (8-cell, 16-cell and early morulae) to resume embryonic development in culture. (5) Repeat the above determination using late morula stages which have been submitted to a microbiopsy procedure (see below). (6) Determine the ability of cryopreserved embryos to implant upon embryo transfer. Ultimately, those embryos should have been determined to be free from intrinsic lethal chromosome abnormalities by microbiopsy procedures.

3. *Screening Out Chromosomally Defective Embryos*

The second and integral part of this research project is to determine the applicability and practicality of methods for performing a microbiopsy on the late morula or blastocyst stage of development. Such methods have already been applied to embryos of laboratory animals (rabbit). Gardner and Edwards [12] have used karyotyping of cells obtained by microbiopsy of the trophoblast to sex rabbit embryos prior to transfer. Prediction of sex by this method has been shown to be 100% accurate, as well as harmless to the embryos. With the refinement of micromanipulative techniques, microbiopsy and karyologic analysis, chromosome morphological and/or numerical abnormalities could be recognized and defective embryos could be selected out. Other quality control procedures must also be applied for the non-invasive monitoring of monospermy, completion of meiosis in the oocyte and normal chronology of preimplantation development. These quality control procedures rest on the combined use of differential inter-ference contrast (Nomarski's) optics, video-intensification microscopy, and time-lapse video recording of significant events. The technology of these procedures has already been worked out [42].

With the development of the above methodologies, the two main objectives of this research project (i.e., transfer of chromosome defect-free embryo in conditions optimal for implantation) should be attained within a reasonable period of time and with a minimum use of preimplantation embryos.

4. *Comments*

Some of the research objectives described above do not involve embryo transfer. For these studies the fertilizable egg donors should be recruited from among patients presenting for elective sterilization. Fully informed consent must be obtained from both egg and sperm donors. Patients presenting an infertility problem cannot be used for such studies. Their informed consent would be much too easy to obtain since they would believe they would reap an immediate benefit from the studies. This would constitute a subtle form of coercion and, from an ethical viewpoint, must be avoided at all costs.

The research proposal described above is in strict conformity with Conclusion No. 2 of the National Ethics Advisory Board in its Report on "HEW Support of Research Involving Human *in Vitro* Fertilization and Embryo Transfer" [11]. Conclusion No. 2 reads as follows: The Ethics Advisory Board finds that it is acceptable from an ethical standpoint to undertake research involving human *in vitro* fertilization and embryo transfer provided that:

A. If the research involves human *in vitro* fertilization without embryo transfer, the following conditions are satisfied:

1. The research complies with all appropriate provisions of the regulations governing research with human subject (45 CFR 46);
2. The research is designed primarily: (A) to establish the safety and efficacy of embryo transfer and (B) to obtain important scientific information toward that end not reasonably attainable by other means;
3. Human gametes used in such research will be obtained exclusively from persons who have been informed of the nature and purpose of the research in which such material will be used and have specifically consented to such use;
4. No embryo will be sustained *in vitro* beyond the stage normally associated with the completion of implantation (14 days after fertilization); and
5. All interested parties and the general public will be advised if evidence begins to show that the procedure entails risks of abnormal offspring higher than those associated with natural human reproduction.

B. In Addition, if the research involves embryo transfer following human *in vitro* fertilization, embryo transfer will be attempted only with gametes obtained from lawfully married couples ([11], pp. 106–107).

[*Reviewer's Note*: The last provision leaves no hope to the infertile couple in which there are factors of both female *and* male origin. This restriction is hard to understand in the light of the widely accepted practice of artificial insemination using donor semen (AID). The situation would be no different in the case of an IVF-ET procedure.]

V. RESEARCH APPLICATIONS OF IVF, NOT INVOLVING ET

Roger V. Short [40], in his report to the Ethics Advisory Board entitled Human *in Vitro* Fertilization and Embryo Transfer, has listed some applications of IVF research, which do not involve embryo transfer. He has characterized those research objectives in the following way: "In contrast to the obvious clinical applications of human IVF-ET for treating infertility in women with bilateral occlusion of the Fallopian tubes, there are significant applications of this technique for fundamental research in a number of areas. Indeed, it seems probable that these fundamental discoveries will far outweigh the rather restricted use of embryo transfer in their ultimate clinical significance". Although this reviewer does not fully agree with the last sentence of Short's statement, he does share some of Short's general views on the overall importance of fundamental research using human IVF alone. To give Short full credit for his views, they are quoted below verbatim. Short's views are identified by an asterisk (*) but some of this reviewer's personal views are also included here and are identified by a double asterisk (**).

The order in which these research objectives are listed below reflects the priority rating they should be awarded in this reviewer's opinion.

1. *Contraceptive Research*

*The mammalian oocyte is surrounded by a glycoprotein 'shell', the zona pellucida. This shell contains specific binding sites for the spermatozoa of closely related species; unless the spermatozoa first bind to the zona, they will not be able to penetrate it and reach the vitelline membrane. If the glycoproteins of the zona pellucida of hamsters are injected into mice, antibodies are formed that render the mice infertile and passive transfer to mice of rabbit antibodies raised against mouse eggs will make the mice temporarily infertile [52]. *In vitro*, it can be shown that the antibody works as predicted by preventing attachment of spermatozoa to the zona pellucida [52]. However, there may be an additional antifertility effect, since even if fertilization did occur, implantation would be prevented because the antibodies around the zona are known to prevent the blastocyst from hatching

[8]. These studies in laboratory animals, therefore, show considerable promise as a novel form of immunologic contraception. If research is to proceed in a logical manner toward the evaluation of this technique for human clinical use, the first step will be to see if antisera raised against the zonal glycoproteins of a variety of species, including primates and the human, are able to block the fertilization of human eggs by human spermatozoa *in vitro*. If this effect can be demonstrated in man, the next step will be to characterize and, if possible, synthesize the zonal glycoprotein, so that enough antigen can be produced for human clinical trials. Antisera raised in human would initially be screened for their antifertility action in an IVF system, before proceeding to clinical trials *in vivo*.

*Another area of contraception research where human IVF can provide an invaluable if not essential test system, relates to the development of male contraceptives. There is now abundant evidence to show that a variety of steroids (synthetic androgens, antiandrogens, or mixtures of androgens and gestagens) can be used to suppress sperm production by the testis [7]. Although it is a relatively easy matter to produce severe oligospermia with sperm densities of less than 5 million per milliliter, it is extremely difficult to produce complete azoospermia. As long as there are still some motile sperm in the ejaculate, it will not be possible to reassure the man that he is indeed sterile. It would seem unethical to put the matter to the test by encouraging the man to have unprotected intercourse with his wife, who would then have to resort to abortion to make up for any failures of the male contraceptive. Yet, one such clinical trial, sponsored by NIH, is currently going on at my own institution. Abortion, not therapeutic, but corrective, in this case, is an officially approved procedure, while human IVF technology is still awaiting routine use in federally funded research projects. If it could be shown beforehand by IVF tests that the few spermatozoa produced by men on steroid suppression therapy were incapable of fertilizing the human egg, this would provide sufficient reassurance, to principal investigators and institutional review boards as well, to allow one to embark on a limited clinical trial. Without some such IVF testing, it is difficult to see how it will ever be possible to develop chemical approaches to male contraception, unless they result in complete azoospermia.

2. *Infertility Research and Diagnostic Research in Idiopathic Infertility*

*In contrast to the great research advances that have been made in the diagnosis and treatment of infertility in women over the past decade, there has been little or no progress in our understanding of male infertility. It is generally accepted that about 10% of married couples have an infertility problem, and although we cannot know for certain, it seems likely that the man is at fault in a significant proportion of such cases. The most useful index of male infertility is still the sperm count, but even this is an extremely imprecise guide. Nobody knows what a 'normal' human spermatozoon looks like, and although a great deal of effort is devoted to scoring the proportion of morphologically 'abnormal' spermatozoa in the ejaculate, we have no idea whether abnormal shape reflects abnormal function, apart from the fact that excessively large spermatozoa are diploid and hence incapable of normal fertilization [37]. However, detailed studies of the chromosomes of early human abortuses show that in 60% of cases there is a grossly abnormal karyotype that is presumably the cause of abortion. These abnormalities are mainly due to errors of gametogenesis, and many are paternally derived [38]. Thus, it must follow that there are many genetically defective spermatozoa in the ejaculate, although with the present techniques we have no way of detecting them. It is also generally believed that if a man is oligospermic, with a sperm density of less than 20 million per milliliter, his fertility is greatly reduced. This is presumably not due to the low sperm count *per se*, since 'bulking' a number of ejaculates in the deep-freezer and inseminating an increased number of spermatozoa at one time rarely seem to improve the fertility of these men. The likely explanation is that whatever factor is responsible for the inhibition of spermatogenesis was also responsible, in most cases, for introducing some genetical, morphological or biochemcial lesions into the few sperm that were produced, thus rendering them infertile. Even considering current advances that make it possible to 'reveal' the karyotype of human spermatozoa by such techniques as their fusion to zona-free hamster ova [35], it is only possible at best to test the karyotype of a few hundred human spermatozoa out of about some 200 million present in the ejaculate. It is not yet known whether such limited sampling will be of statistically significant diagnostic value.

     **In idiopathic infertility, when all diagnostic resources of the art have failed to indicate the cause of the problem, IVF testing may be the last look at the cause of infertility. Trounson *et al.* [51] have conducted some preliminary studies on this aspect of infertility, encountered both in IVF-ET and AI programs. Their preliminary conclusion is that in iodiopathic infertility, IVF testing reveals a high rate of fertilization failure and severe polyspermy, as compared to a control group of patients with tubal infertility, in which 83% of preovulatory ova led to apparently normally developing embryos.

3. Cancer Research

*One of the most fascinating tumors is the hydatidiform mole. It is a benign placental tumor, formed after fertilization of a 'blighted ovum', following which the embryo itself fails to develop at all, while the placenta continues to grow as a cystic, grape-like structure, which secretes, among other things, greatly increased quantities of hCG. The mole usually reveals itself by hemorrhage and if the uterus is not completely evacuated surgically, there is a risk that some of the molar tissue will go on to develop into one of the most malignant tumors, a choriocarcinoma. The incidence of hydatidiform moles varies greatly in different areas of the world (e.g., highest in the Philippines), although the reason for these local differences in incidence rate is completely unknown. Recently, Kajii and Okama [20] made a discovery of the utmost significance in our understanding of the genesis of human cancer. They investigated the karyotype of a number of moles and confirmed that they were invariably diploid and XX. Using chromosome banding techniques, they were able to deduce in a number of cases which of the individual chromosomes in the mole were derived from the father and which from the mother. They made the amazing discovery that *both* sets of chromosomes in the mole are always derived from the *father*, with no maternal contribution to its genotype whatsoever. Therefore, it seems likely that the mole is caused by fertilization of an oocyte with a defective nucleus by a haploid X-bearing spermatozoon. There is then a failure of the first cleavage of the egg, so that the cell becomes diploid and homozygous for all the paternal genes. Since a cell needs at least one X chromosome to survive, no mole would result from a defective oocyte fertilized by a Y-bearing spermatozoon. This exciting discovery opens up many promising lines of investigation. It should be possible to recreate *in vitro* the conditions necessary for the formation of a mole and then to investigate the way in which this bizarre, benign placental tumor eventually becomes malignant. It might be possible to explain the geographic variations in incidence rates in terms of some environmental factor that influences the production of defective ova. The fact that defective human fertilization can give rise to such an unpleasant tumor should sound a note of caution to those who seek to exploit human IVF-ET without adequate safeguards.

4. Basic Research on the Causes of Spontaneous Human Embryonic Wastage

**A most important aspect of IVF research, not involving ET, concerns the elucidation of the causes of massive embryonic wastage characterizing animal

and human reproduction. Chromosomal abnormalities, numerical as well
as morphological, do occur during gametogenesis and affect both spermatogenesis and oogenesis. And these are occurrences over which we have at
present no control whatsoever. The frequent occurrence of chromosomal
aberrations is suspected only by inference, based on the analysis of products
of clinical spontaneous abortion [5] and defective offspring. Spontaneous preclinical abortions, which never come to medical attention, must be extremely
frequent too. The analysis of the cytogenetics of human preimplantation
embryos, obtained by IVF techniques, is the only possible way to gain
knowledge of the true incidence of embryonic wastage in man as well as
of its mechanisms. Detailed metabolic studies on human preimplantation
embryos would also indicate the relative significance of one given chromosome missing from, or supplementary to, the normal chromosome balance.
Such an approach, in the long run, could help clarify the role of each chromosome in the determination of normal embryonic development.

This particular research objective is an integral part of the immediate
research objectives listed in Section IV of this review. It is only repeated
here to emphasize its importance as a basic contribution to our understanding
of human reproductive failure.

5. *Basic Research on Factors Regulating Human Oocyte Maturation*

** Obviously, studies on *in vitro* maturation of human oocytes under various
influences, using IVF and preimplantation development as endpoints, are
needed with a view to improving our understanding of the factors involved
and of their regulatory functions.

6. *Basic Research into Man's Evolutionary Origin*

*Evolutionary biologists have always been fascinated by man's affinities with
his 4 closest living relatives, the chimpanzee, pygmy chimpanzee, orangutang,
and gorilla, and it has recently been suggested that on anatomical and biochemical grounds, the pygmy chimpanzee is most likely the common ancestor
from which man, the chimpanzee, and the gorilla take their origin [57].
However, studies of the morphology of the spermatozoon in the four species,
and spermatozoal DNA content, show that the spermatozoa of man and the
gorilla are virtually indistinguishable from one another, although differing
in a number of important respects from those of the orangutang and the
two chimpanzee species ([37], [57]). Since spermatozoal morphology has

proven to be an excellent taxonomic guide in other, more closely related, species, there is a real possibility that man and the gorilla are far more closely related than has hitherto been suggested. One way of investigating this possibility would be to carry out a series of *in vitro* experiments to assess the ability of spermatozoa from the 4 great apes to bind to the zona pellucida of the human egg, to penetrate the zona, and to effect fertilization. Such an experiment, with its undertones of human-animal hybrids and genetic manipulations in a new sense of the word, would be abhorrent to many, and it is undoubtedly fear of public reaction that has prevented the experiment being performed to date. But the topic is mentioned here as it probably raises the greatest ethical dilemmas and the scientific community at large would appreciate some guidance. The obvious fear would be that if fertilization occurred *in vitro*, somebody would be tempted to implant the human-great ape hybrid embryo back into the uterus of an ape, or even a human, or more simply, to inseminate a female great ape with human semen. Some day, no doubt such experiments will be attempted, and it is impossible to forecast their outcome. The ethical implication could be minimized if the experiment were strictly confined to an *in vitro* situation; a further safeguard would be to use immature human oocytes aspirated from nonovulatory follicles, those that are capable of being fertilized by human spermatozoa *in vitro*, but incapable of subsequent normal development. One could even irradiate the human oocytes prior to fertilization, thereby guaranteeing that no postfertilization development would occur [1], or one could perform the experiment on dead oocytes recovered from a cadaver at autopsy, when fertilization would be impossible but the zonal sperm-binding mechanism would remain intact. Whatever the ethical implications of such experiments, the results would be of utmost significance in the assessment of man's phylogenetic origins.

Despite their obvious interest for the sake of knowledge itself, studies in the phylogenetic origin of man should enjoy only very low priority rating as compared to the other objectives listed in the above section.

VI. POSSIBLE FUTURE RESEARCH INVOLVING IVF AND THE PREIMPLANTATION EMBRYO: A REAPPRAISAL

1. *Genetic Screening and Sexing of Human Embryos*

Under the heading of 'Future Issues', LeRoy Walters [53] listed several possibilities for future research. In the opinion of this reviewer two of these

possibilities deserve immediate consideration, namely: (1) preimplantation
genetic screening; and (2) the sexing of embryos.

From previous discussion in this paper, it should be clear that one of
the two critical conditions for the improvement of the implantation success
rate in the IVF-ET procedure is the screening out of embryos which will
not make it past the end of the first week of implantation. Genetic screening
and embryo sexing are not separate issues since karyotyping by microbiopsy
procedures automatically sexes the embryo. Thus genetic screening and
sexing of human embryos are no longer part of 'Future Issues' but must
and can receive biomedical investigators' immediate and active attention.

2. Other 'Future Issues'

Among other 'Future Issues', Walters [53] also mentioned research on parthenogenesis, cloning, various types of hybridization or chimera-production,
the preimplantation repair of genetic defects, the creation of human-animal
hybrids, and ectogenesis. Among these issues, research on parthenogenesis,
cloning and preimplantation repair of genetic defects deserve further comments here because of very recent developments which were not mentioned
in Walters' review [55].

(a) Research on parthenogenesis and oocyte fusion. Parthenogenesis is
the initiation of early embryonic development without the participation of
a fertilizing spermatozoon. The rationale behind the study of parthenogenetic
activation is twofold: (1) investigation of the sperm contribution to early
embryonic development; (2) a more efficient means of studying spontaneous
or induced mutations since parthenogenones are either haploid or homozyg-
ously diploid. Yet, fertilization and parthenogenetic activation are no longer
the only means of initiating embryonic development in mammals since it
has recently been observed that the experimental fusion of two mammalian
(mouse) oocytes can also initiate early embryonic development ([43], [44]).
This new mode of initiating embryonic development is based on a simulation
of one of the critical phenomena of fertilization, i.e., the membrane fusion
process occurring between male and female gametes which is the usual mode
of delivery of the paternal DNA to the egg. The oocyte membrane fusion
procedure represents a strict analog to fertilization with one major difference:
no Y chromosome is ever present in the system and therefore only female
embryos can be produced. Whether or not these 'oocyte fusion products',
which have at present developed to the blastocyst stage, will result in live
offspring upon transfer remains to be determined. Experimentally, the

oocyte fusion procedure represents a new and promising approach to the study of sperm contribution to embryonic development (by default). If the procedure can be made practical, i.e., lead to live birth of female offspring, and there is no a priori reason why this cannot be achieved, it is bound to have considerable impact of utmost nutritional and economic significance, especially in developing countries where, very often, meat consumption is prohibited by religious beliefs, while that of dairy products is not. Thus, it appears that oocyte fusion technology not only offers considerable potential for broadening our understanding of the regulation of mammalian development, but it is also relevant to the acutely growing problems of world nutrition, since, in animal husbandry, the all-important animal is the female. The possible, although quite uncertain, application of this technology to human ova is bound to open a new and most acute level of ethical debate. The presentation of current results of this technology at scientific meetings has already led, fortuitously but regrettably, to sensational coverage by the news media (*National Enquirer*, November 20, 1979: "U.S. Government backs top scientist who claims . . . WOMEN CAN HAVE BABIES WITHOUT MEN", *The Washington Post*, February 3, 1980: "Life Without Fathers? Men May Ultimately Become Unnecessary for Reproduction"). Such premature sensational media coverage is most undesirable because an unduly alarmed public opinion may interfere with the rapid development of a technology with the potential for alleviating some of the world's nutritional problems. Indeed, such a possibility is already a matter of fact. Outraged and ill-informed constituents were led to believe that their tax money would promote the development of an Amazonian society and have put pressure on their Representatives. Congressmen in turn put pressure on at least one federal funding agency which had previously supported the research effort of this reviewer in the area of oocyte fusion. Although not in writing, it was made quite clear to this reviewer that support would be discontinued owing to what was termed 'bad' publicity. Under such circumstances, one has to seek confort in the fact that, in the history of mankind, political and/or ideological pressures have never been able to curb for long the development of useful knowledge.

(b) Research on cloning. Cloning of a human being is an issue which in the words of R. G. Edwards [9] has been given "false prominence by scientists and commentators alike, for there is little that can be done at present — should anyone wish to do it". The availability of the technology for transplanting a somatic (i.e., diploid) cell nucleus into an enucleated oocyte may not be as remote as suggested by Edwards' statement. Hoppe and Illmensee [17], who demonstrated the viability of microsurgically produced homozygous-diploid uniparental mice, seem to be currently making significant progress in this area. Transplantation of the nucleus of a cell from the blastocyst inner cell mass into an enucleated mouse oocyte seems to initiate embryonic development. However, compelling evidence should be provided that benefit to society would accrue from applying such technology to human ova. To be sure, cloning would provide information concerning the interaction between the nucleus and the surrounding cytoplasm, the process by which genes are activated, and ultimately provide important clues in the search for causes of malignant growth [21]. Yet, that carrying such a process up to the live birth of a human clone would accrue benefit to society remains most doubtful.

(c) Preimplantation repair of genetic defects. The repair of the defect has been presented as an alternative to the discarding of genetically defective early embryos [53]. Although the technology of repairing genetic defects may be more complex than that of discarding defective embryos, it is currently at hand. Early in September 1980 (*Newsweek*, September 15, 1980), Dr. Frank Ruddle, leader of a research team at Yale University, reported that microinjection of foreign genes into mouse eggs induced some of the embryos to incorporate these new genes into their tissues. This new development is bound to reactivate the ethical debate about genetic engineering.

VII. CONCLUSION

The presentation has been prepared using the standard model for writing a research proposal. From background material, one proceeds to the definition of problems, to the description of rational methods of procedure for the solution of these problems and, finally, to an exposé of the significance of the proposed research.

The ethical issues concerning present and future research uses of human embryos revolve around one's concept of the moral status of the human embryo. Because of its human origin the embryo undoubtedly deserves to be paid a high degree of respect when treated as a research object. What higher form of respect could be paid to human embryos than to ask them to provide vital information leading to the alleviation of some types of human infertility, the prevention of birth defects, contraceptive and cancer research, and the actual causes of natural embryonic losses in man? Moreover, and most significantly, all benefits to society expected from such research can be gained without recourse to genetic engineering, so feared by some.

Vanderbilt University School of Medicine,
Nashville, Tennessee

ACKNOWLEDGEMENTS

The preparation of this contribution has been supported by the Department of Obstetrics and Gynecology, Vanderbilt University Medical Center, Nashville, Tennessee 37232. Thanks are due to the skills of Mrs. Angela Sullivan in the careful preparation of this manuscript.

NOTE

[1] On 28 December, 1981, the first child was delivered in the United States who owes her existence to the technique of *in vitro* fertilization. At this point in time, nineteen babies in total have been born – twelve in Australia, six in the United Kingdom, and one in the United States.

BIBLIOGRAPHY

1. Baker, T. G.: 1971, 'Radiosensitivity of Mammalian Oocytes with Particular Reference to the Human Female', *Am. J. Obstet. Gynecol.* **110**, 746–761.
2. Bavister, B. D.: 1980, '*In Vitro* Fertilization: Principles, Practice and Potential', *Arch. Androl.* **5**, 53–55.
3. Beatty, R. A.: 1978, 'The Origin of Human Triploidy: An Integration of Qualitative and Quantitative Evidence', *Ann. Hum. Genet. Lond.* **41**, 299–314.
4. Biggers, J. D.: 1979, '*In Vitro* Fertilization, Embryo Culture and Embryo Transfer in the Human', in U.S. Department of Health, Education, and Welfare, Ethics Advisory Board *Appendix: HEW Support of Research Involving Human in Vitro Fertilization and Embryo Transfer*, Department of Health, Education, and Welfare, Washington, D. C., Essay No. 8.
5. Boué, J. G. and A. Boué: 1976, 'Chromosomal Anomalies in Early Spontaneous Abortions', *Curr. Topics Path.* **62**, 193–204.
6. Croxatto, H. B., S. Diaz, B. Fuentalba, H. D. Croxatto, D. Carillo, and C. Fabres: 1972, 'Studies on the Duration of Egg Transport in the Human Oviduct. I. The Time Interval Between Ovulation and Egg Recovery From the Uterus in Normal Woman', *Fertil. Steril.* **23**, 447–458.
7. Dekretser, D. M.: 1976, 'Toward a Pill for Men', *Proc. R. Soc. Lond.* **195**, 161–176.
8. Dudkiewicz, A. B., I. G. Noske, and C. A. Shivers: 1975, 'Inhibition of Implantation in the Golden Hamster by Zona-precipitating Antibody', *Fertil. Steril.* **26**, 686–694.
9. Edwards, R. G.: 1974, 'Fertilization of Human Eggs *in Vitro*: Morals, Ethics and the Law', *Quarterly Rev. Biol.* **49**, 3–26.
10. Elliott, K. and J. Whelan (eds.): 1977, 'The Freezing of Mammalian Embryos', *Ciba Foundation Symposium No. 52* (New Series), Elsevier–North Holland, New York.
11. Ethics Advisory Board, DHEW: 1979, 'Protection of Human Subjects: HEW Support

of Human *in Vitro* Fertilization: Report of the Ethics Advisory Board', *Federal Register* **44**, p. 35033.

12. Gardner, R. L. and R. G. Edwards: 1968, 'Control of Sex Ratio at Full Term in the Rabbit by Transferring Sexed Embryos', *Nature Lond.* **218**, 346–349.
13. Gomel, V.: 1978, 'Recent Advances in Surgical Correction of Tubal Diseases Producing Infertility', *Curr. Probl. Obstet. Gynecol.* **10**, 231–246.
14. Gomel, V. (ed.): 1980, 'International Symposium on Microsurgical Techniques in the Treatment of Infertility', *Clin. Obstet. Gynecol.* **23**, 554–559.
15. Hertig, A. T. and J. Rock: 1949, 'A Series of Potentially Abortive Ova Recovered from Fertile Women Prior to the First Missed Menstrual Period', *Am. J. Obstet. Gynecol.* **58**, 968–974.
16. Hertig, A. T., J. Rock, E. C. Adams, and W. J. Mulligan: 1954, 'On the Preimplantation Stages of the Human Ovum: A Description of Four Normal and Four Abnormal Specimens Ranging from the Second to the Fifth Day of Development', *Contr. Embryol. Carnegie Inst.* **35**, 199–210.
17. Hoppe, P. C. and K. Illmensee: 1977, 'Microsurgically Produced Homozygous-Diploid Uniparental Mice', *Proc. Natl. Acad. Sci. U.S.A.* **74**, 5657–5661.
18. Hösli, P.: 1977, 'Quantitative Assays of Enzyme Activity in Single Cells: Early Prenatal Diagnosis of Genetic Disorder', *Clin. Chem.* **23**, 1476–1484.
19. Jacobs, P. A. *et al.*: 1978, 'The Origin of Human Triploids', *Ann. Hum. Genet. Lond.* **42**, 49–57.
20. Kajii, T. and K. Okama: 1977, 'Androgenic Origin of Hyatidiform Mole', *Nature Lond.* **268**, 633–634.
21. Karp, L. E.: 1976, *Genetic Engineering: Threat or Promise?*, Nelson–Hall, Chicago, Illinois.
22. Leibo, S. P.: 1980, 'Water Permeability and its Activation Energy of Fertilized and Unfertilized Mouse Ova', *J. Membrane Biol.* **53**, 179–188.
23. Leridon, H.: 1977, *Human Fertility: The Basic Components*, University of Chicago Press, Chicago, Illinois.
24. Lopata, A.: 1980, 'Beginning Human Conception in the Laboratory', in G. Jagiello and H. J. Vogel, (eds.), *Bioregulators of Reproduction*, Academic Press, New York, pp. 83–99.
25. Lopata, A., I. W. H. Johnston, I. J. Hoult, and A. I. Speirs: 1980, 'Pregnancy Following Intrauterine Implantation of an Embryo Obtained by *In Vitro* Fertilization of a Preovulatory Egg', *Fertil. Steril.* **33**, 117–120.
26. Mazur, P.: 1963, 'Kinetics of Water Loss from Cell at Sub-Zero Temperatures and the Likelihood of Intracellular Freezing', *J. Gen. Physiol.* **47**, 347–359.
27. McLeod, J. and R. Z. Gold: 1953, 'The Male Factor in Fertility and Infertility', *Fertil. Steril.* **4**, 10–19.
28. McMullen, J. C.: 1979, 'The Baby Makers', *CBS Reports*, October 30.
29. Mittwoch, U.: 1978, 'Parthenogenesis', *J. Med. Genet.* **15**, 165–181.
30. Moore, K. L.: 1977, *The Developing Human: Clinically Oriented Embryology*, 2nd ed., W. B. Saunders, Philadelphia, pp. 2–4.
31. Mühlbock, O. (ed.): 1976, *Basic Aspects of Freeze Preservation of Mouse Strains*, Fischer, Stuttgart.
32. Pereda, J. and H. B. Croxatto: 1978, 'Ultrastructure of a 7-Cell Human Embryo', *Biol. Reprod.* **18**, 481–489.

33. Rary, J. M. *et al.*: 1980, 'Techniques of *In Vitro* Fertilization of Oocytes and Embryo Transfer in Humans', *Arch. Androl.* **5**, 89–90.
34. Roberts, C. J. and C. R. Lowe: 1975, 'Where Have All the Conceptions Gone?', *Lancet* **1**, 498–509.
35. Rudak, E., P. A. Jacobs, and R. Yanagimachi: 1978, 'Direct Analysis of the Chromosome Constitution of Human Spermatozoa', *Nature Lond.* **274**, 911–913.
36. Schlesselman, J. J.: 1979, 'How Does One Assess the Risk of Abnormalities from Human *In Vitro* Fertilization', *Am. J. Obstet. Gynecol.* **135**, 135–148.
37. Seuanez, D. M., A. D. Carothers, D. E. Martin, and R. V. Short: 1977, 'Morphological Abnormalities in Spermatozoa of Man and Great Apes', *Nature Lond.* **270**, 345–358.
38. Short, R. V.: 1978, 'When a Conception Fails to Become a Pregnancy', *Ciba Foundation Symposium No. 64* (New Series), on Maternal Recognition of Pregnancy.
39. Short, R. V.: 1979, 'Summary of the Presentation by Dr. P. C. Steptoe and Dr. R. G. Edwards at the Royal College of Obstetricians, London, January 26, 1979', in U.S. Department of Health, Education, and Welfare, Ethics Advisory Board, *Appendix: HEW Support of Research Involving Human in Vitro Fertilization and Embryo Transfer*, Department of Health, Education, and Welfare, Washington, D. C., Essay 8.
40. Short, R. V.: 1979, 'Human *in Vitro* Fertilization and Embryo Transfer', in U.S. Department of Health, Education, and Welfare, Ethics Advisory Board, *Appendix: HEW Support of Research Involving Human in Vitro Fertilization and Embryo Transfer*, Department of Health, Education, and Welfare, Washington, D. C., Essay 10.
41. Soules, M. R., G. P. Sutton, C. B. Hammond, and A. F. Haney: 1980, 'Endocrine Changes at Operation under General Anesthesia: Reproductive Hormone Fluctuations in Young Women', *Fertil. Steril.* **33**, 364–371.
42. Soupart, P.: 1979, Recording of the Opening Address Delivered by Dr. P. C. Steptoe to the 1979 Annual Meeting of the American Fertility Society, San Franciso, February 5, 1979. (Reported but unpublished observations) '*In Vitro* Fertilization and Embryo Transfer', in *Current Problems in Obstetrics and Gynecology*, Part I, Vol. III, No. 2, October 1979, Part II, Vol. III, No. 3, November 1979.
43. Soupart, P.: 1978, 'La Fécondation de l'oeuf par l'oeuf', in A. Netter and A. Gorens (eds.), *Actualites Gynécologiques* 9e série, Masson et cie Paris, p. 63.
44. Soupart, P.: 1980, 'Initiation of Mouse Embryonic Development by Octye Fusion', *Arch. Androl.* **5**, 428–436.
45. Soupart, P.: 1980, 'Current Status of *in Vitro* Fertilization and Embryo Transfer in Man', *Clin. Obstet. Gynecol.* **23**, 683–717.
46. Soupart, P. and P. A. Strong: 1974, 'Ultrastructural Observations on Human Oocytes Fertilized *in Vitro*', *Fertil. Steril.* **25**, 11–23.
47. Soupart, P. and P. A. Strong: 1975, 'Ultrastructural Observations on Polyspermic Penetration of Zona Pellucida-Free Human Oocytes Inseminated *in Vitro*', *Fertil. Steril.* **26**, 523–537.
48. Soupart, P., M–L. Anderson, D. H. Albert, J. G. Coniglio, and J. E. Repp: 1979, 'Accumulation, Nature, and Possible Functions of the Malachite Green Affinity Material in Ejaculated Human Spermatozoa', *Fertil. Steril.* **32**, 450–454.

49. Steptoe, P. C. and R. G. Edwards: 1978, 'Birth After Preimplantation of a Human Embryo', *Lancet* **2**, 336.
50. Tayaraman, K. S.: 1978, 'India Reveals Deep-Frozen Test Tube Baby', *The New Scientist*, October 16, p. 159.
51. Trounson, A. O., J. F. Leeton, C. Wood, J. Webb, and G. Kovacs: 1980, 'The Investigation of Idiopathic Infertility by *in Vitro* Fertilization', *Fertil. Steril.* **4**, 29–36.
52. Tsunoda, Y.: 1977, 'Inhibitory Effects of Anti-Mouse Egg Serum on Fertilization *in Vivo* and *in Vitro* in the Mouse', *J. Reprod. Fertil.* **50**, 353–355.
53. Walters, L.: 1979, 'Ethical Issues in Human *in Vitro* Fertilization and Research Involving Early Human Embryos', in U.S. Department of Health, Education, and Welfare, Ethics Advisory Board, *Appendix: HEW Support of Research Involving Human in Vitro Fertilization and Embryo Transfer*, Department of Health, Education, and Welfare, Washington, D. C., Essay 1.
54. Whittingham, D. G.: 1980, 'Principles of Embryo Preservation', in M. J. Ashwood-Smith and J. Farrant (eds.), *Low Temperature Preservation in Medicine and Biology*, Pitman Medical Ltd., Tunbridge Wells, Kent, pp. 65–83.
55. Whittingham, D. G., S. P. Leibo, and P. Mazur: 1972, 'Survival of Mouse Embryos Frozen to −196° and −269°C', *Science* **187**, 411–425.
56. Zamboni, L., D. R. Mishell, Jr., J. H. Bell, and M. Baca: 1966, 'Fine Structure of the Human Ovum in the Pronuclear Stage', *J. Cell Biol.* **30**, 579–587.
57. Zihlman, A. L., J. E. Cronin, D. L. Cramer, and V. M. Sarich: 1978, 'Pygmy Chimpanzee as Possible Prototype for the Common Ancestor of Humans, Chimpanzees and Gorillas', *Nature Lond.* **275**, 744–753.

SECTION II

FETUSES, PERSONS, AND THE LAW

LEONARD GLANTZ

IS THE FETUS A PERSON? A LAWYER'S VIEW

I. INTRODUCTION

Whenever a lawyer is asked to define a term, the first question he should ask is "Why do you want to know?". This question reflects a jurisprudential reality that the same term may have different meanings in different contexts. It also reflects the fact that defining a term in a certain way leads to certain consequences. So if a lawyer is asked if a certain individual is an 'employee', he may want to know whether you mean 'employee' in the context of the National Labor Relation Act, the Occupational Safety and Health Act, the Internal Revenue Code, Worker Compensation Acts or a variety of other contexts. The same problem arises when a lawyer is asked "Is a fetus a person?". In order to answer this question I have looked at the variety of circumstances in which it might be asked. If the fetus is deemed to be a person in a certain circumstance this conclusion might lead to a *requirement* to protect the fetus, but even if the fetus is not deemed to be a person there may be circumstances in which we may *choose* to protect it.

II. CONSTITUTIONAL LAW

Since 1973 the starting point for any discussion of 'fetal rights' is the case *Roe v. Wade* [25]. As is almost universally known, this is the case that held that a woman, in consultation with her physician, may decide whether or not to have an abortion, and that the states may interfere with this decision only in particular circumscribed circumstances. For our purposes, this case is interesting because it points out the dichotomy between a state being required to protect the fetus and the state choosing to do so.

In *Roe v. Wade*, the state of Texas argued that a fetus was a person for purposes of the Fourteenth Amendment to the Constitution. That amendment states that no 'person' shall be deprived of life, liberty or property without due process of law. If Texas' assertion was correct, then the state would be obliged to protect the fetus from deprivation of life, just as it protects all other 'persons'; therefore abortions would be impermissible. The Court in responding to this argument noted that no case could be cited to support

107

William B. Bondeson et al. *(eds.), Abortion and the Status of the Fetus*, 107–117.
Copyright © 1983 *by D. Reidel Publishing Company, Dordrecht, Holland.*

Texas' argument and that although the word 'person' is used in a number of phrases in the Constitution, the use of the word throughout the Constitution is such that it has application only postnatally. Therefore, the Court concludes that "the word 'person' as used in the Fourteenth Amendment, does not include the unborn" ([25], p. 158).

However, this conclusion does not mean that the state does not have an interest in regulating abortions, or in protecting fetal life. The opinion goes on to balance the interests of the woman in being free to choose whether or not to have an abortion, against the interests of the state in regulating this freedom.

The Court found that women have a 'fundamental' Constitutional right to privacy ([25], pp. 152–154). This means that in order for the state to abridge this right it must demonstrate that it has some 'compelling state interest'. The Court realizes that the interests of the state may change as the fetus develops and comes closer to the point of 'personhood'. In the first trimester, the state has essentially no compelling interest in regulating abortions, in the second trimester, the state has a compelling interest in the health of the woman, since the dangers inherent in the abortion procedure increase, and the state may then, "if it chooses, regulate the abortion procedure in ways that are reasonably related to maternal health" ([25], p. 164). After the fetus reaches the point of viability the state — in promoting its interest in the "potentiality of human life" — may, if it chooses, proscribe abortion except in those cases where it is necessary for the preservation of the life or health of the mother. The Supreme Court did *not* say that a fetus becomes a person after reaching the point of viability. What it did say is that after the point of viability, the scale upon which we balance the interests of the woman against the interests of the state tip further toward the state, so that it may abridge a woman's right more at that point than at any other time in the pregnancy. However, the state may not totally obliterate the right of the living person in order to protect its interest in this non-person.

It must be emphasized in the context of this volume that the Court did not say that the state has no interest in protecting fetuses, even in the first trimester. It merely concludes that the state may not protect the fetus at the expense of sacrificing a woman's fundamental right to privacy. The Court also made clear that the term 'fetus' is not specific enough to aid in the delineation of the states' power to protect fetuses, but instead demonstrated its sensitivity to the fact that these interests may change as the fetus develops.

III. CRIMINAL LAW

There is a long line of cases dealing with the issue of whether or not the killing of a fetus is homicide. Homicide has been defined as "the killing of a human being by another human being" ([21], p. 28). Under the common law the killing of a fetus was not homicide. That common-law rule still applies today. In order for a homicide to occur the deceased must have been born alive. Since the critical point in determining 'personhood' in these cases is live birth, there is a good deal of case law trying to define just when this point is reached.

Generally birth requires complete expulsion from the mother, so that the child survives through independent respiration and circulation [2]. These requirements have led to some relatively bizarre results. For example, in one case a woman was tried for murder for decapitating her 'child' during delivery. An examination of the lungs indicated that the child had breathed prior to complete expulsion, but this was still insufficient evidence to convict the woman. The fact that the fetus was clearly viable was not an issue that was even considered. In common law there is a split in the decisions as to whether or not the child was a 'person' for purposes of homicide if it was expelled but the unbilical cord was not cut. An examination of one of these cases shows how one court used medical evidence to arrive at its decision a century ago.

In *State v. Winthrop* [27], a doctor was accused of the murder of a child while attending a woman giving birth. The state claimed that the child had respired and had independent circulation. The trial court instructed the jury that the child could have independent existence even when attached to the mother by the umbilical cord, whether or not it breathed or had independent circulation. The Supreme Court of Iowa reversed the conviction based upon this instruction and pointed out that the evidence demonstrated that the fetus' *ductus arteriosus* was not closed and that this indicated a lack of independent circulation. According to the court this meant the child had a *potential* for independence, but was not at the time of death truly independent. The court, in continuing its scientific analysis, went on to say that:

While the blood of the child circulates through the placenta, it is renovated through the lungs of the mother. In such a sense it breathes through the lungs of the mother ([27], p. 521).

It went on to cite Beck's *Medical Jurisprudence*:

It must be evident that when a child is born alive, but has not yet respired, its condition is precisely like that of the fetus *in utero*. It lives merely because the fetal circulation is still going on. In this case none of the organs undergo any change ([4], Vol. 1, p. 498).

The court completed its opinion by stating that if the child is not independent, the possibility of independence is merely conjecture and not enough to convict a person of murder.

One commentator has pointed out that, due to the state of medicine at the time the common law was developing, there was probably a presumption that a child would not be born alive; therefore the requirement of live birth made some sense [19]. The rule requiring live birth has been criticized because of the startling results to which it can lead [15]. One authority on criminal law has suggested "a more advanced view" that a viable 'child' should be considered to be born alive for the purposes of homicide law after the birth process has begun. A child would be considered stillborn only in those instances when it was dead before birth starts ([21], p. 30, Note 5). A California court adopted this view in the case *People v. Chavez* [20]. In this case a woman was accused of killing her newborn child, in that there was evidence of breathing and independent heart action. The defense established that both of these functions could have started prior to complete explusion from the mother. The court stated that there is not a meaningful difference between a child the moment before birth and the moment after birth, and went on to state.

[A] viable child in the process of being born is a human being within the meaning of the homicide statute, whether or not the process has been fully completed. It should at least be considered a human being where it is a living baby and where in the natural course of events a birth which is already started would naturally be successfully completed ([20], p. 94).

There are two requirements that this court sets down. The first is viability and the second is that the birth process has begun. A later California Supreme Court case, *Keeler v. Superior Court*, decided that viability alone is not sufficient to establish 'personhood' for purposes of the homicide statute.

In this case, *Keeler v. Superior Court* [14], Mrs. Keeler had received an interlocutory decree of divorce from her husband and was living with another man. She became pregnant; when Mr. Keeler discovered this fact, he sought out Mrs. Keeler and said to her, "I'm going to stomp it out of you", and proceeded to kick her repeatedly in the abodomen. Mrs. Keeler, who was between thirty-one to thirty-six weeks pregnant, was taken to the hospital and a casearean section was performed. The fetus, which weighed

5 pounds, was stillborn, the cause of death being a fractured skull. Mr. Keeler was indicted and convicted of murder, the trial court finding that a viable fetus is a 'person' for purposes of the homicide statute ([13], p. 868). The Supreme Court of California reversed the conviction, relying on the common-law rules discussed above and distinguishing this case from *Chavez* in that the birth process had not begun.

There is a strong dissenting opinion in *Keeler* which argues that changes in medicine must be followed by changes in the law. It points out that we would all agree that shooting a corpse is not murder, but that our concept of what constitutes a corpse is continually modified by advances in medicine. The dissent goes on to ask rhetorically,

Would this court ignore the developments and exonerate the killer of an apparently 'drowned' child merely because the child would have been pronounced dead in 1648 or 1850? Obviously not. Whether a homicide occurred in that case would be determined by medical testimony regarding the capability of the child to have survived prior to the defendant's acts. And that is precisely the test which this court should adopt in the instant case ([14], p. 632).

In discussing the policy issues involved, the dissenting judge asks, "what justice will be promoted, what objects effectuated" by not considering this child a human being for the purposes of the homicide statute? He argues that this fetus, with "its unbounded potential for life", must be protected.

Following *Keeler*, the California legislature amended the homicide statute to include the killing of fetuses regardless of age [8]. However, it is clear that, in the absence of a special statute, the killing of a fetus is not murder.

As recently as 1976, the Massachusetts Supreme Judicial Court had to confront these issues in a case in which a physician was accused of killing a fetus in the course of performing an abortion via hysterotomy [9]. The Court readily applied the rules requiring independence from the mother, and the rule that the death of a fetus *in utero* is not manslaughter. There was a great deal of evidence concerning whether or not the fetus had breathed, and the prosecution argued that there is independence when the placenta is removed from the uterine wall, even though the fetus is still *in utero*. Although five of the six justices voted to acquit the physician on a variety of grounds, there were a number of separate opinions in which three of the six justices agreed that it would be permissible to base a conviction for manslaughter on the defendant's prenatal acts. That is to say that although live birth is a prerequisite for a homicide conviction, if the live born child dies as a result of the defendant's reckless and wanton prenatal acts, these acts may be sufficient to satisfy a manslaughter conviction. In this regard a fetus may be subject to some protection *in utero* by the homicide law. This rule also seems to be in accordance with common law ([21], p. 30, Note 5).

IV. TORT LAW

Recently courts have begun to re-examine the issues surrounding compensation of fetuses for prenatal injuries. This has taken the form of 'wrongful life', 'wrongful birth', and 'wrongful conception' cases. Because our attention has recently been called to this issue we tend to think of it as novel. But the first case in point arose in Massachusetts in 1884 when a woman who was four to five months pregnant slipped and fell due to a defect in the road [10]. As a result, the woman gave birth prematurely to a fetus that lived for 10–15 minutes. In ordinary cases of this sort a favorable outcome for the plaintiff is usually based on a finding that the defendant owed a duty of care to the plaintiff and breached that duty, which caused the resulting injury. In this particular case, Justice Holmes held that a fetus is not a person in being and thus no one could owe a duty to it. This is based on his understanding that the fetus and the mother constitute one person, and although a duty is owed to her, there can be no separate duty owed to the fetus. Additionally, Justice Holmes held that this rule would not be affected by the "degree of maturity reached by the embryo at the moment of the organic lesion or act".

Although this rule was to be followed by all courts until 1946, Justice Boggs, in a powerful dissent in the 1920 case, *Allaire v. St. Luke's Hospital* [1], foreshadowed what future cases would bring. He argued that the viable fetus is not merely a part of the mother's body since "her body may die in all of its parts and the child remain alive and capable of life ... " ([1], p. 641). Therefore, Boggs argued, if a fetus is injured after it reaches the point of viability, and is thereafter born alive, the live born child should be entitled to compensation for its prenatal injuries.

The 1946 case that changed the direction of this line of cases is *Bonbrest v. Kotz* [6]. In that case a child was injured by a physician during delivery and subsequently sued the doctor for malpractice. The court readily conceded that in common law a child *en ventre sa mère* has no judicial existence and therefore could not successfully bring suit. The court referred to the *Dietrich* case but distinguished from it by pointing out that in the present case the court was dealing with a direct injury to a *viable* child. The court claimed that the child's viability was proved by its existence at the time of the suit. It then flatly stated that a viable fetus is not part of the mother, as the mother could die but the fetus could continue to live. The court attempted to outline the significance of viability – the viable fetus has its own bodily form and members, manifests all of the anatomical characteristics of individuality, possesses its own circulatory, vascular, and excretory systems and is now capable of living.

The court argued that as a matter of policy the fetus must be allowed to recover for damage which it will suffer for the rest of its life. If the child is not allowed to recover, then a wrong will have been inflicted for which there is no remedy. Quoting a Canadian decision the court found:

If a right of action be denied to the child it will be compelled without any fault on its part, to go through life carrying the seal of another's fault and bearing a very heavy burden of infirmity and inconvenience without any compensation therefore. To my mind it is but natural justice that a child, if born alive and *viable* should be allowed to maintain an action in the courts for injuries wrongfully committed upon its person while in the womb of its mother ([6], pp. 141–142, quoting [18]).

Thus we have a court trying to utilize scientific facts to show the separate nature of the fetus from the mother, and struggling with notions of natural justice.

In the post-1946 cases a number of courts have decided that for a fetus to recover for prenatal injuries after it is born alive, the injury had to occur while it was viable [22]. This is because the courts hold that the injury must be done to a 'person', and prior to viability there is no person in existence. A number of courts have decided that the viability of the infant at the time of the injury is an irrelevant factor as long as the fetus is born alive. In *Hornbuckle v. Plantation Pipe Line* [12], it was decided that if a child born after an injury sustained at any period of its prenatal life can prove the ill effect, it would have the right to recover. One justice of the court stated that he believed the fetus had to be quick at the time of the injury to recover. The law, he argued, requires injury to be done to a person and no such person exists prior to quickening ([12], p. 729).

In 1960 the New Jersey Court also decided that the child could recover for injuries occurring at any time after conception [26]. In this case the court recognized that recovery for such injuries was generally not allowed because the child was a part of the mother and not an independent person to whom a duty could be owed. It then discussed the scientific basis for disputing this proposition. The court stated that medical authorities have

recognized that a child "is in existence" at the moment of conception and is
not merely a part of its mother's body. The unborn child has its own circulatory system, a heartbeat not in tune with the mother's but more rapid,
and having no dependence on the mother except for sustenance, which is
also true after birth. It scorns the 'semantic argument' on whether or not
an unborn child is a person. The court found that from the *moment of
conception* a process is placed in motion that will produce a person if left
undisturbed, and that "a child has a legal right to begin life with a sound
mind or body" ([26], p. 503). While the court admits that most courts
require viability at the time of injury as a precondition for recovery, it
states that the "viability rule is impossible of practical application" since
viability is so difficult to ascertain ([26], p. 504).

Today, most courts that have addressed the issue have decided that the
point of fetal development at which the pre-natal injury occurred is irrelevant
as long as one can prove a causal connection between the wrongful act and
the damage incurred [24].

The fact that courts permit live born infants to recover damages for
prenatal injuries does not mean that courts view the unborn as 'persons'.
Instead, the courts are interested in protecting the interests of the damaged
live born person. The courts are not compensating fetuses but are instead
compensating children who need special medical treatment, schooling,
or other services because of the acts of some tortfeasor. The point in the
pregnancy when those acts occur does not serve to deflect the courts from
their rightful goal of compensating the injured *child*. This is most strongly
indicated by those courts that permit recovery for preconception wrongful
acts.

In *Renslow v. Mennonite Hospital* [23], the defendants negligently
transfused a 13-year-old girl who had Rh-negative blood with Rh-positive
blood. Eight years later, without knowledge that she had been improperly
transfused, she became pregnant. Her sensitization led to the premature
birth of her child, who also suffered from permanent damage to her brain,
nervous system and other organs. A lawsuit was filed on behalf of the newborn alleging that the defendants owed a duty to her even though she did not
exist at the time of the wrongful acts that caused her injury. The court held
that the defendants could be liable in this circumstance since the defendants
could have foreseen that their breach of duty to a teenager could injure her
yet to be conceived child. From this case we can clearly see that the court's
purpose is to compensate a live-born child suffering from injuries caused by
the defendants, even though there was clearly no person in existence at the

time of the wrongful act. This type of case can be distinguished from the 'wrongful life' cases (see, e.g., [5]), in which the plaintiff argues that it would not have been born at all but for the defendant's negligence. A typical 'wrongful life' case would involve a child with Down's Syndrome, who would argue that had its 45-year-old mother been told by her obstetrician that amniocentesis could be used prenatally to diagnose Down's Syndrome, its mother would have undergone the diagnostic procedure, the defect would have been discovered, and the pregnancy aborted. The child essentially argues that it would have been better off had it been aborted. In such a case the difficult issue of balancing non-existence against existence with handicaps has prevented courts from allowing the child to recover, although the parents may be compensated for the additional expenses they will incur raising a handicapped child. In this type of 'wrongful life' case, the physician's negligence is not the cause of the defect, but is the cause of the birth. The best that the child can argue is that its very existence constitutes injury to it. This is quite different from the *Renslow* type of case where the child can prove that its injury was *caused* by the negligent physician, and, but for this negligence, it would have been a healthy child. This latter type of case conforms quite well with traditional theories of tort law, as discussed above, and is therefore much more likely to be successful than cases in which it is argued that the tortfeasor caused the birth but not the defect.

A similar issue has arisen in 'wrongful death' cases. 'Wrongful death' cases may be brought because of the existence of state statutes that permit recovery for the death of a 'person'. Thus, if a fetus injured *in utero* were then live born and subsequently died as a result of the prenatal injury, a 'person' died as a result of such injuries (see, e.g., [16]). However, a different issue arises when the fetus is stillborn. In such cases the courts must decide if the legislature desired to include fetuses in its use of the term 'person'. Although the courts are split on this issue, the majority of jurisdictions permit recovery even in the absence of live birth ([24], p. 1423, Note 34). However, it appears that the fetus must be viable at the time of its death to recover under the 'wrongful death' statutes. Again, the courts are not so much interested in establishing the 'personhood' of the fetus, as they are in compensating parents for their loss or punishing the wrongdoer who caused this loss.

From the foregoing we can conclude that although live born children may be compensated for prenatal injuries, this is not due to courts concluding that fetuses are persons.

V. OTHER ISSUES

The question of personhood has arisen in other circumstances. Under the Aid to Families with Dependent Children statute, 'dependent children' are given certain rights in order to receive welfare payments. In one case it was argued that the term 'dependent child' included unborn children. The Supreme Court, in interpreting the statute, decided that Congress used the word 'child' to refer to an individual already born with an existence separate from its mother [7]. Once again the resolution of the question depended on legislative intent, and not the fetus's 'personhood'.

The issue of property rights of fetuses has also arisen in numerous instances. In common law, if an unborn child's father dies prior to its birth, that child may inherit from its father upon its being live born. The fetus had an inchoate property interest that vested at its birth ([17], p. 421). Trust law also recognizes the right of unborn children to be trust beneficiaries. This, however, does not mean that such unborn children are 'persons', especially given the fact that unconceived children may also have such an interest [11]. The interest being protected in these cases does not devolve from the fetus's personhood, but instead has to do with fulfilling the wishes of the testator or settlor of the trust.

VI. CONCLUSION

Although the law rarely lends itself to blanket statements, it can be clearly stated that a fetus is not a person under the law. However, this does not mean that we may not offer it certain protections or rights. This conclusion means, instead, that fetuses are not required to be protected. As demonstrated above, we can give the fetus certain property rights. We may also punish those who injure the fetus, and federal regulations and state statutes regulate or prohibit research on fetuses. Of course, certain protections have also been extended to animals, and human corpses. It is therefore possible to give fetuses rights with the limitation that these rights do not abridge the rights of persons now existing. Indeed, the lesson of *Roe v. Wade* [25] is that a state may not subjugate a woman's right to decide whether or not to carry a pregnancy to term to the rights of a fetus, a constitutional non-person. But with this exception the law clearly permits us to protect the fetus — and the issue of when and to what extent we choose to do this presents us with the difficult problems.

Boston University Medical Center,
Boston, Massachusetts

BIBLIOGRAPHY

1. *Allaire v. St. Luke's Hospital*, 184 Ill. 359, 56 N.E. 638 (1920).
2. *American Law Report Annotations* 159:525 (1945).
3. Annas, G., L. Glantz, and B. Katz: 1977, *Informed Consent to Human Experi-mentation: The Subject's Dilemma*, Ballinger, Cambridge, Massachusetts.
4. Beck, T. R.: 1863, *Medical Jurisprudence*, I. B. Lippincott, Philadelphia.
5. *Becker v. Schwartz*, 46 N.Y. 2d 401, 386 N.E. 2d 807 (1978).
6. *Bonbrest v. Kotz*, 63 F. Supp. 138 (D.D.C. 1946).
7. *Burns v. Algala*, 420 U.S. 575 (1975).
8. California Penal Code, Section 187.
9. *Commonwealth v. Edelin*, 371 Mass. 497 (1976).
10. *Dietrich v. Inhabitants of Northhampton*, 138 Mass. 14 (1884).
11. Holder, A.: 1977, *Legal Issues in Pediatrics and Adolescent Medicine*, John Wiley and Sons, New York.
12. *Hornbuckle v. Plantation Pipe Line*, 212 Ga. 504, 93 S.E. 2d 727 (1956).
13. *Keeler v. Superior Court*, 80 Cal. Rpt. 865 (1969).
14. *Keeler v. Superior Court*, 87 Cal. Rpt. 481, 470 P. 2d 617 (1970).
15. 'The Killing of a Viable Fetus is Murder' (Note), *Maryland Law Review* 30: 140 (1970).
16. *Lecesse v. McDonough*, 361 Mass. 64, 279 N.E. 2d 339 (1972).
17. Means, C.: 1968, 'The Law of New York Concerning Abortion and the Status of the Fetus, 1664–1968: A Case of Cessation of Constitutionality', *New York Law Forum* 14, 411–515.
18. *Montreal Tramways v. Leveille*, 4 Dom. L.R. 337 (1933).
19. 'The Non-Consensual Killing of an Unborn Infant: A Criminal Act' (Comment), *Buffalo Law Review* 20: 563 (1970–1971).
20. *People v. Chavez*, 176 P. 2d 92 (Cal. App. 1947).
21. Perkins, R.: 1970, *Perkins on Criminal Law*, 2nd. ed., Foundation Press, Mineola, New York.
22. Prosser, W.: 1971, *Handbook of the Law of Torts*, 4th ed., West Publishing Co., St. Paul, Minn.
23. *Renslow v. Mennonite Hospital*, 67 Ill. 2d 348, 367 N.E. 2d 1250 (1977).
24. Robertson, H.: 1978, 'Toward Rational Boundaries of Tort Liability for Injury to the Unborn: Prenatal Injuries, Preconception Injuries, and Wrongful Life', *Duke Law Review* 197, 1401.
25. *Roe v. Wade*, 410 U.S. 113 (1973).
26. *Smith v. Brennan*, 31 N.J. 353, 157 A. 2d 497 (1960).
27. *State v. Winthrop*, 43 Iowa 519 (1876).

PATRICIA D. WHITE

THE CONCEPT OF PERSON, THE LAW,
AND THE USE OF THE FETUS IN BIOMEDICINE *

There are two distinct ways in which an analysis of the concept of person —
as used in the law — might prove useful to the general inquiry into the relationship between the concept of person and the proper use of the fetus in
biomedicine. One is its examination with regard to determining whether a
coherent concept of person has evolved which will allow us to predict the
legal prospects for the use of the fetus in biomedical research, *in vitro* fertilization, embryo transplantation, and abortion.[1] The other is its examination
with regard to determining whether a coherent concept of person has been
developed which can be used with profit in the broader context of addressing
the ethical questions that surround this area of medicine.

At the outset, it is appropriate to ask why the concept of person is thought
to be crucial to either of the two sorts of examinations that I have just
described. The answer to this question in the first instance is, I think, relatively straightforward. Our laws both prescribe and proscribe the behavior of
individuals and institutions toward persons. To the extent that a fetus is a
person within the meaning of some legal stricture,[2] that stricture will apply to
the behavior of its subjects toward fetuses. The answer in the second instance,
however, is neither straightforward nor clear, although it seems frequently
thought to be both. Moral strictures, like legal ones, set standards for human
behavior. Thus it is often thought that to the extent that a fetus is a person,
a moral injunction that applies generally to the treatment of persons will
apply to the treatment of a fetus. We ought therefore, according to this
view, to analyze the concept of person as fully as possible to see if, and
to what extent, fetuses belong within it.[3] The following argument, for
example, is often implicit, and sometimes expressed, in the context of the
seemingly endless literature on abortion: it is a fundamental moral principle
that it is wrong intentionally to kill an innocent person. If a fetus is a person,
then — since a fetus is innocent — it is wrong intentionally to kill (or abort)
a fetus. The analogy between legal rules and moral principles is clear. It
is not obvious that it is justified.

In an ideal legal system, legal rules would never conflict with one another.
A citizen would never necessarily violate one law in order to comply with
another. Cases of apparent conflict might well arise, but the system would

119

William B. Bondeson et al. *(eds.), Abortion and the Status of the Fetus*, 119–157.
Copyright © 1983 by D. Reidel Publishing Company, Dordrecht, Holland.

provide for an adjudicatory process by which to resolve the conflict — either by overturning one of the rules or by establishing a new rule which would determine what should be done in such circumstances. However, moral principles undoubtedly function somewhat differently; to ask just how differently is to raise many of the most fundamental and difficult questions in moral philosophy. Is moral action governed by rules at all? If so, how are those rules derived? How are they applied? Can they conflict? How are conflicts to be resolved? If moral action is not governed by rules, how are moral standards expressed, and how are they applied? Because these questions are so substantial, it should not be surprising that in morals it is obvious that it is not sufficient to define the terms which together express a moral principle in order to determine its scope, whereas it is often sufficient to do so with legal rules.

To put the same point more specifically in the context of my earlier example: even if the fetus is a person, and even if it is a fundamental moral principle that it is wrong intentionally to kill an innocent person, it does not obviously follow that it is a fundamental moral principle that it is wrong intentionally to kill (or abort) a fetus. It is not obvious, for example, that to the extent that there are moral rules, their strength is invariable across the full scope of each rule. For instance, it is often thought, and sometimes argued, by those who maintain both that a fetus is (at least at some stage *in utero*) a person and that it is a fundamental moral principle that it is wrong intentionally to kill innocent persons, that if a doctor can save the life of only the mother *or* the fetus, he should save the mother — even if the chances of saving the fetus if he tries are greater than those of saving the mother if he tries.[4] Similarly, it is not obvious that the relative importance of different rules remains constant across their full range of mutual application. For example, although I believe that, in a hierarchy of moral principles, the general injunction not intentionally to kill innocent persons *would* override the general injunction not intentionally to inflict serious injury upon innocent persons, I would not be prepared simply to assert, without argument, that it therefore follows that it is more important that a women not abort her healthy fetus than that she not take thalidomide during her pregnancy.[5]

Thus, despite the considerable body of writing that focuses on the question whether the fetus is a person, and which seems to find the answer to that question somehow determinative of the question of the moral permissibility of abortion, I remain genuinely puzzled about the implications of the concept of person for the ethical questions which surround not only abortion, but the use of the fetus in biomedicine generally.

I suspect, then, that if there is a coherent concept of person to be found in the law, it will more immediately serve our predictive aims than our ethical ones. This is not to say, of course, that the personhood of the fetus *is* irrelevant to the ethical questions raised by its use in biomedicine. Rather, it is to say that a claim for its relevance requires substantial argument.

The law in the United States with respect to the fetus varies somewhat from jurisdiction to jurisdiction and from one area of the law to another.[6] Moreover, the relevance of the question of the fetus's status as a person to its juridical status varies as well.[7] Together these facts serve to illustrate an important feature of our law: it tends to develop in a somewhat *ad hoc* fashion, and the key terms can have their meaning and scope stipulated in the course of that development. As a consequence, it is often less fruitful than might be hoped to look to the law for insight about the proper analysis of general concepts (as opposed, of course, to specifically legal concepts).

The law encounters the problem of how to treat the fetus in a variety of contexts. In property law, for example, such questions arise as whether a fetus *in utero* inherits a share of property left by its deceased father to his "surviving children";[8] whether a fetus *in utero* inherits through the laws of succession when its relative dies intestate;[9] and whether others may inherit from a fetus *in utero* after it is stillborn.[10] In criminal law, one question has been the extent, if any, to which the law of homicide applies to the death of a fetus.[11] A similar set of concerns arises in connection with criminal abortion.[12] A third area of law which must determine how to treat the fetus is tort law. Can a fetus recover for harm that accrues to it as a consequence of the reckless, negligent, or even careful act of someone?[13]

The answers that have been fashioned to these questions reveal that the fetus has traditionally been accorded a different legal status from that given someone after birth [14]; but they also suggest that for the most part this difference is not to be explained historically by a self-conscious determination that a fetus is not a person (in any interesting sense). Rather, the law in this area has tended to evolve — until recently — without even focusing directly on when a fetus becomes a person (in any interesting sense). By no means do I intend to claim that the law's evolution does not reflect a commonly held perception that a fetus is importantly different from someone who has emerged from the womb. My claim is simply that the philosophical question, "Is the fetus a person?", has not usually been treated as determinative of the juridical status of the fetus.

This point is well illustrated by the history of criminal abortion law in the United States. As everyone interested in this subject knows, the current state of the law *is* intimately connected with the public debate concerning whether or not a fetus is a person. The Supreme Court reflected the prominence of this debate when it held in *Roe v. Wade* ([204], pp. 159–160) that "the unborn have never been *recognized in the law* as persons in the whole sense" ([204], p. 162), and that "the word 'person', as used in the Fourteenth Amendment, does not include the unborn" [emphasis added] ([204], pp. 157–158).

The Court explicitly declined to speculate as to whether the fetus *is* a person "in the whole sense", noting only that those trained in medicine, philosophy, and theology have been unable to arrive at any consensus ([204], pp. 159–160).[15] Despite this, the Court in *Roe* went on to conclude that the states may place such a high value on the life of the fetus that they may proscribe the abortion of a viable fetus except in circumstances when the procedure is necessary to preserve the life or health of the mother ([204], pp. 163–164). Whatever one thinks of the quality of the general argument offered in the *Roe* opinion – and most commentators appear, justly, to think very little of it (e.g., [47], [56], [90], [105]) – it is interesting to note that even though the Court focused on the fetus's ontological status, it did not regard legal (much less genuine) status as a person "in the whole sense" as a prerequisite to a very substantial degree of fundamental legal protection. Indeed, the Court was prepared to say that the states could give such protection to the fetus even if life (much less personhood) does not begin before birth:

Logically, of course, a legitimate state interest in this area need not stand or fall on acceptance of the belief that life begins at conception or at some other point prior to live birth ([204], p. 150).

The Court was right to acknowledge the independence of the two issues. The protection of the law has never been limited to persons "in the whole sense" nor, for that matter, to living beings ([47], p. 926). Even constitutionally protected activity may be prohibited by a state if certain state interests are sufficiently threatened. This is why, to borrow Professor Ely's example, a state could prohibit the burning of draft cards although it is claimed to be an exercise of the First Amendment right of political protest ([47], p. 926). Thus, although the *Roe* Court looked at some length at the question whether the fetus is a person "in the whole sense" ([204], pp. 159–162), its answer to that question is limited to the claim that the law has not recognized the fetus as a person "in the whole sense" and this claim does not determine the case it had to decide.

What if the Court had concluded that from the moment of conception the fetus *is* a person "in the whole sense"? Would it then have been compelled to prohibit abortion absolutely? The Court felt that it would have been if it had found that the "fetus is a 'person' within the language and meaning of the Fourteenth Amendment" because "the fetus's right to life would then be guaranteed specifically by the Amendment" ([204], p. 162). But the Court clearly did not think that a person "in the whole sense" is necessarily a person for purposes of the Fourteenth Amendment, since it was prepared to say that the unborn are *not* persons in the sense intended by the Fourteenth Amendment and it was not prepared to suggest that the fetus is *not* a person "in the whole sense". The crucial point for my present purpose is that, even taking the *Roe* opinion at face value, we do not find the philosophical question, "Is the fetus a person?", to be determinative of the fetus's legal status.

The evolution of criminal abortion law in the United States before *Roe* makes a fascinating tale. And it is one in which concern for the personhood of the fetus plays a surprisingly small role. Until *Roe* was decided in 1973, abortion had been regulated at the state, rather than at the federal, level.[16] After 1821, when Connecticut's became the first American legislature to enact a statute that dealt with the question of abortion,[17] the states began to address abortion legislatively. Until then the legal status of the practice was determined by the common law.[18] At common law, abortion performed before quickening[19] was not criminal. After quickening abortion was criminal, though the crime was considered to be different from murder. Later in this paper, I shall look briefly at the role the question of the fetus's status as a person played in the common law treatment of abortion.[20] For the moment, however, I want to focus on the role that question played in the growth of anti-abortion legislation in America.

James C. Mohr has argued very convincingly in his book, *Abortion in America*, that the shift in the abortion policies of the states from uniform acceptance of the common law in 1820, to the passage, by 1900, of detailed criminal statutes in which abortion was proscribed, was "inextricably bound up with the history of medicine and medical practice in America" ([17], p. 31). Physicians, it seems, were roughly divided into two camps by the late 1820s — those who were highly educated men of some social standing, and those who were not ([17], p. 34). The latter group included self-taught practitioners of folk medicine as well as those who had attended one of the many anti-establishment medical schools which had to compete among themselves for tuition paying students. Members of the former group were known as "regulars" ([17], p. 33). Between 1820 and 1850, many regulars found that the proliferation of irregulars practicing medicine was causing a substantial drop in their incomes, with a consequent loss of social standing ([17], p. 34). In reaction they sought state legislation to regulate various elements of the practice of medicine.[21] It was in this context that anti-abortion legislation was first enacted ([17], p. 43).

According to Mohr, the regular physicians were especially interested in opposing abortion for a number of reasons:

Ideologically, one of the things that distinguished the regulars was their adherence to the Hippocratic Oath, and the Hippocratic Oath condemned abortion. . . . [I]t had become one of the touchstones of regular medicine in the United States by the early nineteenth century, and the oath was considered the basic platform upon which the regulars were attempting to upgrade the ethical standards of their profession in a host of different areas, not just in regard to abortion. . . . Scientifically, regulars had realized for some time that conception inaugurated a more or less continuous process of development, which would produce a new human being if uninterrupted. Consequently, they attacked the quickening doctrine on the logical grounds, that quickening was a step neither more nor less crucial in the process of gestation than any other . . . . [Their] moral opposition to abortion [had another dimension as well.] . . . The nation's regular doctors, probably more than any other identifiable group in American society during the nineteenth century, including the clergy, defended the value of human life per se as an absolute. . . . And once they had decided that human life was present to some extent in a newly fertilized ovum, however limited that extent might be, they became the fierce opponents of any attack upon it. . . . Practically, . . . [a]s more and more irregulars began to advertise abortion services openly, especially after 1840, regular physicians grew more and more nervous about losing their practices to healers who would provide a service that more and more American women after 1840 began to want. . . . The best way out of these dilemmas was to persuade state legislators to make abortion a criminal offense ([17], pp. 35–37).

Indeed, by 1841 the regulars had begun to experience some measure of legislative success. Ten of the 26 states had passed anti-abortion legislation,[22] though none of them made it illegal for a woman to have an abortion. Five of the ten prohibited abortion before quickening.[23] However, none of the ten provisions was a separate bill. Each was merely a part of larger criminal legislation ([17], p. 42). Such success as the regulars had had was quiet. Abortion was not a publicly debated issue and the legislators had not acted because of great pressure to resolve the moral issues that it raised ([17], p. 43).

During the period between about 1840 and 1870, abortion became increasingly common ([17], p. 50). In part, this was the result, no doubt, of its commercialization. Abortion services sprang up in many parts of the country and they advertised freely — if somewhat obliquely by modern standards.[24] Some of these services were economically very successful and it is clear that substantial numbers of women were procuring and paying for abortions.[25] There is evidence from the estimates given during this period by various physicians and pharmacists that abortion was being used as a method of birth control, and that a significant number of pregnancies (estimates frequently ranged as high as twenty percent of all pregnancies) were being intentionally aborted ([17], p. 82; [24], pp. 15–64). This evidence is corroborated, to some extent at least, by the fact that the birth rate in America dropped dramatically between 1840 and 1850 and continued to fall sharply thereafter ([17], pp. 82, 91).

Although such claims are hard to verify, there is considerable evidence that abortions during the period after 1840 were being procured by middle and upper class, married, Protestant, American-born women for the first time in any great number ([17], p. 90; [24], pp. 67–69). This represented a shift from the first part of the century when abortion was largely restricted to unmarried, usually poor, and frequently very young women. This shift in clientele provided an important impetus for much of the anti-abortion legislation that was passed in the second half of the nineteenth century. The physicians who led the campaign often wrote and spoke of their fears that unchecked abortion would cause native-born Protestants to lose their position as the dominant social class in the United States, simply by virtue of being outbred by various Catholic immigrant groups ([17], p. 167; [24], pp. 74–75, Note 2).

Anti-abortion legislation made some strides during the period between 1840 and 1860, but abortion was still not an issue which occasioned much public debate. In 1845, Massachusetts became the first state to pass legislation that dealt exclusively with abortion policy.[26] The measure was passed in the wake of a much publicized and rather horrifying case in which a woman had died as the result of an abortion.[27] The legislation provided that *any* attempted abortion was a heavily punishable misdemeanor which would become a felony if the woman died as a result of the attempt. New York and New Hampshire passed anti-abortion statutes soon after, and by 1850 they had become the only two states to make it illegal for a women either to seek or to obtain an abortion.[28] By 1860, according to Mohr,

[a] bortion carried some onus, but not enough to damage irreparably a woman's social standing. Legislators had been annoyed at the flagrant commercialization of abortion that arose during the 1840's and continued into the 1850's, and were fearful about the possibility of incompetent abortionists wreaking serious harm, even death, to the nation's women. But these factors by themselves had not produced forceful new policies ([17], p. 145).

In fact, by 1860 only 20 of the 33 states had passed any legislation dealing with abortion ([17], pp. 145–146). You will recall that ten states had already passed such legislation by 1841.

The real impetus toward strong anti-abortion legislation seems to have come from the American Medical Association, which was founded in 1847 ([17], p. 147). For the first time, the regulars had an organizational framework within which they could effectively press for their legislative and social goals.

The AMA campaign against abortion relied on at least three sorts of claim. One was undeniably moral. The physicians who led the campaign wrote frequently and fervently about the evils of abortion generally, and in particular about the "unwarrantable destruction of human life" that had been spawned by the quickening doctrine ([101], p. 75–78, cited in [17], p. 157, Note 35). Another was directed at exposing the grave danger to women that abortionists represented. They were the "vilest of quacks" and women should not put their lives and health into the hands of such people ([94], cited in [17], p. 179). The third sort of claim has already been described. Native Americans – i.e., white, Protestant, middle class people – would lose their dominance if abortion were allowed to keep their numbers down.

Which of these sorts of claim had the most influence on the legislatures that, between 1860 and 1880, passed some forty anti-abortion statutes?[29] This burst of legislative activity, the culmination of the regulars' efforts, resulted in a fundamental shift in American law from the predominant acceptance of the quickening doctrine to its predominant rejection. All three prongs of the AMA's attack on abortion argued for eliminating the quickening distinction. Not surprisingly, it is difficult – if not impossible – to determine whether any of the three in fact had a greater effect than the others on the legislatures that did eliminate the distinction.[30]

We can, however, find in the histories of the anti-abortion statutes passed during this period, examples that indicate evidence of the acceptance of each of the three claims.[31] What we do not find, even in the contexts where the predominant concern seems to be with the moral problems associated with the intentional taking of life, is evidence that the question, "Is the fetus a person?" was being answered in the affirmative. We find acceptance of the regulars' assertions that life begins at conception, and that it is no more or less present at quickening than it was soon before.[32] Similarly, we find widespread acceptance of the regulars' conclusion that therefore abortion is morally wrong.[33] But at the same time we see the resultant legislation. Nowhere was the intentional abortion of a fetus made first degree murder, and in many jurisdictions it remained a misdemeanor.[34] Only in New York could the mother who voluntarily procured an abortion be guilty of the same crime as the person who performed it [35] — and in most states the woman was guilty of no crime at all.[36]

Although the view that life begins at conception and therefore ought not to be aborted is certainly perceived to be related to the question, "Is the fetus a person?", it is just as certainly not an *answer* to that question. On the one hand, since we are examining the actions of legislatures, it is crucial to recall that as the *Roe* Court rightly indicated, the law can (and, most would agree, often should) provide legal protection to those who are not persons "in the whole sense".[37] We cannot infer from the fact that legal protection was given the prequickened fetus, that the legislatures regarded it as a person (in any sense at all). Indeed, the fact that abortion legislation generally treated the fetus differently from the way the homicide statutes treated victims who clearly were persons (in some important sense) is evidence that the fetus was not considered to be a person "in the whole sense". And, perhaps of equal importance to my claim that we have no evidence that the legislatures were answering the question, "Is the fetus a person?", is the observation that here is a respect in which morality is analogous to the law. We can have moral obligations to living beings who are not persons "in the whole sense" — to our pets, for example (see, e.g., [21], pp. 48–50). Whether their simply being alive is the source of that obligation is another matter altogether, but we cannot, simply as a matter of logic, conclude that if someone believes that abortion is morally wrong because *life* begins at conception, he is committed to the view that the fetus is a person "in the whole sense".

As this rather lengthy summary has indicated, until the Supreme Court decided *Roe* in 1973, criminal abortion in this country was governed first by the common law, and then largely by state statute. The majority of the anti-abortion statutes, whose constitutionality was thrown into doubt by the *Roe* decision, were enacted during the period from 1860 to 1900 and they were in significant measure the result of a vigorous campaign by the AMA to outlaw abortion. The factors which led to the formation of the AMA and to its anti-abortion zeal are various, and undoubtedly more complex than my summary reveals, but the forms that the crusade took and the reasons that the AMA gave for its position are open to public inspection. I think that I have fairly summarized them. If I have, then we are led to the conclusions that anti-abortion legislation in the United States did not reflect an actual determination by the various state legislatures that the fetus is a person "in the whole sense" and that the statutes themselves imply nothing whatsoever about the fetus's status as a person.

It might still be suggested that the anti-abortion legislation's rejection of the common law distinction between the abortion of a fetus before quickening and that of one after quickening, can be explained as at least a tacit determination that quickening does not mark the beginning of personhood. Such a suggestion would have some appeal if it turned out that the common law distinction were grounded in the notion that a fetus becomes a person at quickening. Then the argument could be made that the rejection of the distinction is itself evidence that the anti-abortion legislation enables us to say something about the development in the law of a concept of person "in the whole sense", which in turn might enable us to say that the legislation had some bearing on the question, "Is the fetus a person?".

Currently there is some debate about the precise antecedents of the common law distinction. Some scholars have claimed that the importance of the distinction dates from a deliberate misrepresentation by Coke of the state of the law. In fact, they argue, there is strong evidence that it was not a crime to abort even a quickened fetus.[38] Other scholars accept Coke's report that the abortion of a woman "quick with child" is "a great misprison [sic], and no murder" ([9], p. 50), as genuinely reflective of the law at the time ([14], p. 433; [15], p. 94). But whichever view of Coke's role is correct, the facts remain that more than 100 years later, Blackstone accepted Coke's description as accurate ([3], Vol. 1, p. 125) and that the abortion of a fetus after quickening was clearly a crime in both England and the United States.

Although abortions after quickening were crimes, they were not murders. They were, and under any account had always been, treated as different from the intentional killing of someone *ex utero*.[39] Quickening was held by some to mark the actual beginning of life[40] and by others to represent the first time at which anyone could be certain that a woman was pregnant, and hence that another life had begun.[41] But once again (and this simple point cannot be stressed too often) to say that life begins at quickening, or at conception, or even at birth, is *not* to say that an entity becomes a person at quickening, or at conception, or even at birth.

The great jurists whose commentaries did so much to determine what was applied as the common law, simply did not address either the question, "Is the fetus a person?" or the question, "When does personhood begin?". Blackstone certainly implies that someone becomes a person at birth, when he says:

Natural persons are such as the God of nature formed us. . . . By the absolute rights of individuals we mean those which are so in their primary and strictest sense; such as would belong to their persons merely in a state of nature, and which every man is intitled to enjoy whether out of society or in it. . . . For the principal aim of society is to protect individuals in the enjoyment of those absolute rights, which were vested in them by the immutable laws of nature; . . . the absolute rights of man, considered as a free agent, endowed with discernment to know good from evil, . . . are usually summed up in one general appellation, and denominated the natural liberty of mankind. This natural liberty consists properly in a power of acting as one thinks fit, without any restraint or control, unless by the law of nature: *being a right inherent in us by birth*, and one of the gifts of God to man at his creation, when he endued him with the faculty of free will. . . . In these several articles consist the rights, or, as they are frequently termed, the liberties of Englishmen . . . [a] nd we have seen that these rights consist, primarily, in the free enjoyment of personal security, of personal liberty, and of private property. . . . And all these rights and liberties *it is our birthright* to enjoy entire. . . . [emphasis added] ([3], pp. 119–40).

But Blackstone does not, and does not need to, focus on the aforementioned questions about personhood. The law he was describing simply did, in general, treat fetuses differently from persons *ex utero*. More importantly, he was concerned to give an account of the law. As he conceived it, the law "is a rule of civil conduct, commanding what is right, and prohibiting what is right, and prohibiting what is wrong" ([3], p. 118), life is "a right inherent by nature in every individual" ([3], p. 125), and the right which a person has to personal security includes his "legal and uninterrupted enjoyment of his life . . . " ([3], p. 125). And in fact, life "begins in contemplation of law as soon as an infant is able to stir in the mother's womb" ([3], p. 125). Unless he had wanted to argue that a fetus *is* a person in some whole sense, Blackstone had no need to come to grips with when personhood was achieved, and it should not surprise us, therefore, that he did not.

If Blackstone did not base his account of the quickening distinction on the claim that it is at that point that a fetus becomes a person, it is highly likely that the distinction as it evolved in the application of the common law in the United States was not grounded in the view that personhood begins at quickening. Thus we are left with the conclusion that the anti-abortion legislation of the nineteenth century, like the *Roe* decision, fails to provide us with a concept of person in the law, coherent or otherwise.

As I suggested earlier, there are other areas of the law in which the problem of how to treat the fetus has been addressed. The question of personhood has been even less compelling in those contexts than in the context of criminal abortion. Intentional abortion represents the action in which, in some fundamental sense, the fetus has the most at stake. If the law has not focused *and has not needed to focus* on whether the fetus is a person in fashioning answers to the question how to treat intentional abortion, it should not surprise us that the juridical status of the fetus is not a function of its status as a person (see also [65]).

The period between the time that this paper was written and the time that it appeared in page proof was one during which, for the first time, there was significant Congressional interest in addressing the philosophical question 'Is the fetus a person?' and making its answer determinative of the fetus's juridical status. This interest arose in the context of the efforts of some members of Congress to overcome the effect of *Roe v. Wade* and to outlaw abortion altogether (except perhaps to save the life of the mother).

Some 18 proposals to amend the Constitution to prohibit abortion were introduced in Congress during the first half of 1981. Some of these explicitly provided that a fetus from the moment of conception is a 'person' for purposes of the Fifth and Fourteenth Amendments (see, e.g., S. J. Res. 17, H. J. Res. 125, 97th Cong., 1st Sess.). In addition, various bills were proposed which would have the effect of undermining *Roe* by declaring that, for example, Congress finds that the "life of each human being begins at conception" and that for purposes of the States' enforcement of the Fourteenth Amendment, " 'person' shall include all human life" as so defined (S. 158, H. R. 900, 97th Cong., 1st Sess.). Despite the enormous public debate which these proposals have occasioned, none of them has gained Congressional approval.

We can now return to the comment with which I began this paper. I indicated that there were two reasons why someone interested in the relationship between the concept of person and the proper use of the fetus in biomedicine might undertake an analysis of the concept of person in the law. On the one hand, he might seek to discover whether a coherent concept had evolved which would enable him to predict how the law will deal with the questions it will inevitably face in connection with the use of the fetus in biomedicine. On the other hand, he might harbor hopes that, having found a coherent concept of person in the law, he might bring it profitably to bear in addressing the moral issues that abound in this area. Whatever our hopes, they are disappointed, because what we have seen is that the law has not developed, and has not needed to develop, a coherent concept of person "in the whole sense" (or in *any* interesting sense).

There may yet be something instructive to be gleaned from this exercise, although the theme of the suggestion is somewhat gloomy. There are no shortcuts to deciding the answers to the increasingly difficult moral questions that the phenomenal growth of biomedical capability has thrust so urgently upon us. Some of the very best minds in the history of thought have been devoted to trying to discover the foundations of morality. That there is still no consensus is testimony to the difficulty of the enterprise. The crisis that is fast upon us should cause us to redouble our investigation of the foundations, not to abandon that job in favor of looking elsewhere for the answers.

Georgeton University Law Center,
Washington, D.C.

EDITORS' NOTE

Though none of the proposals to amend the Constitution in order to forbid abortions have been adopted, they have raised serious legal and moral issues. From a legal point of view, they would not only restrict the right of women to abortion, but might engender unforeseen legal problems. A good study of these possible difficulties has been provided by David Westfall in a recent study of proposed constitutional amendments and right to life bills. ('Beyond Abortion: The Potential Reach of a Human Life Amendment', *American Journal of Law and Medicine* [Summer 1982], pp. 94–135.) As Westfall argues, such right-to-life legislation might have the threatening consequence of forbidding women from "skiing, working in hazardous environments, flying, and riding in automobiles" on the ground of protecting the conceptus. Indeed, "restricting the activities of potentially pregnant women might similarly be justified on the ground that such classification is necessary to protect the conceptus during the period between conception and proof of pregnancy" (*ibid.*, p. 111). In addition, the use of intrauterine contraceptive devices, the mini-pill, and the morning-after pill, which may act through impeding implantation, could be proscribed along with abortions (*ibid.*, p. 117). Other even more bizarre consequences might follow as well, including conceptuses qualifying as dependents for federal income tax purposes, and as persons to be counted in the apportionment of legislators.

These consequences flow from the attempt to forbid abortion through expanding the notion of persons and imputing personhood to fetuses. The proposed Ashbrook amendment to the Constitution, for example, states:

Section 1. With respect to the right to life guaranteed in this Constitution, every human being, subject to the jurisdiction of the United States, or of any state, shall be deemed, from the moment of fertilization, to be a person and entitled to the right to life. (J. R. J. Res. 13, 97th Cong., 1st Sess. [1981].)

One finds somewhat similar wording in the more detailed proposal by Garn-Rhodes:

Section 1. With respect to the right to life the word 'person', as used in this article and in the fifth and fourteenth articles of amendment to the Constitution of the United States, applies to all human beings, irrespective of age, health, function, or condition of dependency, including their unborn offspring at every stage of their biological development.

Section 2. No unborn person shall be deprived of life by any person: Provided, however, that nothing in this article shall prohibit a law permitting only those medical procedures required to prevent the death of the mother. (S. J. Res. 17, 97th Cong., 1st Sess. [1981].)

In addition to such proposed amendments to the Constitution, there have been attempts to change the meaning of 'person' through Congressional action alone. The Helms-Hyde human life bill, for example, proposes that:

Section 1. The Congress finds that present day scientific evidence indicates a significant likelihood that actual human life exists from conception. The Congress further finds that the fourteenth amendment to the Constitution of the United States was intended to protect all human beings. Upon the basis of these findings, and in the exercise of the powers of the Congress, including its power under section 5 of the fourteenth amendment to the Constitution of the United States, the Congress hereby declares that for the purposes of enforcing the obligation of the states under the fourteenth amendment not to deprive persons of life without due process of law, human life shall be deemed to exist from conception, without regard to race, sex, age, health, defect, or condition of dependency: and for this purpose 'person' shall include all human life as defined herein. (S. 158, 97th Cong., 1st Sess. [1981].)

The Helms-Hyde bill curiously adds the premise that it is modern scientific evidence that sustains the notion that fetal life is human life. As papers in this volume argue, this is at best a confusion of the concept of human life with the concept of personhood. There is no doubt that the zygote of two humans is a human zygote, and therefore human life, just as human sperm and ova are examples of human life, albeit human haploid life. What is at stake are the grounds for holding that fetal life should be accorded the standing of persons. This confusion runs through the Senate hearings on the human life bill. For example, Dr. Jerome Lejeune begins by recognizing that the central question is "when does a person begin" but ends by arguing that 'life' begins at conception. (Testimony by Dr. Jerome Lejeune on The Human Life Bill: Hearings before the Subcommittee on Separation of Powers of the Committee of the Judiciary, 97th Congress, U.S. Government Printing Office, Washington, D.C., 1982, Vol. 1, pp. 7–13.) The testimony by most witnesses is a web of semantic and conceptual confusion.

Given the continuing disapproval of abortion on request by many individuals, it is quite likely that such controversies will continue, even if they are not successful to the point of amending the Constitution. One finds already in 1983 further attempts as a new 'Hatch amendment' (S. J. Res. 3, 98th Cong., 1st Sess. [1983], as well as S. J. Res. 4, 98th Cong., 1st Sess. (1983), S. J. Res. 9, 98th Cong., 1st Sess. (1983), and S. J. Res. 59, 98th Cong., 1st Sess. (1983), to name only a few.

NOTES

* I am very grateful to Nancy L. Schimmel for her invaluable research assistance and her work on the Appendix to this paper.

[1] *"In vitro* fertilization" refers to the fertilization of the female ovum outside the mother's body. Once fertilization in the test tube or petri dish is achieved, the zygote – or fertilized egg – is implanted into the mother's uterus where, it is hoped, it will develop normally until birth ([59], pp. 548–558).

"Embryo transplantation", or artificial embryonation, involves the transfer of a newly formed embryo from one female's uterus to that of another. Although this procedure has not yet been successfully performed on human beings, it is becoming an increasingly common practice among livestock breeders. Semen from a prize bull is used to fertilize a prize cow's egg. The embryo is then transplanted to another female to be carried to term. Because their estrus cycles are not interrupted by gestation, the prize cows are – at least theoretically – able to conceive once each cycle, and the "surrogate mothers" give birth to genetically superior offspring.

"Abortion" is the premature termination of a pregnancy. When it occurs naturally or spontaneously, this process is usually referred to as "miscarriage". When it is artificially induced – whether by vacuum extraction, dilation and curettage ("D & C"), injection of hypertonic saline into the uterus, or any or the more primitive techniques – the law has sought to intervene. For general discussion of the legal issues surrounding artificial insemination, see [97], [71], [99], and [108].

[2] I use the word "stricture" here, rather than the word "rule", in order to emphasize that these observations do not presuppose the truth of any of the various metaethical positions which hold that moral action is governed by rules. See pp. 119–120 of this essay.

[3] Much of the contemporary philosophical writing on abortion has followed this general line. For fairly explicit examples which represent widely disparate views, see [19], pp. 51–59; [110]; [103]; and [6].

[4] This phenomeon is most striking perhaps among theologians who have argued against abortion at *any* stage of fetal development. See, e.g., [2], pp. 414–416.

It is worth noting, as well, that the idea that a physician has a greater duty to save the life of the mother than that of the fetus is apparent in the widely recognized "therapeutic abortion" exception to most criminal abortion statutes. Long before the Supreme Court's 1973 decision in Roe v. Wade [204], most states permitted abortion when it was necessary to preserve either the life or the health of the mother. The trend began in 1829, when New York passed its first abortion law, N.Y. Rev. Stat. ([87], tit. 2, art. 1, Section 9, p. 661; [187], tit. 6, Section 21, p. 264) cited in ([204], p. 138).

In 1974, the Pennsylvania Legislature enacted an Abortion Control Act which attempted to impose on physicians performing abortions, including therapeutic abortions, a duty to use the technique most likely to result in the fetus's survival "so long as a different technique would not be necessary to preserve the life or health of the mother". In holding this statute to be impermissibly vague, the United States Supreme Court wrote:

"... [I]t is uncertain whether the statute permits the physician to consider his duty to the patient to be paramount to his duty to the fetus, or whether it requires the physician to make a 'trade-off' between the woman's health and additional percentage points of fetal survival. Serious ethical and constitutional difficulties, that we do not address, lurk behind this ambiguity. We hold only that where conflicting duties of this magnitude are involved, the State, at the least, must proceed with greater precision before it may subject a physician to possible criminal sanctions" (Colautti v. Franklin [132], p. 400).

It is unclear after the *Colautti* decision whether the states could constitutionally draft a statute which equates the duty owed to a viable fetus with that owed to the mother. Although I am not persuaded, at least one commentary has suggested that the Court in *Colautti* did limit the states' abilities to protect their compelling interest in the preservation of potential life. See [114], p. 404.

5 The thalidomide tragedy was probably one of the most publicized pharmacological disasters in recent medical history. Preliminary testing had indicated that thalidomide was something of a wonder-drug among sedatives: it was fast-acting, produced little or no "hangover" effect, and did not appear to be lethal if taken in excess. In 1960, the drug was widely prescribed in West Germany, and a United States manufacturer, Richardson-Merrell, solicited the Food and Drug Administration's approval for its sale in this country. Early in 1961, while the Food and Drug Administration was considering Richardson-Merrell's application, reports were received from Europe that indicated that thousands of deformed babies had been born to women who had taken thalidomide during pregnancy. Not surprisingly, the drug was never approved for sale here.

Experts disagree about how strong the correlation between thalidomide and fetal abnormality actually is. Most reports tend to indicate that approximately twenty percent of the women who took the drug during pregnancy had abnormal babies. See [28], p. 624. However, Dr. Widukind Lenz of West Germany believes that the risk exceeds fifty percent when the drug is ingested during a particular two-week period in the first trimester of pregnancy. Lenz notes further that a one hundred percent rate of damage during certain sensitive periods has been produced experimentally in monkeys ([70], pp. 104–105).

Whatever the precise statistical risk, it was against these odds that in 1961 one American woman, Sherri Finkbine, who had taken thalidomide during pregnancy and feared that her baby would be affected, determined to obtain an abortion. Mrs. Finkbine petitioned the Arizona courts for immunity from prosecution under the state's abortion law. The law permitted abortion only when the procedure was necessary to save the life of the mother. Her petition was denied. She then traveled to Sweden to seek the approval of the Royal Swedish Medical Board for an abortion in that country. After lengthy deliberation, the Board approved her request. As she had feared, the fetus was defective.

In 1962, in another highly publicized outgrowth of the thalidomide tragedy, Suzanne van de Put was tried in Belgium for the murder of her infant daughter. Madame van de Put had taken the drug during her pregnancy, and her child had been born with severe limb deformities. The mother, who was acquitted by a jury, admitted killing the baby but claimed to have acted in order to save her child from a miserable life [13], p. 91.

It was no doubt the fear of events such as these that prompted the American Law Institute to include a "eugenic abortion" exception in its Model Penal Code:
(2) *Justifiable Abortion.* A licensed physician is justified in terminating a pregnancy if:

(a) he believes ... that the child would be born with grave physical or mental defects... (Section 207.11).
See generally [107], pp. 226–230; see also [68].
6 For a discussion that illustrates the jurisdictional variations within tort law alone, see the Appendix to this paper.
7 For the suggestion that the fetus's status as a person (in some fundamental sense) is irrelevant to whether it should have legal protection, see [65], p. 1687.
8 The law is clear that a potential or "unperfected" interest in property may be created in an unborn child and that the right of possession vests upon the infant's live birth. As the Illinois Supreme Court explained in 1922:

"A child *en ventre sa mère* is capable of taking by legacy or devise. The only requisite for such child taking in the same manner as other children is that it shall be afterward born. If it be born dead, or in such early stage of gestation as to be incapable of living, it is as if it had never been born or conceived" (Tomlin v. Laws [226], p. 618).

Thus, devises "to my surviving heirs" or "to my children living at the time of my death" are held to include children born posthumously but in gestation at the time of the testator's death. See, e.g., Tomlin v. Laws [226]; Kimbro v. Harper [116]; Barnett v. Pinkston [122]; In re Well's Will [160].
9 The English rule that the unborn fetus, so long as it is subsequently born alive, has the right to take under the Statute of Distributions, has been carried over to the American law of intestate succession. Thellusson v. Woodward [225]; see [22], p. 57.
10 A stillborn child does not enjoy an estate. If property is devised to a fetus that is subsequently stillborn, the property does not pass through to the infant's heirs, but instead reverts to the grantor as if the fetus had never been conceived. See, e.g., Tomlin v. Laws [226]; In re Roberts' Estate [159] (a stillborn fetus has no right to an estate administrator because the fetus never had legal existence and the underlying property right was never perfected).
11 At common law, the killing of an unborn child was not murder unless the child was first born alive. See, e.g., Rex v. Poulton [202]; Rex v. Enoch [201]; and Rex v. Pritchard [203]. In accordance with this tradition, most of the early American decisions required evidentiary proof that the child was "fully born, and born alive, having an independent circulation and existence separate from the mother ... " before the court would sustain an indictment for murder (State v. Winthrop [220], p. 520). See also Morgan v. State [179]; Shedd v. State [209]; Jackson v. Commonwealth [165].
Although in recent years a growing number of jurisdictions have enacted feticide statutes that treat the killing of an unborn fetus as manslaughter (see generally [35], p. 365, Note 118), the common law view that a fetus cannot be the victim of homicide has endured. As recently as 1970, the California Supreme Court held that a fetus was not a "human being" within the meaning of the state's murder statute. The case involved a stillbirth that resulted from a fractured skull that the fetus suffered when its mother was savagely beaten during her eighth month of pregnancy. See Keeler v. Superior Court of Amador County [166]. The decision prompted the California Legislature to amend its homicide statute to include within the definition of "murder" the killing of a fetus. The statute provides for a variety of exceptions, most notably any abortion

"solicited, aided, abetted or consented to by the mother of the fetus" ([130], Section 187).

12 The evolution of early abortion legislation in this country is discussed on pp. 123–127 of this essay. Prior to 1840 the abortion of a prequickened fetus (see Note 27) was not an indictable offense, either under state criminal statutes or under the common law. See, e.g., Smith v. Gaffard ([213], p. 51); Abrams v. Foshee ([115], p. 278); Mitchell v. Comm'r ([177], p. 210); Commonwealth v. Luceba Parker [135]; Commonwealth v. Gangs ([134], p. 388); State v. Cooper ([217], p. 57); Conn. Stat. (1821) [137] quoted at Note 17; Ark. Rev. Stat. (1838) [121]; Ill. Rev. Code (1827) [158]; Iowa (Terr.) Stat. (1838) [162]; N.J. Rev. Stat. (1838) [181]; N.Y. Rev. Stat. (1828–1835) [187]; and Ohio Gen Stat. (1841) [190]. See [87], p. 447–520 (reprinting statutes).

Beginning in 1840 with the state of Maine [(Me. Rev. Stat. (1840) [174]) reprinted in [87], p. 478], a growing number of state legislatures began to pass measures which made it criminal to perform an abortion at any stage of gestation. However, it was not until the latter part of the nineteenth century that the abortion of a prequickened fetus was made a felony. See, e.g., Pa. Laws (1860) [192] reprinted in [87], p. 507. By 1960, 49 states and the District of Columbia had declared all abortions – or, at the least, all 'nontherapeutic' abortions – to be felonies. See statutes cited in [46], p. 102, Note 174.

In 1850 the Supreme Court of Pennsylvania became the first state court to depart from the common law rule when it sustained an indictment for the abortion of a prequickened fetus in Mills v. Commonwealth [175]. Dismissing the great weight of authority to the contrary, the *Mills* court wrote that requiring the woman to be quick with child "is not ... the law in Pennsylvania and never ought to have been the law anywhere. It is not the murder of a living child which constitutes the offense, but the destruction of gestation ... " ([175], p. 632). The decision rendered in State v. Slagle ([219], p. 545) accorded with this.

In Griswold v. Connecticut [150], the United States Supreme Court struck down a state statute which prohibited the use of contraceptives by married and unmarried people alike. In so doing, the Court recognized, for the first time, a constitutional right to privacy. Subsequent decisions have extended that right to other areas of personal and familial relationships, culminating in Roe v. Wade [204] (discussed at pp. 122–123 of this essay), where the Court recognized, within the right to privacy, a woman's qualified right to have an abortion ([26], pp. 41–48). See also [32].

Roe established that a woman's right to privacy includes the right to decide, absent a compelling state interest to the contrary, whether or not to terminate her pregnancy ([204], p. 155). It invalidated a state statute that permitted abortion only to save the life of the mother, and it fixed viability as the point at which a state's legitimate interest in potential life arises ([204], p. 160). Its companion case, Doe v. Bolton [143], invalidated the procedural steps required to obtain an abortion under Georgia law [146], a statute based largely on the Model Penal Code. And three years later in Planned Parenthood v. Danforth [196], the Court addressed other restrictive statutes under which the availability of abortion turned on some form of consent and physician reporting requirements. The constitutional issues surrounding abortion continue to generate litigation on a wide range of topics [46].

13 Tort law poses a variety of questions concerning the legal claims of the fetus. Among them: Does the fetus have a cause of action for harm negligently inflicted on it prior

to or during its birth? Can its survivors maintain an action for the wrongful death of a stillborn fetus? Does a deformed or defective infant have a cause of action for wrongful life when its impairment could have been, but was not, detected prior to its birth? Does such an infant have a cause of action when the impairment is the result of someone's negligence prior to the infant's conception? For a brief summary of the juridical status of the fetus in tort law, see the Appendix to this paper.

14 The significance that the law has placed on live birth cannot be over-emphasized. See, e.g.,[38].

15 The Supreme Court noted in Roe v. Wade [204]:

"We need not resolve the difficult question of when life begins. When those trained in the respective disciplines of medicine, philosophy and theology are unable to arrive at any concensus, the judiciary, at this point in the development of man's knowledge, is not in a position to speculate as to the answer. It should be sufficient to note briefly the wide divergence of thinking on this most sensitive and difficult question. There has always been strong support for the view that life does not begin until live birth" ([204], pp. 159–160).

16 A survey of state abortion laws can be found in [46] and [87].

17 Conn. Stat. (1821) ([137], p. 152):

"Section 14. Every person who shall, willfully and maliciously, administer to, or cause to be administered to, or taken by, any person or persons, any deadly poison, or other noxious and destructive substance, with an intention him, her or them, thereby to murder, or thereby to cause or procure the miscarriage of any woman, then being quick with child, and shall be thereof duly convicted, shall suffer imprisonment, in newgate prison, during his natural life, or for such other term as the court having cognizance of the offence shall determine" (reprinted in [87], p. 453).

18 See, e.g., Allaire v. St. Luke's Hosp. [117]; Gorman v. Budlong [148]; Buel v. United Rys. Co. [129].

19 'Quickening' is defined as the point at which the mother first perceives fetal stirring in the womb. It may occur at any time between the sixteenth and twentieth weeks of gestation. See [12], Para. 311.20.

20 See pp. 128–129 of this essay.

21 [17], p. 37; see also East River Medical Association:

"Your committee deem the unrestrained practice of medicine as the main cause for the existence of professional abortionists, and the want of proper laws to regulate the practice of medicine as encouraging knaves to assume and practice under titles which institutions duly chartered by the State alone have the right to confer. Our laws know no distinction between the duly authorized physician and the imposter" ([10], p. 1).

22 Alabama, Arkansas, Illinois, Indiana, Iowa, Maine, Mississippi, Missouri, New York, and Ohio.

23 Indiana, Maine, Missouri, New York, and Ohio.

24 Examples of early abortion advertisements appear in [17], pp. 51, 52, 54, 197.

25 One of the most successful entrepreneurs of the abortion business in the mid-nineteenth century was Madame Restell (née Ann Lohman). Although her business was based in lower Manhattan, she used such marketing techniques as traveling salesmen and newspaper advertisements to enable her to open offices in other cities. ([17], p. 50).
26 [17], p. 121, Note 8. Mass. Acts and Resolves (1845) [173], reprinted in [87], p. 481:

"... Whoever maliciously or without lawful justification, with intent to cause and procure the miscarriage of a woman then pregnant with child, shall administer to her, prescribe for her, or advise or direct her to take or swallow, any poison, drug, Medicine or noxious thing ... and whosoever maliciously and without lawful justification, shall use any instrument or means whatever with the like intent, and every person, with the like intent, knowingly aiding and assisting such offender or offenders, shall be deemed guilty of felony, if the woman die in consequence thereof, and shall be imprisoned not more than twenty years, nor less than five years in the State Prison; and if the woman doth not die in consequence thereof, such offender shall be guilty of a misdemeanor, and shall be punished by imprisonment not exceeding seven years, nor less than one year, in the state prison or house of correction, or common jail, and by fine not exceeding two thousand dollars" (Approved by the Governor, Jan. 31, 1845).

27 Commonwealth v. Luceba Parker [135], cited in [17], p. 120, Note 1.
28 [17], pp. 123–124; N. Y. Laws (1845) [183] as here stated:

"Section 3: Every woman who shall solicit of any person any medicine, drug, or substance or thing whatever, and shall take the same, or shall submit to any operation, or other means whatever, with intent thereby to procure a miscarriage, shall be deemed guilty of a misdemeanor, and shall, upon conviction, be punished by imprisonment in the county jail, not less than three months nor more than one year, or by a fine not exceeding one thousand dollars, or by both such fine and imprisonment."

"Section 4: Any woman who shall endeavor privately, either by herself or the procurement of others, to conceal the death of any issue of her body, which if born alive would by law be a bastard, whether it was born dead or alive, or whether it was murdered or not, shall be deemed guilty of a misdemeanor, and shall, on conviction thereof, be punished by imprisonment in a county jail, not exceeding one year" (reprinted in [87], p. 500).

N. H. Laws (1848) [180] as here stated:

"Section 4: Any woman who shall voluntarily submit to the violation of the provisions of this act upon herself, shall be punished by imprisonment in the county jail not exceeding one year or by fine not exceeding one thousand dollars, or by both said fine and imprisonment at the discretion of the Court" (reprinted in [87], p. 494).

29 These statutes are discussed in [17], Ch. 8, p. 220ff. and cited in [46], p. 101, Note 172.

30 Although a few states, such as New York, did maintain reports of the two houses of their legislatures, none systematically kept transcripts of floor debates or detailed reports of committee deliberations and hearings.

31 The criminal abortion statutes passed by the Connecticut and Pennsylvania legislatures in 1860 were both seemingly aimed at the protection of women. Section 3 of the Connecticut Act made it a felony for a woman either to solicit an abortion or to perform one on herself. [Conn. Pub. Acts (1860) [136], reprinted in [87], p. 454.] Applying this section in the case of State v. Carey [216], the Connecticut court attributed the provision to both the legislature's opposition to the destruction of human life and its desire to protect women from a variety of evils:

"[T]he legislature ... for the purpose of further promoting the public policy which regards all unnecessary miscarriage as a public evil, created two new and distinct offenses, ... one limiting the power of a woman over her own person and punishing an attempt to produce unnecessary miscarriage ....

The public policy which underlies this legislation is based largely on protection due to the woman, protection against her own weakness as well as the criminal lust and greed of others" ([216], p. 352; see also [17], p. 201).

The Pennsylvania Act went even further in the direction of the protection of women. It made the attempt to produce the miscarriage of a woman an indictable offense, *whether or not she was indeed pregnant.* (Pa. Laws (1860) [192], reprinted in [87], p. 507; see also [17], p. 202; and Roe v. Wade [204], p. 149). And commenting on the New Jersey abortion statute, that state's Supreme Court wrote that its purpose "was not to prevent the procuring of abortions, so much as to guard the health and life of the mother against the consequences of such attempts" (State v. Murphy [218], p. 114).

Ohio's 1867 abortion statute appears to have been based on the desire to preserve the supremacy of the white, Protestant class in America:

"Do [our native women] realize that in avoiding the duties and responsibilities of married life, they are, in effect, living in a state of legalized prostitution? Shall we permit our broad and fertile prairies to be settled only by the children of aliens?" ([165]; quoted in [17], pp. 207–208).

32 See, e.g., N. Y. Laws (1869) [185], p. 1502, reprinted in [87], p. 500, punishing the abortion of "any woman with child". See also N. Y. Laws (1846) [184], p. 19, reprinted in [87], p. 500, punishing the abortion of "any woman with a *quick* child" (emphasis added). According to Mohr, the 1869 amendment followed by only one year a resolution by the New York State Medical Society that noted the existence of a living creature from the first moment of conception ([17], p. 216, Note 54).

33 See, e.g., Ore. Gen. Laws Crim. Code [191], p. 528, reprinted in [87], p. 505, discussed in [17], p. 203; and Foster v. State [145].

34 See, e.g., Ala. Rev. Code (1867) [116] (fine to $500 and possible imprisonment of three to twelve months); Colo. Gen. Laws, Joint Res., mem., and Priv. Acts of the Terr. of Colo. Legis. Asm. (1861) [133], pp. 296–297 (punished essentially as manslaughter);

Ill. Pub. Laws (1867) [157], p. 89 (high misdemeanor to cause miscarriage; murder if woman dies); and N. Y. Gen. Stats. (1872) [182], p. 71 (four to twenty years imprisonment if fetus or woman dies).

35 N. Y. Laws (1845) [183], p. 285, reprinted above in Note 36; N. Y. Laws (1872) [186], p. 71, reprinted in [87], p. 501.

36 It was not until the 1880s that other states began to punish women for seeking an abortion. See, e.g., Ariz. Rev. Stat. (1887) [120] (one to five years); Cal. Pen. Code [131] (one to five years); Idaho Rev. Stat. (1887) [156] (one to five years); Ind. Laws (1881) [161] ($10–$50 fine and 30 days to 12 months); Minn. Stat. (1873) [176], p. 987 (three months to two years and/or $300–$1000). Most state statutes merely punished the abortionist and any person who advertised either the instruments or potions used to perform abortions.

37 See Note 7 above.

38 See, e.g., [76]; see Roe v. Wade [204], pp. 134–136; and [87], pp. 430–432; but see [5], Vol. 2, p. 341.

39 See Note 11 above.

40 "Life . . . begins in contemplation of law as soon as an infant is able to stir in the mother's womb" ([3], Vol. 1, p. 125); see also [13], p. 386, Note 13 quoting Evans v. The People:

"Although there may be life before quickening, all the authorities agree that a child is not "quick" until the mother has felt the child alive within her. "Quick" is synonymous with "living" . . . . The woman is not pregnant with a living child until the child has become quick. If the child is a living child from the instant of conception, then all the authorities, medical and legal, are sadly at fault in their attempts to distinguish between mere pregnancy and pregnancy with a quick child . . . " ([144], p. 90).

41 In differentiating between the terms 'pregnant' and 'quick with child', the Massachusetts Supreme Court in Commonwealth v. Luceba Parker noted:

"In the case of Rex v. Phillips, 3 Campb. 73, . . . it was held . . . that . . . the words 'quick with child' must be taken to be according to the common understanding . . . that a woman is not considered to be *quick* with child, till she has herself felt the child alive and quick within her" ([135], pp. 266–267, emphasis added).

APPENDIX

The Status of the Fetus Under the Law of Torts

The common law provided no basis for an action in tort for prenatal injury. Although the fetus had long been granted at least some independent legal status in property law and in criminal law,[1] the courts refused to recognize it as a distinct legal entity in tort.

Injuries to the Fetus in Utero

Oliver Wendell Holmes, writing in 1884 for the Supreme Judicial Court of Massachusetts in *Dietrich v. Northampton* [142] held that a fetus was not a "person" within the meaning of the Commonwealth's wrongful death statute. The case involved a pre-viable fetus born prematurely after its mother had fallen on a negligently maintained road. The child survived its birth for several minutes ([142], pp. 14–15). Holmes held that a fetus is merely a part of its mother until it is actually born, and thus that the defendant owed it no separate duty of care ([142], p. 17).

The 'no-duty' rule of *Dietrich* was given a somewhat different justification in the context of negligence claims against a public carrier, but it was applied nonetheless. In both *Walker v. Grt. No. Ry. of Ireland* [230] and *Nugent v. Brooklyn Hghts. Railroad Co.* [189], the courts accepted the defendant railroads' argument that any liability that they might have for injuries arising out of their negligent conduct was a consequence of the contractual relationship existing between them and their passengers. Because the infant plaintiffs were *in utero* when the purported negligence occurred, no contract ever existed with them, and no duty or liability could be imposed ([230], pp. 672–673; [189], p. 371).

In a concurrence to the *Walker* opinion, one justice expressed concern about the speculative nature of causal proof in cases claiming fetal damage. To recognize an infant's right of action might be to invite a rash of unmeritorious claims ([230], p. 82). Although *Walker* turned on the lack of duty owed to the fetus *in utero*, the suggestion in the concurring opinion was adopted by other courts as an independent justification for dismissing actions for prenatal injury.[2]

Largely out of deference to the doctrine of *stare decisis*,[3] these precedents remained undisturbed in Anglo-American courts for nearly half a century. The only note to the contrary was sounded in 1900 by Justice Boggs' vigorous dissent to *Allaire v. St. Luke's Hospital* [117]. Boggs did not believe that the no-duty rule ought to apply to preclude an infant from recovering for injuries he received when his pregnant mother had ridden in a negligently maintained hospital elevator:

A fetus in the womb of the mother may well be regarded as but a part of the bowels of the mother during a portion of the period of gestation; but if, while in the womb, it reaches that prenatal age of viability when the destruction of life of the mother does not necessarily end its existence also, and when, if separated prematurely, and by artificial means, from the mother, it would live and grow, mentally and physically, as other children generally, it is but to deny a palpable fact to argue there is but one life, and that the life of the mother ([117], p. 641).

The first real break with the lack of duty doctrine occurred in 1933, when the Supreme Court of Canada permitted a deformed infant to recover for prenatal injuries. *Montreal Tramways v. Leveille* [178] involved a pregnant woman who was thrown from a tram car because of the negligence of its operator. Two months later she gave birth to a baby with club feet ([178], p. 338). While acknowledging that the child had not yet been born when the injury occurred, the court nonetheless concluded that when the baby "was subsequently born alive and viable, it was clothed with all the rights of action which it would have had if actually in existence at the date of the accident" ([178], p. 344).

The *Tramways* decision arose under the Quebec Civil Law, and was there-fore technically not binding on either the common law provinces or the American courts ([109], p. 652). However, in 1946 its lead was followed by the United States District Court for the District of Columbia in *Bonbrest v. Kotz* [128]. The plaintiff in *Bonbrest* was an infant who had been harmed when a doctor removed it from its mother's womb in a negligent manner. By focusing on the plaintiff's viability at the time of the injury — as the *Tramways* opinion had done — and on the unusual fact that the injury involved direct contact between the fetus and the defendant, the court was able to circumvent the *Dietrich* rule to hold that the fetus was a distinct legal entity to whom a duty of care was owed.[4] Moreover, the court summarily dismissed the difficulty of proof argument that had been raised in the con-curring opinion to *Walker*:

The law is presumed to keep pace with the sciences, and medical science certainly has made progress since 1884. We are concerned only with the right and not its implementa-tion ([128], p. 143).

The judicial recognition of a duty of care to the fetus represented a milestone in the evolution of negligence law. The duty was held by many state courts to arise only with respect to a viable fetus[5] and to be enforceable only when the injured fetus was subsequently born alive.[6] All 34 of the jurisdictions that have considered negligence claims for prenatal injury have recognized a duty of care to a viable fetus and although a few have extended that duty to cover earlier stages of gestation, a majority continue to require that the fetus be viable at the time of injury.

The viability requirement is frequently criticized on several grounds.[7] It is impossible to determine the precise point at which the fetus becomes viable. Current estimates generally place viability at between 24 and 28 weeks of gestation, but as technologically superior life-support systems are developed, this standard will surely change. Moreover, it is now universally recognized that an embryo develops as an independent organism from the moment of implantation in the uterine wall. While it is dependent upon the mother for oxygen and nourishment, its limbs and organs are distinctly its own. Thus it is scientifically inaccurate to consider a developing fetus as merely a part of its mother until it becomes viable. Some state courts have felt uncomfortable about premising a legal right of action on a misconception of fact and have gradually permitted the viability prerequisite to erode.[8] A few jurisdictions have settled on quickening as a preferable standard.[9] Quickening typically occurs several weeks prior to viability,[10] so its use produces an increased class of potential tort plaintiffs. But quickening is, of course, less satisfying than viability as a scientific standard.

One consequence of the law's adoption of the viability standard has been the preclusion from recovery of a sizable class of seriously deformed infants. As the thalidomide [11] and more recent Bendectin [12] controversies graphically illustrate, fetal sensitivity to teratogenic pharmaceuticals is greatest during the first trimester of pregnancy. The mother's legal remedies in drug cases do not compensate her child for its injury. She may be able to recover for her emotional distress, but she has no remedy for the physical harm done to her child.

Negligence Prior to Conception

Despite the tenacity of the viability standard, a new line of negligence claim is beginning to emerge wherein relief is sought for injuries that are brought about by negligence that predates conception. Central to this development has been the view that the function of the law of negligence is largely compensatory and, therefore, the timing of the wrongdoing is of relatively little importance.[13]

Actions for negligence prior to conception typically take one of two forms.[14] On the one hand, parents sometimes bring action for the *wrongful birth* of a child where, for example, a physician had allegedly performed a sterilization operation [15] or an abortion,[16] or where they had received allegedly negligent genetic counseling.[17] More interestingly, children have claimed a cause of action for their own *wrongful life* in two kinds of circumstance. Illegitimate children have sued their parents for causing them to suffer the stigma of bastardy,[18] and children with serious defects have brought actions against their mothers' negligent physicians.[19] Although courts have, in general, been more receptive to the wrongful birth claims of parents than to the wrongful life claims of their children,[20] the notion that in some circumstances there is a duty of care owed to future conceptuses has taken definite, albeit tenuous, hold in a few jurisdictions.

The issue of negligence prior to conception was squarely confronted for the first time in 1977, by the Supreme Court of Illinois. In *Renslow v. Mennonite Hospital* [200],[21] the Illinois trial court had dismissed the complaint of a child whose birth defects were the alleged result of improper Rh-factor blood transfusions that had been administered to his mother eight years before his birth [198]. The Court of Appeals then reversed [199]. In upholding the appellate court's decision, the State Supreme Court took the position that its principal inquiry in deciding a case of negligence prior to conception ought to be directed toward ascertaining the scope of the defendant's legal duty ([200], pp. 354 and 1253–1254). Noting that "duty is not a static concept" ([200], pp. 357 and 1254), the court went on:

The cases allowing relief to an infant for injuries incurred in its previable state make it clear that a defendant may be held liable to a person whose existence was not apparent at the time of his act. We therefore find it illogical to bar relief for an act done prior to conception where the defendant would be liable for this same conduct had the child, unbeknownst to him, been conceived prior to his act. We believe that there is a right to be born free from prenatal injuries foreseeably caused by a breach of duty to the child's mother . . . . Logic and sound policy require a finding of legal duty in this case ([200], pp. 357 and 1255).[22]

A similar theme was sounded in 1978 by the Eighth Circuit. In *Bergstresser v. Mitchell* [125] a child sought recovery under Missouri law for the permanent brain damage that he suffered during his delivery by emergency ceasarean section ([125], p. 24). The child alleged that his emergency delivery had been necessitated by the damage done to his mother's womb by an earlier, and negligent, caesarean section. Missouri courts had already established that an infant born alive had the right to recover for prenatal injuries, and the Eighth Circuit felt that it was a logical extension of that right to allow a child to recover for injuries that he suffered as a consequence of negligence prior to conception ([125], p. 25). To decide otherwise would have permitted "a wrong [to be] inflicted for which there is no remedy" ([125], p. 25).

In June of 1980, in *Curlender v. Bio-Science Labs. and Automated Lab. Sciences* [138], the California Court of Appeals explicitly recognized an action for wrongful life. The complaint alleged that the defendant laboratory negligently misinformed the Curlenders that they did not carry the genes for Tay-Sachs disease, a degenerative condition of the nervous system which is generally fatal within four or five years. The Curlender's daughter was later born with Tay-Sachs disease. In upholding the child's right to sue, the Court said:

The reality of the 'wrongful life' concept is that such a plaintiff both exists and suffers, due to the negligence of others. It is neither necessary nor just to retreat into meditation on the mysteries of life . . . . The certainty of the genetic impairment is no longer a mystery. A reverent appreciation of life compels recognition that an impaired child has come into existence as a living person with certain rights ([138], p. 811).[23]

Wrongful Death

For years after *Bonbrest* [128], courts had uniformly held that the right of a fetus to recover for harm suffered before birth was contingent upon its subsequent live birth. The effect of this rule, of course, is to permit recovery for minor injuries and to deny relief for fatal injuries. In large measure because of discomfort with this result, the states have recently begun to recognize wrongful death actions on behalf of the stillborn.

No action for wrongful death existed at common law ([20], pp. 898–899). As they have interpreted the various statutory remedies that have evolved to allow recovery for negligence that causes death, the courts have been especially deferential to the intent of the legislatures.[24] Because legislative intent is sometimes not clear, courts have been compelled nonetheless to decide certain interpretive issues; whether, for example, either a stillborn fetus or a deceased newborn is a 'person' within the contemplation of a given death statute.

Wrongful death statutes have traditionally taken one of two forms. A minority of states have 'survival acts' that allow a decedent's right of action for negligent harm to survive his death. In other words, the estate is permitted to bring the tort action that the decedent could have maintained had he not died ([20], p. 910). Where live birth is a precondition to a claim for prenatal negligence, recovery under a survival act for the death of a fetus *in utero* is apparently precluded.[25] The majority of jurisdictions, however, have enacted 'death acts', that create a new cause of action in the decedent's personal representative for the benefit of certain designated beneficiaries ([20], p. 902). These acts seek to compensate the survivors for their loss, rather than to preserve some right of the decedent's.[26] Live birth, therefore, would seem to be irrelevant to the existence of the action (though not, perhaps, to the measure of damages).

Where there are wrongful death statutes of either sort, the overwhelming majority of courts that have considered the question have construed them as applying to fetuses only when the fetus was viable when the fatal injury was inflicted.[27] This policy stands in contrast to the current trend in prenatal negligence cases to reject the viability standard.[28] One commentary has suggested that the viability requirement in wrongful death cases may serve as something like the functional equivalent of the live birth element in fetal injury claims ([38], p. 830). Whatever the rationale, it seems clear that the courts are determined to require that some demonstrable degree of life be present before the loss of life can be compensated.[29]

PATRICIA D. WHITE
NANCY L. SCHIMMEL

NOTES TO THE APPENDIX

[1] See Notes 8—11 above.

[2] See, e.g., Stanford v. St. Louis—San Francisco Ry. [215]; Bliss v. Passanesi [127]; Magnolia Coca-Cola Bottling Co. v. Jordan [170].

[3] Some courts professed to be deferring to the authority of the legislature when they dismissed claims for prenatal injury. See, e.g., Allaire v. St. Luke's Hospital ([117] at pp. 367—368); Newman v. City of Detroit ([188], pp. 63 and 711); Stemmer v. Kline ([221], pp. 456 and 489). Nonetheless the operative rule of law had been laid down by Justice Holmes in *Dietrich* [142] when he had construed the statute's use of the word 'person' to exclude an unborn fetus. See [31], p. 1244.

[4] The *Bonbrest* [128] court went to considerable length to distinguish the facts before it from those in *Dietrich* [142]:

"[B]ut on the assumed facts here we have not, as those in the *Dietrich* case, "an injury transmitted from the actor to a person through its own organic substance, or through its mother, before he became a person" . . . but a direct injury to a *viable* child — the distinction is an important one — by the defendants in their professional capacities" ([128], p. 140, footnote omitted).

[5] See, e.g., Alabama (Huskey v. Smith [155]); Connecticut (Tursi v. New England Winsor Co. [229]); District of Columbia (Bonbrest v. Kotz [128]); Ohio (Peterson v. Nationwide Mut. Ins. Co. [194]); Oregon (Mallison v. Pomeroy [171]); South Carolina (Hall v. Murphy [152]); and Tennessee (Shorsha v. Matthews Drivurself Service, Inc. [210]).

[6] See, e.g., cases cited in Note 24 above; California (Scott v. McPheeters [207]); Georgia (Hornbuckle v. Plantation Pipe Line Co. [153]); Maryland (Damasiewicz v. Gorsuch [140]); Massachusetts (Keyes v. Construction Serv. Inc. [168]); Michigan (Womack v. Buchhorn [232]); New Hampshire (Bennett v. Hymers [124]); New Jersey (Smith

v. Brennan [212]); New York (Kelly v. Gregory [167]); Pennsylvania (Sinkler v. Kneale [211]); Rhode Island (Sylvia v. Gobeille [224]); Texas (Yandell v. Delgado [233]); and Washington (Seattle–First Nat'l Bank v. Rankin [208]).

7 For criticism of the viability standard, see generally Babin ([31], pp. 1247–1248); Crockett and Hyman [38]; Ellman *et al.* ([46], pp. 130–133); Estrep and Forgotson [48]; Gordon [54]; White [111]; Rodger [92]; Willia [112]; see also Prosser ([20], pp. 335–338); [61]; [118]; and [119].

8 The states that no longer require viability as a condition precedent to recovery for prenatal injuries include: California (Scott v. McPheeters [205]; Florida (Day v. Nationwide Mut. Ins. Co. [141]); Georgia (Hornbuckle v. Plantation Pipe Line Co. [153]); Maryland (Damasiewicz v. Gorsuch [140]); Massachusetts (Keyes v. Constuction Serv. Inc. [168]); Michigan (Womack v. Buchhorn [232]); New Hampshire (Bennett v. Hymers [124]); New Jersey (Smith v. Brennan [210]); New York (Kelly v. Gregory [167]); Pennsylvania (Sinkler v. Kneale [209]); Rhode Island (Sylvia v. Grobeille [202]); Texas (Yandell v. Delgado [231]); and Washington (Seattle–First Nat'l Bank v. Rankin [206]).

9 See, e.g., Georgia (Porter v. Lassiter [197]); Maryland (Damasiewicz v. Gorsuch [140]); see also Babin ([31], p. 1248, Note 69).

10 Quickening usually occurs between the 16th and 20th weeks of gestation ([12], 311.20).

11 See the discussion of thalidomide in Note 5 above.

12 For a summary of the current controversy over Bendectin, see de St. Jorre in [4].

13 See Prosser ([120], p. 9).

14 For an interesting discussion of actions for preconception torts, see generally [31]; [45]; [82]; and [104].

15 Most courts now recognize a wrongful birth action in this context, See, e.g., Custodio v. Bauer [139]; Sard v. Hardy [206]; Martineau v. Nelson [172]. Cf. Green v. Sudakin [149]. But see Rogala v. Silva [205]. Suits have also been brought against pharmacists for allegedly misfilling a birth control prescription (e.g., Troppi v. Scarf [228]).

16 E.g., Stills v. Gratton [223].

17 E.g., Curlender v. Bio-Science Labs. and Automated Lab. Sciences [138] (lab negligently told parents they did not carry Tay-Sachs genes); Becker v. Schwartz [123] (37-year-old pregnant woman with greater chance of giving birth to deformed child not tested by physician); Park v. Chessin [193] (negligent genetic counseling regarding hereditary kidney disease); Jacobs v. Theimer [164] (physician failed to diagnose rubella in pregnant woman). But see Gleitman v. Cosgrove [147] (no cause of action where physician fails to inform pregnant woman with rubella of risk of birth defects to fetus); but cf. Howard v. Lecher [154] (no cause of action where parents uninformed of risk that their child would be born with Tay-Sachs disease; duty owed only to child not to parents). Wrongful births are discussed in Morris [79]; Munson [81]; Randall [88]; and Sweeney [102].

18 These suits have consistently been dismissed because of the difficulty of ascertaining the damages suffered. See, e.g., Pinkney v. Pinkney ([195] at pp. 53–54); Zepada v. Zepada ([234] at pp. 245–246); Williams v. State [231] (illegitimate child of mentally-deficient mother sued state because conception occurred when mother was raped while a patient at state institution). For discussion of 'wrongful life', see generally [36]; Kashi [62]; Randall [88]; and Mullen [80].

[19] Where a deformed child has sought recovery from its mother's physician for his failure to warn the parents of the increased possibility of birth defects, the courts have dismissed the infant's complaint. See, e.g., Berman v. Allen [126] (physician failed to warn middle-aged woman of likelihood of Down's Syndrome or mongolism; recovery allowed only by parents); see also [88]; Smith v. United States [212]; Gleitman v. Cosgrove [147]; Becker v. Schwartz [123]; discussed in [102]. The gravaman of the infants' complaints in these cases is fairly simply stated – even if not successful. Had the defendant fully informed the parents of the risk of having their child, they would, in order to spare the child its suffering, either not have conceived or have aborted the fetus.

[20] E.g., in both Berman v. Allen [126] and Becker v. Schwartz [123], the parents' claims for relief were upheld. See Randell [88].

[21] See generally Steefel [100]; Slattery [98]; see also Ross [93].

[22] The court was careful to distinguish the facts before it from the self-perpetuating genetic defects that might result from a nuclear explosion or from a chemical accident.

[23] For a discussion of the legal issues surrounding amniocentesis, see generally Friedman [51]. For a brief introduction to the scientific implications of genetic amniocentesis, see Fuchs [52].

[24] See, e.g., Toth v. Goree ([229], p. 302) where the court said:

"If Michigan is to become the first jurisdiction to allow recovery under the wrongful death act on behalf of an unborn three-month-old nonviable fetus, it is a determination for the legislature."

[25] This result was well expressed by the Ohio Court of Appeals in Stidam v. Ashmore ([222], p. 108):

"The test of the existence of that right is that the injury "would have entitled the party injured to maintain an action and recover damages if death had not ensued". If death had not ensued, the child in our present case would have been entitled to maintain an action. We are unable to reconcile the two propositions, that if the death occurred after birth there is a cause of action, but that if it occurred before birth there is none".

[26] See, e.g., Hale v. Hale ([151], p. 683):

"An action under the survival statute is for injury to the person of the deceased, and is in behalf of his estate; whereas an action under the wrongful death statute is for pecuniary loss sustained by the surviving spouse and children (or next of kin) of the deceased and is solely for their benefit".

See also Roe v. Wade ([204], p. 162).

"Such an action [wrongful death], however, would appear to be one to vindicate the parents' interest and is thus consistent with the view that the fetus, at most, represents only the potentiality of life".

[27] Twenty-five jurisdictions now recognize a cause of action for the death of an unborn fetus. All but two (Georgia and Louisiana) require that the child be viable at the time

of the fatal injury. Five jurisdictions impose the additional requirement that the child have been born alive. A few jurisdictions have continued to deny recovery altogether. See cases cited in Crockett and Hyman ([38], pp. 828–829, Notes 142, 143, 146); see generally Cherken [37]; Del Tufo [39]; and Denton [40].

28 See Notes 25 and 26 above. Although the point is obvious, it is probably worth noting that when the infant lives, its damages may·well be susceptible of economic measurement. When it is stillborn,,they are surely not. See generally Hartye ([55], pp. 291–292).

29 Only Georgia has permitted recovery when the fetus was both pre-viable *and* stillborn (Porter v. Lassiter [197]).

BIBLIOGRAPHY

Books and Pamphlets

1. *The Abortion Problem – Proceedings of the Conference Held Under the Auspices of the National Committee on Maternal Health, Inc. at the New York Academy of Medicine* (June 19 and 20, 1942), Williams and Wilkins Co., Baltimore.
2. Barth, K.: 1961, *Church Dogmatics*, Vol. 3, Pt. 4, *The Doctrine of Creation*, T. and T. Clark, Edinburgh, Scotland.
3. Blackstone, W.: 1979, *Commentaries on the Laws of England*, Vols. 1 and 4, University of Chicago Press, Chicago.
4. Blackstone, W. T. (ed.): 1974, *Philosophy and Environmental Crisis*, University of Georgia Press, Athens, Georgia.
5. Bracton, H. de: 1968, *On the Laws and Customs of England* (Woodbine, ed.), The Belknap Press of Harvard University Press, Cambridge, Massachusetts.
6. Brody, B.: 1975, *Abortion and the Sanctity of Human Life: A Philosophical View*, The MIT Press, Cambridge, Massachusetts.
7. Calderone, M. S. (ed.): 1958, *Abortion in the U.S.* (A Conference Sponsored by the Planned Parenthood Federation of America, Inc. at Arden House and the New York Academy of Medicine), Hoeber–Harper Publishers, New York.
8. Cohen, M. *et al.* (eds.): *The Rights and Wrongs of Abortion*, Princeton University Press, Princeton, New Jersey.
9. Coke, E.: 1797, *Institutes of the Laws of England*, Vol. III, E. and R. Brooke, Bell–Yard, England.
10. East River Medical Association: 1871, *Report of Special Committee on Criminal Abortions*, S. W. Green (Printer), New York (from the collection of the National Library of Medicine, Rockville, Md.), cited in Mohr ([17], p. 160).
11. Feinberg, J. (ed.): 1973, *The Problem of Abortion*, Wadsworth Publishing Co., Inc., Belmont, California.
12. Gordy, L. and R. Gray: 1950, *Attorney's Textbook of Medicine*, (3rd ed. and 1977 Supp.) Vol. 4B, Matthew Bender, New York.
13. Grisez, G.: 1970, *Abortion: The Myths, the Realities and the Arguments*, Corpus Books, New York.
14. Hale, M.: 1847, *The History of the Pleas of the Crown* (First American Edition), Vol. 1, Robert H. Small, Philadelphia, Pennsylvania.

15. Hawkins, W.: 1978, *A Treatise of the Pleas of the Crown*, Vol. 1, Garland Publishing, Inc., New York.

16. Huser, R. J.: 1942, *The Crime of Abortion in Canon Law* (The Catholic University of America Canon Law Studies No. 162), Catholic University Press, Washington, D.C.

17. Mohr, J.: 1978, *Abortion in America: The Origins and Evolution of National Policy, 1800–1900*, Oxford University Press, New York.

18. Nolen, W. A.: 1978, *The Baby in the Bottle*, Coward, McCann and Geoghegan, Inc., New York.

19. Noonan, J. T. (ed.): 1970, *The Morality of Abortion: Legal and Historical Perspectives*, Harvard University Press, Cambridge, Massachusetts.

20. Prosser, W. L.: 1971, *Handbook of the Law of Torts* (4th ed.), West Publishing Co., St. Paul, Minnesota.

21. Ross, W. D.: 1930, *The Right and The Good*, Oxford University Press, Oxford.

22. Scoles, E. F. and E. C. Halbach, Jr.: 1973, *Problems and Materials on Decedent's Estates and Trusts*, Little, Brown and Co., Boston, Massachusetts.

23. Smith, D. T. (ed.): 1967, *Abortion and the Law*, The Press of Western Reserve University, Cleveland.

24. Storer, H. R.: 1868, *Criminal Abortion: Its Nature, Its Evolution, and Its Law*, Little, Brown and Co., Boston.

25. Tribe, L. H.: 1978, *American Constitutional Law*, The Foundation Press, Inc., Mineola, New York.

26. White, G. E.: 1978, *Patterns of American Legal Thought*, The Bobbs–Merrill Company, Inc., Charlottesville, Virginia.

27. Wilkerson, A. E. (ed.): 1973, *The Rights of Children – Emergent Concepts in Law and Society*, Temple University Press, Philadelphia, Pennsylvania.

Articles

28. Apgar, V.: 1966, 'The Drug Problem in Pregnancy', *Clinical Obstetrics and Gynecology* 9, 623–630.

29. Arnold, L. C.: 1969, 'Prenatal Injuries: A Treatment and Prognosis of the Law', *DePaul Law Review* 18, 439–457.

30. Atkinson, G. M.: 1977, 'Persons in the Whole Sense', *American Journal of Jurisprudence* 22, 86–117.

31. Babin, P. B.: 1979, 'Note – Preconception Negligence: Reconciling an Emerging Tort', *Georgetown Law Journal* 67, 1239–1261.

32. Baker, T.: 1974, '*Roe* and *Paris*: Does Privacy Have a Principle?', *Stanford Law Review* 26, 1161–1189.

33. Boyle, J. M.: 1979, 'That the Fetus Should be Considered a Legal Person', *American Journal of Jurisprudence* 24, 59–71.

34. Boyle, L. E.: 1971, 'Comment: The Fetus as a Legal Entity – Facing Reality', *San Diego Law Review* 8, 126–137.

35. Byrn, R. M.: 1970, 'Abortion-on-Demand: Whose Morality?', *Notre Dame Lawyer* 46, 5–40.

36. Byrn, R. M.: 1970, 'A Cause of Action for "Wrongful Life": [A Suggested Analysis]', *Minnesota Law Review* 55, 58–81.

37. Cherken, H. S., Jr.: 1975–1976, 'Recent Development: Torts – Wrongful Death-Recovery for Wrongful Death of a Stillborn Fetus Examined', *Villanova Law Review* **21**, 994–1005.
38. Crockett, K. G. and M. Hyman: 1976, 'Note – Live Birth: A Condition Precedent to Recognition of Rights', *Hofstra Law Review* **4**, 805–836.
39. Del Tufo, R. J.: 1960, 'Recovery for Prenatal Torts: Actions for Wrongful Death', *Rutgers Law Review* **15**, 61–80.
40. Denton, D. O.: 1972, 'Torts: Recovery for Prenatal Injury and the Wrongful Death of a Stillborn Fetus', *Tulsa Law Journal* **8**, 84–101.
41. de St. Jorre, J.: 1980, 'The Morning Sickness Drug Controversy', *The New York Times Magazine* (October 12), 113ff.
42. Destro, R. A. *et al.*: 1976–1977, 'A Symposium: On the Report and Recommendations of the National Commission for the Protection of Human Subjects of Biomedical and Behavioral Research', *Villanova Law Review* **22**, 297–417.
43. Devlin, P.: 1962, 'Law, Democracy, and Morality', *University of Pennsylvania Law Review* **110**, 635–649.
44. Diller, W.: 1968, 'Note – The Unborn Child: Consistency in the Law?', *Suffolk Law Review* **2**, 228–243.
45. Duven, D. R.: 1977, 'Note – Torts Prior to Conception: A New Theory of Liability', *Nebraska Law Review* **56**, 706–722.
46. Ellman, I. M. *et al.*: 1980, 'Special Project: Survey of Abortion Law', *Arizona State Law Journal*, 70–216.
47. Ely, J. H.: 1973, 'The Wages of Crying Wolf: A Comment on *Roe v. Wade*', *The Yale Law Journal* **82**, 920–949.
48. Estep, S. D. and E. H. Forgotson: 1963, 'Legal Liability for Genetic Injuries from Radiation', *Louisiana Law Review* **24**, 1–53.
49. Francis, J. J.: 1968, 'Law, Morality, and Abortion', *Rutgers Law Review* **22**, 415–445.
50. Friedman, J. M.: 1977, 'The Federal Fetal Experimentation Regulations: An Establishment Clause Analysis', *Minnesota Law Review* **61**, 961–1005.
51. Friedman, J. M.: 1974, 'Legal Implications of Amniocentesis', *University of Pennsylvania Law Review* **23**, 92–156.
52. Fuchs, F.: 1980, 'Genetic Amniocentesis', *Scientific American* **242**, 47–53.
53. Gerber, R. J.: 1970, 'Abortion: Two Opposing Legal Philosophies', *American Journal of Jurisprudence* **15**, 1–24.
54. Gordon, D. A.: 1965, 'The Unborn Plaintiff', *Michigan Law Review* **63**, 579–627.
55. Hartye, F. J.: 1976–1977, 'Tort Recovery for the Unborn Child', *Journal of Family Law* **15**, 276–299.
56. Heymann, P. B. and D. E. Barzelay: 1973, 'The Forest and the Trees: *Roe v. Wade* and its Critics', *Boston University Law Review* **53**, 765–784.
57. Holper, R. D.: 1969, 'Note – Abortion: Due Process and the Doctor's Dilemma', *Journal of Family Law* **9**, 300–308.
58. Hopkins, W. R., Jr.: 1974, '*Roe v. Wade* and the Traditional Legal Standards Concerning Pregnancy', *Temple Law Quarterly* **47**, 715–738.
59. Hudock, G. A.: 1973, 'Gene Therapy and Genetic Engineering: Frankenstein is Still a Myth, But it Should be Reread Periodically', *Indiana Law Journal* **48**, 533–558.

60. Huser, R.: 1948, 'The Meaning of "Fetus" in Relation to the Crime of Abortion', *The Jurist* 8, 306–322.
61. Huser, R.: 1949, 'Infants – Unborn Children – Liability for Injuries Negligently Inflicted on Viable Unborn Child', *Harvard Law Review* 63, 173–175.
62. Kashi, J. S.: 1977, 'The Case of the Unwanted Blessing: Wrongful Life', *University of Miami Law Review* 31, 1409–1432.
63. Kidder, J.: 'Metaphysics of the Unborn', unpublished paper (Professor Kidder is Professor of Philosophy, Syracuse University).
64. King, J. L.: 1967, 'Note: Criminal Law – Abortion – The "Morning-After Pill" and Other Pre-Implantation Birth-Control Methods and the Law', *Oregon Law Review* 46, 211–218.
65. King, P. A.: 1979, 'The Juridical Status of the Fetus: A Proposal for Legal Protection of the Unborn', *Michigan Law Review* 77, 1647–1688.
66. Knecht, J. A.: 1972, 'A Survey of the Present Statutory and Case Law on Abortion: The Contradictions and the Problem', *Illinois Law Forum*, 177–197.
67. Krimmel, H. T. and M. J. Foley: 1977, 'Abortion: An Inspection into the Nature of Human Life and Potential Consequences of Legalizing its Destruction', *Cincinnati Law Review* 46, 725–821.
68. Leavy, Z. and A. F. Charles: 1967, 'California's New Therapeutic Abortion Act: An Analysis and Guide to Medical and Legal Procedure', *U.C.L.A. Law Review* 15, 1–31.
69. Lenhardt, W. A.: 1974, 'Abortion and Pre-Natal Injury: A Legal and Philosophical Analysis', *Western Ontario Law Review* 13, 97–123.
70. Lenz, W.: 1966, 'Malformations Caused by Drugs in Pregnancy', *American Journal of Diseases in Children* 112, 99–106.
71. Lombard, J. F.: 1968, 'Artificial Insemination – Civil Law and Ecclesiastical Views', *Suffolk Law Review* 2, 137–155.
72. Louisell, D. W.: 1969, 'Abortion, the Practice of Medicine and the Due Process of Law', *U.C.L.A. Law Review* 16, 233–254.
73. Lovell, P. A. and R. H. Griffith–Jones: 1974, ' "The Sins of the Fathers" – Tort Liability for Pre-Natal Injuries', *Law Quarterly Review* 90, 531–558.
74. Martin, M. M.: 1975, 'Ethical Standards for Fetal Experimentation', *Fordham Law Review* 43, 547–570.
75. Means, C. C., Jr.: 1968, 'The Law of N. Y. Concerning Abortion and the Status of the Foetus, 1664–1968: A Case of Cessation of Constitutionality', *New York Law Forum* 14, 411–515.
76. Means, C. C., Jr.: 1971, 'The Phoenix of Abortional Freedom: Is a Penumbral of Ninth Amendment Rights About to Arise from the 19th Century Legislative Ashes of a 14th Century Common-Law Liberty?', *New York Law Forum* 17, 335–410.
77. Meldman, J. A.: 1968, 'Legal Concepts of Human Life', *Marquette Law Review* 52, 105–115.
78. Moore, E. C.: 1971, 'Abortion and Public Policy: What are the Issues?', *New York Law Forum* 17, 411–436.
79. Morris, K. L.: 1976, 'Note: Wrongful Birth in the Abortion Context – Critique of Existing Case Law and Proposal for Future Actions', *Denver Law Journal* 53, 501–520.

80. Mullen, M. J.: 1980, 'Wrongful Life: Birth Control Spawns a Tort', *The John Marshall Law Review* **13**, 401–420.
81. Munson, J. W.: 1975–1976, 'Fetal Research: A View from Right to Life to Wrongful Birth', *Chicago-Kent Law Review* **52**, 133–156.
82. Muse, W. T., and N. A. Spinella: 1950, 'Right of Infant to Recover for Prenatal Injury', *Virginia Law Review* **36**, 611–624.
83. Noonan, J. T., Jr.: 1967, 'Abortion and the Catholic Church: A Summary History', *Natural Law Forum* **12**, 85–131.
84. Noonan, J. T., Jr.: 1968, 'Deciding Who is Human', *Natural Law Forum* **13**, 134–140.
85. 'Obstetrical Malpractice – *Friel v. Vineland Obstetrical and Gynecological Professional Ass'n.*', Comment, 1979–1980, *Journal of Family Law* **18**, 425–431.
86. Paul, E. W. and P. Schaap: 1980, 'Abortion and the Law in 1980', *New York Law School Law Review* **25**, 497–525.
87. Quay, E.: 1961 (Part 2): 'Justifiable Abortion – Medical and Legal Foundations', *Georgetown Law Journal* **49**, 395–538.
88. Randall, K. C.: 1979, 'Comment: *Berman v. Allen* – Wrongful Birth and Wrongful Life', *Hofstra Law Review* **8**, 257–272.
89. Reback, G. L.: 1974, 'Fetal Experimentation: Moral, Legal and Medical Implications', *Stanford Law Review* **26**, 1191–1207.
90. Regan, D. H.: 1979, 'Rewriting *Roe v. Wade*', *Michigan Law Review* **77**, 1569–1646.
91. Robinson, W. T., III: 1970, 'Comment: Criminal Law – Abortion – Man, Being Without a Legal Beginning: *People v. Belous*', *Kentucky Law Journal* **58**, 843–850.
92. Rodger, A.: 1974, 'Case and Comment: Report of the Scottish Law Commission on Antenatal Injury', *Juridical Review*, 83–90.
93. Ross, J. L.: 1978, 'Torts – Negligence – Infant May Maintain a Cause of Action for Prenatal Injuries Resulting from a Negligent Act Prior to Infant's Conception – *Renslow v. Mennonite Hospital*', *Texas Tech. Law Review* **9**, 715–732.
94. St. Clair, A.: 1871, 'The Evil of the Age', *The New York Times* (August 23).
95. Schroeder, O. C., Jr., *et al.*: 1965, 'Symposium: Abortion and the Law', *Western Reserve Law Review* **17**, 366–568.
96. Shaffer, T. L.: 1967, 'Abortion, the Law and Human Life', *Valparaiso University Law Review* **2**, 94–106.
97. Shaman, J. M.: 1979–1980, 'Legal Aspects of Artificial Insemination', *Journal of Family Law* **18**, 331–351.
98. Slattery, M. K.: 1977, 'Note – *Renslow v. Mennonite Hospital*: Prenatal Injuries and a Pre-Existence Duty', *John Marshall Journal of Practice and Procedure* **10**, 417–436.
99. Smith, G. P., II: 1968, 'Through a Test Tube Darkly: Artificial Insemination and the Law', *Michigan Law Review* **67**, 127–150.
100. Steefel, D. S.: 1977, 'Comment – Preconception Torts: Foreseeing the Unconceived, *Renslow v. Mennonite Hospital*', *University of Colorado Law Review* **48**, 621–649.
101. Storer, H. *et al.*: 1859, 'Report on Criminal Abortion', *Transactions of the American Medical Association* **XII**, 75–78.

102. Sweeney, G. W.: 1979, 'Medical Malpractice: Wrongful Birth − Preconception Torts − Duty to Inform of Genetic Risks − *Becker v. Schwartz*', *Akron Law Review* 13, 390−400.
103. Tooley, M.: 1972, 'Abortion and Infanticide', *Philosophy and Public Affairs* 2, reprinted in Cohen *et al.* ([8], pp. 52−84).
104. 'Trial Lawyers Address New Practice Methods', *1979 American Bar Association Journal*, p. 1300.
105. Tribe, L. H.: 1973, 'Foreward: Toward a Model of Roles in the Due Process of Life and Law', *Harvard Law Review* 87, 1−53.
106. 'The Unborn Child and the Constitutional Conception of Life', Note, 1971, *Iowa Law Review* 56, 994−1014.
107. Vukowich, W. T.: 1971, 'The Dawning of the Brave New World − Legal, Ethical and Social Issues of Eugenics', *Illinois Law Forum*, 189−231.
108. Wangard, R. E.: 1968, 'Note: Artificial Insemination and the Law', *Illinois Law Forum*, 203−231.
109. Weiler, K. M. and K. Catton: 1976, 'The Unborn Child in Canadian Law', *Osgoode Hall Law Journal* 14, 643−659.
110. Wertheimer, R.: 1971, 'Understanding the Abortion Argument', *Philosophy and Public Affairs*, reprinted in Cohen *et al.* ([8], pp. 23−51).
111. White, A. A.: 1952, 'The Right of Recovery for Prenatal Injuries', *Louisiana Law Review* 12, 383−406.
112. Willia, R.: 1973, 'Comment − Negligence and the Unborn Child: A Time for Change', *South Dakota Law Review* 18, 204−220.
113. Winfield, P. H.: 1942, 'The Unborn Child', *The University of Toronto Law Journal* 4, 278−295.
114. Wood, M. A. and L. B. Hawkins: 1980, 'State Regulation of Late Abortion and the Physician's Duty of Care to the Viable Fetus', *Missouri Law Review* 45, 394−422.

Cases and Statutes

115. *Abrams v. Foshee*, 3 Iowa 274 (1863).
116. Ala. Rev. Code, Pt. 4, Tit. 1, Ch. 5, Section 3605 (1867).
117. *Allaire v. St. Luke's Hospital*, 184 Ill. 359, 56 N.E. 638 (1900).
118. *Annot.*, 40 A.L.R.3d 122 (1971).
119. *Annot.*, 70 A.L.R.3d 315 (1976).
120. Ariz. Rev. Stat. (Pen. Code) Section 455 (1887).
121. Ark. Rev. Stat. Ch. 44, Div. III, Art. II, Section 6 (1838).
122. *Barnett v. Pinkston*, 238 Ala. 327, 191 So. 371 (1939).
123. *Becker v. Schwartz*, 46 N.Y.2d 401, 386 N.E.2d 807, 413 N.Y.2d 895 (1978).
124. *Bennett v. Hymers*, 101 N.H. 483 A.2d 108 (1958).
125. *Bergstresser v. Mitchell*, 577 F.2d 22 (8th Cir. 1978).
126. *Berman v. Allen*, 80 N.J. 421, 404 A.2d 8 (1981).
127. *Bliss v. Passanesi*, 326 Mass. 461, 463, 95 N.E.2d 206 (1950).
128. *Bonbrest v. Kotz*, 65 F. Supp. 138 (D.D.C. 1946).
129. *Buel v. United Rys. Co.*, 248 Mo. 126, 154 S.W. 71 (1913).

130. Cal. Penal Code Section 187 (West Supp. 1979).
131. Cal. Penal Code Section 275 (Deering 1886).
132. *Colautti v. Franklin*, 439 U.S. 379 (1979).
133. Colo. Gen. Laws, Joint Res., mem., and Priv. Acts of the Terr. of Colo. Legis. Asm., 1st Sess., Section 42 (1861).
134. *Commonwealth v. Bangs*, 9 Mass. 387 (1812).
135. *Commonwealth v. Luceba Parker*, 50 Mass. (9 Met.) 263 (1845).
136. Conn. Pub. Acts Ch. LXXXI, Section 3 (1860).
137. Conn. Stat. Tit. 22, Section 14 (1921).
138. *Curlender v. Bio-Science Labs. and Automated Lab. Sciences*, 106 Cal. App. 3d 811 (1980).
139 *Custodio v. Bauer*, 251 Cal. App. 2d 303, 59 Cal. Rptr. 463 (1967).
140. *Damasiewicz v. Gorsuch*, 197 Md. 417, 79 A.2d 550 (1951).
141. *Day v. Nationwide Mut. Ins. Co.*, 328 So. 2d 560 (Fla. Dist. Ct. App. 1976).
142. *Dietrich v. Northhampton*, 138 Mass. 14 (1884).
143. *Doe v. Bolton*, 410 U.S. 179 (1973).
144. *Evans v. The People*, 49 N.Y. 86 (1892).
145. *Foster v. State*, 182 Wis. 298, 196 N.W. 233 (1923).
146. Ga. Code Ann., Section 26–1201–03 (1971).
147. *Gleitman v. Cosgrove*, 49 N.Y. 22, 227 A.2d 689 (1967).
148. *Gorman v. Budlong*, 23 R.I. 169, 49 A. 704 (1901).
149. *Green v. Sudakia*, 81 Mich. App. 545, 265 N.W.2d 411 (1978).
150. *Griswold v. Connecticut*, 381 U.S. 479 (1965).
151. *Hale v. Hale*, 426 P.2d 681 (Okla. 1976).
152. *Hall v. Murphy*, 236 S.C. 257, 11 S.E.2d 790 (1960).
153. *Hornbuckle v. Plantation Pipe Line Co.*, 212 Ga. 504, 93 S.E.3d 727 (1956).
154. *Howard v. Lecher*, 42 N.Y.2d 109, 366 N.E.2d 64, 397 N.Y.S.2d 363 (1977).
155. *Huskey v. Smith*, 289 Ala. 52, 265 So. 2d 596 (1972).
156. Idaho Rev. Stat. (Pen. Code) Section 6795 (1887).
157. Ill. Pub. Laws Sections 1 and 2 (1867).
158. Ill. Rev. Code Section 46 (1827).
159. *In re Roberts' Estate*, 158 Misc. 698, 700, 286 N.Y.S. 476, 478 (Sur. Ct. N.Y. Cy. 1963).
160. *In re Well's Will*, 129 Misc. 447, 221 N.Y.S. 714 (Sur. Ct. Westchester Cy. 1927).
161. Ind. Laws Ch. XXXVIII, Section 23 (1881).
162. Iowa (Terr.) Stat. 1st Legis., 1st Sess., Section 18 (1838).
163. *Jackson v. Commonwealth*, 256 Ky. 295, 96 S.W.2d 1014 (1936).
164. *Jacobs v. Theimer*, 519 S.W.2d 846 (Tex. 1975).
165. *Journal of the Senate of the 57th Gen'l Ass'y of the State of Ohio*, App. 233–235 (1867).
166. *Keeler v. Superior Ct. of Amador County*, 2 Cal. 3d 619, 470 P.2d 617, 87 Cal. Rptr. 481 (1970).
167. *Kelly v. Gregory*, 282 App. Div. 542, 125 N.Y.S.2d 696 (3d Dep't. 1953).
168. *Keyes v. Construction Serv. Inc.*, 340 Mass. 633, 165 N.E.2d 912 (1960).
169. *Kimbro v. Harper*, 113 Okla. 46, 238 P. 840 (1925).
170. *Magnolia Coca-Cola Bottling Co. v. Jordan*, 124 Tex. 347, 78 S.W.2d 944 (1938).
171. *Mallison v. Pomeroy*, 205 Ore. 690, 291 P.2d 225 (1955).

172. *Martineau v. Nelson*, 311 Minn. 92, 247 N.W.2d 409 (1976).
173. Mass. Acts and Resolves Ch. 27 (1845).
174. Me. Rev. Stat. Ch. 160, Sections 13 and 14 (1840).
175. *Mills v. Commonwealth*, 13 Pa. 631 (1850).
176. Minn. Stat. at large Vol. II, Ch. 54, Section 29, Para. 3 at 987 (1873).
177. *Mitchell v. Comm'r*, 78 Ky. 204 (1879).
178. *Montreal Tramways v. Leveille*, 4 D.L.R. 337 (1933).
179. *Morgan v. State*, 148 Tenn. 417, 256 S.W. 433 (1923).
180. N. H. Laws Ch. 743, Section 4 at 708 (1848).
181. N. J. Rev. Stat. Section 3 (1838).
182. N. Y. Gen. Stats. Ch. 181, Section 181, Para. 1 at 71 (1872).
183. N. Y. Laws Ch. 260, Sections 3 and 4 at 285 (1845).
184. N. Y. Laws Ch. 22, Section 1 at 19 (1846).
185. N. Y. Laws Ch. 631, Section 1 at 502 (1869).
186. N. Y. Laws Ch. 181, Section 2 at 71 (1872).
187. N. Y. Rev. Stat. Pt. IV, Ch. 1 (1828–1835).
188. *Newman v. City of Detroit*, 281 Mich. 60, 274 N.W. 710 (1937).
189. *Nugent v. Brooklyn Hghts. Railroad Co.*, 154 A.D. 667, 139 N.Y.S. 367 (1913).
190. Ohio Gen. Stat. Sections 111 (1), 112 (2) (1841).
191. Ore. Gen. Laws Crim. Code, Ch. 43, Section 509 (1845–1864).
192. Pa. Laws No. 374, Sections 87–89 (1860).
193. *Park v. Chessin*, 60 A.D.2d 80, 400 N.Y.S.2d 110 (2d Dept. 1977); *modified* 46 N.Y.2d 401, 386 N.E.2d 807, 413 N.Y.S.2d 895 (1978).
194. *Peterson v. Nationwide Mut. Ins. Co.*, 175 Ohio St. 551, 197 N.E.2d 194 (1964).
195. *Pinkney v. Pinkney*, 198 So. 2d 52 (Fla. Dist. Ct. App. 1967).
196. *Planned Parenthood v. Danforth*, 428 U.S. 52 (1976).
197. *Porter v. Lassiter*, 91 Ga. App. 712, 87 S.E.2d 100 (1955).
198. *Renslow v. Mennonite Hospital*, 10 Ill. Dec. 484 (1976).
199. *Renslow v. Mennonite Hospital*, 40 Ill. App. 3d 234, 351 N.E.2d 870 (1976).
200. *Renslow v. Mennonite Hospital*, 67 Ill. 2d 348, 367 N.E.2d 1250 (1977).
201. *Rex v. Enoch and Pulley*, 5 Carr. and Pay. 539, 24 E.C.L.R. 696 (1833).
202. *Rex v. Poulton*, 5 Carr. and Pay. 329, 24 E.C.L.R. 590 (1832).
203. *Rex v. Pritchard*, 17 T.L.R. 310 (1901).
204. *Roe v. Wade*, 410 U.S. 113 (1973).
205. *Rogala v. Silva*, 16 Ill. App. 3d 63, 305 N.E.2d 571 (1973).
206 *Sard v. Hardy*, 281 Md. 432, 379 A.2d 1014 (1977).
207 *Scott v. McPheeters*, 33 Cal. App. 2d 629, 92 P.2d 678, *hearing denied*, 33 Cal. App. 2d 640, 93 P.2d (1939).
208. *Seattle-First Nat'l Bank v. Rankin*, 59 Wash. 2d 288, 367 P.2d 835 (1962).
209. *Shedd v. State*, 178 Ga. 653, 173 S.E. 847 (1934).
210. *Shorsha v. Matthews Drivurself Service, Inc.*, 210 Tenn. 384, 358 S.W.2d 471 (1962).
211. *Sinkler v. Kneale*, 401 Pa. 267, 164 A.2d 93 (1960).
212. *Smith v. Brennan*, 31 N.J. 353, 157 A.2d 497 (1960).
213. *Smith v. Gaffard*, 31 Ala. 45 (1857).
214. *Smith v. United States*, 392 F. Supp. 654 (N.D. Ohio 1975).

215. *Stanford v. St. Louis–San Francisco Ry.*, 214 Ala. 611, 108 So. 566 (1926).
216. *State v. Carey*, 76 Conn. 342 (1904).
217. *State v. Cooper*, 22 N.J.L. 52 (1849).
218. *State v. Murphy*, 17 N.J.L. 112 (1858).
219. *State v. Slagle*, 83 N.C. 544 (1880).
220. *State v. Winthrop*, 43 Iowa 519, 22 Am. Rep. 257 (1876).
221. *Stemmer v. Kline*, 128 N.J.L. 455, 26 A.2d 489 (1942).
222. *Stidam v. Ashmore*, 108 Ohio App. 431, 167 N.E.2d 106 (1959).
223. *Stills v. Gratton*, 55 Cal. App. 3d 698, 127 Cal. Rptr. 652 (1976).
224. *Sylvia v. Gobeille*, 101 R.I. 73, 220 A.2d 222 (1966).
225. *Thellusson v. Woodward*, 4 Ves. 322, 31 Eng. Rep. 117 (1799).
226. *Tomlin v. Laws*, 301 Ill. 616, 134 N.E. 24 (1922).
227. *Toth v. Goree*, 65 Mich. App. 296, 237 N.W.2d 297 (1975).
228. *Troppi v. Scarf*, 31 Mich. App. 240, 187 N.W.2d 511 (1971).
229. *Tursi v. New England Windsor Co.*, 19 Conn. Supp. 242, 111 A.2d 14 (1955).
230. *Walker v. Grt. No. Ry. of Ireland*, 28 L.R. Ir. 69 (Q.B. 1891).
231. *Williams v. State*, 18 N.Y.2d 481, 482–84, 223 N.E.2d 342, 343–44, 276 N.Y.S. 2d 885, 886–87 (1966).
232. *Womack v. Buchhorn*, 384 Mich. 718, 187 N.W.2d 218 (1971).
233. *Yandell v. Delgado*, 468 S.W.2d 475 (Tex. Civ. App. 1971).
234. *Zepada v. Zepada*, 41 Ill. App. 2d 240, 245–46, 262, 190 N.E.2d 849, 851, 859 (1963), *cert. denied*, 379 U.S. 945 (1964).

GERALD T. PERKOFF

TOWARD A NORMATIVE DEFINITION OF PERSONHOOD

When is a person a person? How does a society provide an answer to this serious and challenging question? What place does the law have in the definition of such important states of man that all else which flows subsequent to the definition is changed? These are only a few of the questions occasioned by the two preceding essays. As I discuss this subject it will be evident immediately that I am not a lawyer, a philosopher, or a theologian. My comments, therefore, will be those only of an interested clinical observer who has tried to understand the reasoning of others who have considered this difficult topic.

My task was not easy. I had hoped to find the law clear on one or two definitions of personhood so that we might have been able to adopt one or another view. However, it turns out that this is not the case. Both Professors Glantz [9] and White [24] agree that the concept of personhood has not been dealt with directly in legal precedent. Indeed, most often it is not even mentioned. Instead the subject has been dealt with in more general ways by defining the rights of the fetus in various circumstances under criminal and civil law. Therefore, we cannot depend completely upon the law to guide us.

For my remarks, therefore, I will draw upon other major views about the person which might assist physicians and others who make decisions about fetal life, termination of such life, and fetal experimentation. Such views come not from the law, but from philosophic, theologic, anthropologic, and modern lay literature and are useful both in their own right and to help us see functional roles for the law and for physicians in this complex arena.

Several key papers on personhood are cited by almost all philosophers and non-philosophers alike. Like the theologic and cultural views to be cited below, these papers are remarkably varied and range from the most conservative to the most radical. For example, Noonan [17] considers that the historical basis for what he calls the 'Christian position' is

a refusal to discriminate among human beings on the basis of their varying potentialities. Once conceived, the being was recognized as man because he has man's potential. The

159

William B. Bondeson et al. *(eds.), Abortion and the Status of the Fetus,* 159–166.

criterion for humanity, thus, was simple and all embracing: if you are conceived by human parents, you are human ([17], p. 53).

Noonan never mentions personhood *per se* but by implication he includes this in the concept 'human'. He discusses various other criteria which have been used to distinguish the non-human (or non-person) from the human and then discards them all. He recognizes, however, a substantial Christian tradition, which held that taking the life of a fetus early in gestation was not murder, i.e., not the taking of a life of a human, a concept evidently in rough synonymity with 'person'. Noonan holds that being 'of humans' makes one human, or in other words, a person. Ramsey [19] makes this scientifically explicit, reasoning that each specific genetic code is unique and identifies that 'human individual', a term he nevertheless distinguishes from human person.

At the other extreme of the spectrum is Tooley [23] who makes such a strict definition that even an extra-uterine baby may not be considered a person. Tooley's single criterion for personhood is that to be a person one must have a "serious moral right to life" as determined by the "self-con-sciousness requirement", i.e., the individual can "experience" and is capable of "desiring to exist as a subject of experiences and other mental states" ([23], p. 44). Since such a definition excludes newborns as well as fetuses, Tooley uses this concept as a basis for justifying *infanticide* as well as abor-tion. Another aspect of his work is noteworthy: he clearly differentiates between human (a biologic term), and a person (a social term), and in so doing contributes a conceptual refinement to Noonan's reflections. Others take an intermediate view, identifying the fetus either as something other than a person, or alternatively, as something deleterious to the mother on any of several grounds, entitling her to abortion on the grounds of 'self defense'. The conception of the fetus as an 'aggressor' is part of the history both of Catholic and Jewish tradition as well ([8], [14], [16], [20]). Although these views comprise only a small sample, we can see already that philosophic writings on this subject are extremely varied.

Theologic views about personhood also have changed over time. The current view of the Catholic Church is that from the moment of fertilization the fetal material is human, it has the complete potential of becoming a person, that it is thus alive or, perhaps better stated, is a life. Therefore, it cannot be treated in any way different from an extra-uterine person.

As well known and as absolute as this view is, it arises from a Catholic history in which respected authorities held different views. St. Thomas

Aquinas believed killing an ensouled embryo was homicide [22], but that ensoulment did not take place at conception [21]. Other writers placed a stigma only on the abortion of a 'formed or animated fetus', animation occurring from 40 to 90 days after conception [11]. The modern statement of church doctrine as it exists today dates only from 1869 [18]: as late as 1860, abortion still was occurring frequently among Catholic women [15].

The situation with the Orthodox Jewish faith is somewhat, but not entirely, different. Like other aspects of Orthodoxy, the teaching about abortion has been consistent throughout the ages and is unchanged today. The Talmud clearly gives the mother precedence over the baby in the instance of a medical crisis involving birth until the baby's head emerges. When that happens, the precedence shifts immediately to the child, even though the entire baby's body may yet be contained within the birth canal. Until that moment, even dismemberment of the baby is considered acceptable if it is essential to save the mother's life [14]. Jewish law also contains other citations consistent with the view that ensoulment may occur at varied times, implying the fetus before that time is not a person [13].

While no specific statement about personhood is made in these rules, placing the mother first is strong evidence that the baby and the mother were not considered equal in classical Orthodox Jewish teaching. Further, neither Orthodox nor other branches of Judaism give full status to the fetus until 30 days after birth (*Kitzur Shulhan Arukh*, Section 203, paragraph 3). During this period, one which is longer than the ten day wait for circumcision and the formal naming ceremony, or 'bris', one is not obliged to observe laws of mourning if the child dies. The concepts of life, humanness, and person somehow are different under Jewish law, though the subtle meanings are hotly disputed [1].

Other, later branches of the Jewish religion take a more liberal view, reflecting the more secular society in which the members of those sects find themselves [3]. They hold that the fetus is not a full human person. Such divergent views have special importance for us as we consider defining personhood. Even theologic teachings within single religions give examples and rules subject to extremely varied interpretations.

Protestant teachings show a similar dichotomy. Joining together, several churches as recently as September 11, 1980, shared a full-page advertisement in the *Columbia Daily Tribune* (Missouri) which asserted that 'babies' are 'alive' from the moment of conception, and that abortion is the same as euthanasia and/or infanticide after birth [6]. More moderate Protestant views also exist, analogous in every way to the Orthodox-Reform dichotomy just described for the Jewish religion. In each instance different positions have been taken by branches of churches which see themselves differently in relation to society.

Variations in major cultural determinants of what we are here calling personhood also may give us pause as we try to decide upon any firm relationship between fetus and personhood. I will cite several examples. The first fits the commonly held belief that primitive tribes recognize the fragility of a newborn infant by waiting a bit before naming it, giving it rights, and accepting it into the tribe. J. W. Hamilton, of the University of Missouri, studied the Pwo Karen, a tribe located in northern Thailand [10]. In that culture a series of ritually defined life-cycle states signal changes in role and status in the society. The first, conception-birth, extends into the first few days after birth when the child is not yet considered human. This is because life is so precarious and the chance of survival is so slim. However, there is more to it than this, because the second stage, baby-child, does not just happen by time lapse. It is signaled by a ritual involving the capturing of a soul, which is enticed into the body of the child. Only after this ceremony is the child considered human, and by implication, a person.

Thomas Rhys Williams, in his book on Borneo's Dusun people, describes a culture which does not name babies until they are two years of age [25]. At that point a series of rituals is carried out expressly to create character in the baby. This ultimately leads to the naming itself. These rituals are performed by a specialist with the express purpose of shaping and directing the maturation of the infant's character and reason, i.e., to "build a person". Even more striking is the quote from one Dusun who stated that, "If I give the infant a name and he dies, we have lost him". Thus, the unnamed, unformed being is considered less than a full human person, and a loss before naming is considered less of a loss than the loss of a named infant. At age two everyone in our culture would consider a child a person in every sense of that word.

Jocano describes the difference between a baptized and unbaptized child in a Philippine culture as follows: Unbaptized children "are considered half-human, their popular nickname being Muritu (not yet human). Such babies are viewed as constitutionally weak and are susceptible to illness. They do not yet enjoy the protective concern of their guardian angels. Should they die, their soul cannot enter heaven" [12]. In this group, the baptized child is considered strong and prepared for heaven. If a baptized child dies, the parents are assured they have done all they can do for the child. If the unbaptized child dies, in this culture, there is more concern and grief, for the parents may believe they have committed a mortal sin by not preparing the child.

Also striking is Indian Hindu Vedic law which describes a tradition more than 1500 years old in which naming, age, and personhood are separated. For example, naming ceremonies may take place anywhere from the 10th to the 21st day of life in a formal sacramental rite not dissimilar to the 10th day circumcision rite of the Jewish faith. If a child dies before being named, the funeral does not require libations or even cremation, an important ceremony accorded the named [4]. Such an unnamed death is of a different kind of entity. Even more interesting is the practice of conducting ritual teaching for a child up to age 12, 13, or even 16 or more years before permitting initiation of the child as a member of the parent's caste. This is a legal procedure without which the child cannot participate in rituals and does not have rights [5]. Again, though personhood is not mentioned *per se*, the clear implication is that until initiation takes place the individual is less than a full person in the eyes of his or her culture and laws.

Thus the arguments of philosophers and physicians notwithstanding, anthropologic and theologic evidence suggests that notions of what constitutes a person in the strict sense range all the way from assignment of rights to zygotes on the basis of the potential for later development of full personhood to the withholding of that designation until an individual has had formal teachings designed to make him or her a person at or near the age of puberty. Such a wide range of practices, all of them supported by hundreds to thousands of years of precedent, to use the legal term, tell us that there is no likely agreement to be found about the definition of personhood.

To underscore the difference of opinion which this brief review reveals, I offer a citation from a recent media presentation [2]. Last year a one hour program was broadcast nationally on commercial television in which the structure and function of the human eye was presented in beautiful detail. Each point was illustrated with imagination and creativity. As part of the explanation of the function of the eye, a fiberoptic endoscope was introduced into the uterus of a pregnant woman to view the reactions of a 12 week fetus to the bright light and to show the stage of development of the eye at that point in pregnancy. The fetus was pale and clearly visible. The eyes, which as yet had no lids, were obvious, as were the ear slits, still located low on the neck before migration upward to the permanent location they would later occupy. The fetus's hands, still encased in an enveloping membrane, showed well demarcated fingers and thumbs. And every time the bright light from the fiberoptic scope shone on the fetus's face, the head turned away, and the hands were raised to cover the lidless eyes. This happened not once but several times. Despite beliefs about abortion and personhood, almost no one from our modern Western culture could avoid the instinctive conclusion that what was being shown was a small person, even though they might believe in an abstract or intellectual view that what they were seeing was only a human body.

Thus it seems to me that as long as we have many groups of many different backgrounds making up our culture, that we should expect controversy about this issue. Only in social groups which hold a single set of views and practices, such groups as small tribes or single religious sects or groups, is there agreement about what a person is.

Can the law help us as physicians to deal with this complex issue? Our essayists tell us that the law has made only general statements about personhood and that legal decisions about the fetus have been made without dependence on the issue of fetus's personhood. What then is the function of the law? As indicated by these attorneys, that function is to set limits which define what can and cannot be done in a society and to monitor those doings. In this sense, the law is an expression of the culture in which it exists. That this should be so for personhood is appropriate and functional. For the law establishes reasonably consistent rules for behavior in the general area of the person without having to define personhood formally. This leaves the law open to modification either because the majority view changes or because a society may exceed boundaries generally held to be acceptable for related kinds of behavior.

One can be reasonably comfortable with this approach in a society in which all have a free opportunity to speak, argue, discuss, persuade and where all have equal access to the courts. To a great extent, though not completely, our own society qualifies on these counts. However, the poor and the minorities in our country have much less access to free forums for discussion, financial support, and legal assistance in this area than do others. And current attempts to legislate a definition of the start of life, particularly when viewed against the remarkably varied social background I have described, are disquieting. We may be seeing abrogation of the limit-setting and monitoring roles of the law despite opinion opposing such a move.

What of the physician now faced with a body of experts failing to agree on a universally held definition of personhood? How should he or she behave when faced with clinical and research decisions which depend in part upon one's concept of personhood? Here is where such deliberations as ours can help. Together with our legal, philosophic, anthropologic, and theologic colleagues, we must develop a step-wise reasoning system which we can follow to help patients and ourselves come to agreement about which concept of personhood should prevail for any given situation. The beliefs of the patient and physician must be tested for a match/mismatch. If a serious mismatch exists and there is no way to correct it, the physician should exclude him or herself from participation in that patient's decision-making process or get assistance from others for that process. There are two methods for doing just that in medicine. The first involves the careful and imaginative use of the consultant-referral process which is a basic part of medicine whenever the knowledge or opinion upon which the physician bases his or her recommendations is incomplete or inappropriate to the immediate situation. The second involves the culturally and socially aware physician in a process of advocacy for the patient. The physician must identify in his or her own community the various people sympathetic to various theological and cultural views. Priests, ministers, and rabbis exist in most communities who are interested both in doctrinal thought and in sensitive, humane counseling. Social workers who know different cultures must be involved; patients themselves may serve in this role for other patients. The physician may find it possible to guide action and assuage guilt by reviewing with patients applicable parts of the very information assembled for this commentary so as to assure the patient that her action fits with norms of the culture from which she comes. The law must be made clear to the patient as well. The physician has the responsibility to build the support system which can serve as a surrogate culture for the patient in need. Such an approach has been tried in other sensitive circumstances with benefit [7] .

We frequently argue for more personal involvement of physicians with patients. In contrast here, the doctors' personal beliefs about personhood are not critical, those of the patient are. Personhood is one area in which the physician must partially remove him or herself from the fray, avoiding imposition of his or her personal value system on the patient. In this way we can, indeed must, take advantage of our strength in diversity.

University of Missouri–Columbia,
Columbia, Missouri

BIBLIOGRAPHY

1. Bleich, J. D.: 1975, 'Critique of Brickner, B., Judaism and Abortion', *Sh'ma* 5, 85.

2. *The Body Human Series: The Magic Sense*, 1980, Columbia Broadcasting System (September 8).
3. Brickner, B.: 1974, 'Judaism and Abortion', Testimony before the Bayh Senate Subcommittee on Constitutional Amendments, March 7.
4. Buhler, G. (trans.): 1969, *The Laws of Manu*, V, 68, 69, 70, Dover Publications, Inc., New York, p. 180.
5. Buhler, G. (trans.): 1969, *The Laws of Manu*, II, 36, 37, 38, Dover Publications, Inc., New York, p. 36–37.
6. *Columbia Daily Tribune*, September 11, 1980, p. 5.
7. Duff, R. S. and A. G. M. Campell: 1973, 'Moral and Ethical Dilemmas in a Special-Care Nursery', *New England Journal of Medicine* 189, 890–894.
8. English, J.: 1975, 'Abortion and the Concept of Person', *Canadian Journal of Philosophy* 5, 233–243.
9. Glantz, L. H.: 1982, 'Is the Fetus a Person: A Lawyer's View', in this volume, pp. 107–117.
10. Hamilton, J. W.: 1976, *Pwo Karen at the Edge of Mountain and Plain*, West Publishing Co., St. Paul Minnesota.
11. Innocent III, 1211.
12. Jocano, F. L.: 1969, *Growing Up in a Philippine Barrio*, Holt, Rhinehart, and Winston and Co., New York, p. 15.
13. Midrash T'hallim, *ad loc*, 25.
14. Mishnah Ahiloth 7: 6.
15. Mohr, J. C.: 1978, *Abortion in America: The Origins and Evolution of National Policy*, Oxford University Press, Inc., Oxford, England, p. 243.
16. Noam, Vol. VII (1964), pp. 36–56.
17. Noonan, J. T., Jr.: 1970, 'An Almost Absolute Value in History', in J. T. Noonan, Jr. (ed.), *The Morality of Abortion: Legal and Historical Perspectives*, Harvard University Press, Cambridge, Mass., pp. 51–59.
18. Pius IX, *Ineffabilis Deus*, Denzinger, Note 113.
19. Ramsey. P.: 1968, 'The Morality of Abortion', in D. H. Labby (ed.), *Life or Death: Ethics and Options*, University of Washington Press, Seattle, Wash., pp. 60–93.
20. Sanchez, T.: 1737, *De Sancto Matrimonia Sacramento*, Venice, 9.22.
21. St. Thomas Aquinas, *Libros Sententiarum* 3.1.3.
22. St. Thomas Aquinas, *Summa Theologica* (Leonine ed.) 2.2. 64. 8.
23. Tooley, M.: 1971, 'Abortion and Infanticide', *Philosophy and Public Affairs* 2, 37–65.
24. White, P. D.: 1982, 'The Concept of Persons in the Law: Its Implications for the Use of the Fetus', in this volume, pp. 119–157.
25. Williams, T. R.: 1969, *A Borneo Childhood: Enculturation in Dusun Society*, Holt, Rhinehart, and Winston and Co., New York, p. 87.

SECTION III

HUMANHOOD, PERSONHOOD, AND THE CONCEPT
OF VIABILITY

ROLAND PUCCETTI

THE LIFE OF A PERSON

When one reflects on the life of a person, it becomes immediately apparent that this can be done in two very different ways. One way is to look upon the person as a particular organism with a spatiotemporal history of its own; there the identity question is approached from the outside, so to speak, and differs not at all from questions about the identity of material objects though time. The other way is to look upon the person's life history as the total span of conscious experience that this person has had; here identity is approached from the inside, whether it be your own life you are reflecting on, or that of another person. It was Lucretius' contention, in Book III of *De Rerum Natura*, that since good or harm can accrue only to a subject of conscious experiences, the latter is the correct view and the former leads to superstition.

I am inclined to think Lucretius was right about this, that personal life is ineluctably shorter at both ends than the life of the organism which is the biological substrate of the person, because developmental processes at the beginning and degenerative processes at the end of organic life are insufficient to support conscious functions, and without these nothing done to the living tissue has personal value or disvalue. But to bring out the intuitive force of Lucretius' position, consider the following parable.

1. THE GENIE'S BARGAIN

Suppose that one day a genie appears before you and convincingly displays magical powers. Now he tells you that he will, if you want, expand your brain so that you will have an IQ of 400. This means that whatever you're interested in achieving will come within easy grasp, whether it be leadership of state, heading a conglomerate, outpainting Picasso or getting a Nobel Prize in medicine. However, he explains, there is one hitch. If you want him to do this for you, you will at the moment of brain expansion cease forever to have conscious experience. No one will know this, for he will program your brain to make all the correct responses to questions, etc. Nevertheless the great future achiever will be an automaton and no more. Would you accept this offer?

169

William B. Bondeson et al. *(eds.), Abortion and the Status of the Fetus*, 169–182.
Copyright © *1983 by D. Reidel Publishing Company, Dordrecht, Holland.*

I have tried this out on several groups of students and it is amazing how uniform the reaction has been. A few say they would accept the bargain, but upon probing it turns out they have in mind an altruistic act that might lead to discovering a cure for cancer or building world government. They, as well as the majority who refused, all agreed that accepting would be tantamount to personal annihilation, at least in this world, and that one could indeed doubt that wholly unconscious achieving automata with their bodies would still be *them*. But if this is correct, and given that the one and same living organism persists from conscious to permanently unconscious activity, it appears bodily continuity through time is not a sufficient condition of personal identity, whereas continuity of consciousness is, and that without even a capacity for conscious experience there is no person any more.

Let us now apply the same lesson to the other end of the life spectrum. Suppose the genie tells you that you are the reincarnation of Napoleon Bonaparte, whose life you happen to admire greatly. You protest that this can't be, since you have no recollection of doing the things Napoleon did, or experiencing his triumphs and defeats. The genie replies that of course you do not because as a young man Napoleon accepted the genie's bargain and thus did all he is remembered for in the history books quite unconsciously. Just supposing you believed this, would you feel proud of Napoleon's deeds as if they had been yours? I think not, because without any sense of those deeds being included in your personal conscious history, they could just as well be the past deeds of anyone else around. Once again it is psychological continuity which underlies the strand of personal identity, and in its absence there is no clear notion of being one and the same person.

But if so, how vain it seems to extend personhood beyond the loss of a capacity for conscious experience, and equally so to thrust it back in time to a stage of organic life before that capacity existed. Yet, as we shall now see, this is exactly what many people tend to do.

2. POSSIBLE PERSONS

I begin with a notion Lucretius would certainly have found strange, namely that of *possible* persons. Here the reference is not to something so general as, say, persons who will live five generations from now, but to *specific* as yet unconceived humans. R. M. Hare [6], for example, asks whether a life-saving operation for an abnormal child might not be denied so that the parents, facing the burden of caring for such an offspring, will not be discouraged from having normal, healthy children later on. He invites us to imagine "the next child in the queue", whom he christens "Andrew", and asks if a full, constructive and probably happy life for this possible person is not a better moral outcome than sustaining the abnormal child and risking Andrew's future nonexistence. Hare grants that since Andrew is only a possible person he cannot be *deprived* of life, but suggests that he can be harmed by *withholding* life from him. And Derek Parfit [11], commenting on Hare's remarks, apparently concurs. He asks why, if it can be in a person's interest to have his life prolonged, it cannot be in his interest to have it started.

To this the Lucretian response would surely be that life cannot be *withheld* from a nonexistent subject any more than this nonexistent subject can be deprived of it. Similarly, a nonexistent subject cannot have his life *started* by anyone. To talk this way is to imagine there are ghostly persons somewhere just waiting to be given flesh and blood, but there are none. For suppose one agreed with Hare that it is unjust to withhold life from Andrew. In that case, how could one make restitution to him? Where would we go to find this possible person and give him, at last, the life he deserves? All one can do is imagine that the parents of the abnormal child, once it is gone, might conceive a healthy child two years down the road and, when it is born, baptize him "Andrew". It is only by retroactively predating this latter child's existence beyond the point of conception that we get the notion of him, quite illicitly, as a specific possible person awaiting conception. There are no such persons (except in the barren sense of a *logically* possible combination of genes occurring in the conceptus), and thus no harm can be done them.

3. POTENTIAL PERSONS

When I was writing on this topic many years ago [14], I used the term *potential* persons to refer to human children, for reasons I shall make clear later. However, I now find the term has been preempted in the literature to refer to fetuses, and shall follow that usage here. Fetuses have an advantage over possible persons in that they exist; the question is whether they are really the sorts of entities that qualify as having a right to life (assuming there are *any* such entities) by virtue of their potential for becoming human persons.

Michael Tooley [15] has argued strongly against the potentiality principle as follows. Most of us would agree that it is not morally wrong, or only slightly so, to destroy surplus newborn kittens. Now if a chemical were discovered that, when administered to newborn kittens, led to their developing into rational, language-using animals and hence candidate persons, would it become grossly immoral to continue destroying newborn kittens? If not, and if artificial vs. natural potentiality for becoming persons is not a morally relevant distinction, then naturally potential persons have no more right to life than such kittens would have.

What is it like to *be* a potential person, i.e., from the inside of that stage of life? None of us knows, not because we have forgotten what it is like, but because our conscious personal lives had not begun yet. I do not deny that it is possible a fetus has crude sensations of pressure, temperature, etc. But zygotes, morulae, blastocysts, embryos and even (in the technical sense) early 'fetuses' do not have the neural complexes necessary to sustain believably a conscious and therefore, by Lucretius' criterion, a personal life. If not, no *person* begins his or her personal life before late term in the intra-uterine environment, and only barely then. Terminating a human life before that stage is not, therefore, killing an innocent *person*. It is destruction of at most the organic blueprint of a future person.

For suppose we had the means, technically, of saving life and promoting normal development of a spontaneously aborted fetus at *any* stage whatever. Would the zygote have *more* of life ahead than a near neonate? Biologically, yes. Does that mean more personal value accrues to the saved zygote than to the premature baby? Surely not, for if they both lived a normal human life span and had equal enjoyment of it, it matters not at all that the zygote's organic life was saved seven or so months earlier; that was time at which its personal life had not yet begun and nothing in the events of those months adds to that future person's enjoyment of life. If so, can any event detract from it?

Many would say yes, for abortion constitutes an abrupt cancellation of the promise of a future personal life. My point is that cancellation of a promise is not cancellation of the thing promised. Take a young couple who have two healthy, happy children. It may be that at the time of the second pregnancy they gave serious thought to terminating it as inopportune, but relented and now are glad they did, for he is a wonderful child who shows every sign of enjoying a long and prosperous life. The temptation is to say they are glad not only to have him as a son but glad they did not deprive *him* of his life. But on the Lucretian stance I am developing here, the latter source of self-contentment is confused. He did not exist as a *person* until shortly before his birth. Abortion of the fetus from which his personal life ensued would have prevented someone with his particular genetic throw of the dice from getting launched as a person, but could not have ended a personal life, for this had not yet begun. Blueprints and miniature models are not edifices. What is more, all those early formative experiences in his personal life, comparable to the architect's dabbling with the original design to secure improvements as it actually takes shape, are indispensable ingredients in the individuation of the growing structure of a conscious human, and none of those could have taken place before extra-uterine life, so the *particular person* he is would not have lost this actual life.

4. BEGINNING PERSONS

I will speak now of *beginning* persons, as a term to replace the pre-empted 'potential persons' I used to designate human neonates and infants more than a decade ago. The reason I did this was that I then wanted to reserve 'person' as co-extensive with *moral agent*. A moral agent, I said, is both moral subject and moral object, and while small human children are moral objects, as are other higher forms of animal life, by virtue of being able to suffer, they are not yet moral subjects but only potentially so. Adapting now to the terminological shift, I would say that potential persons, meaning fetuses before late term, are not even moral objects[1], whereas beginning persons are, just as they are potential moral subjects as well.

But Tooley [15] has questioned even this. He holds that it is only when an organism becomes *self*-conscious and has a concept of itself as a continuing subject of experiences that it qualifies as a person with a right to life. Such a view, if correct, could be used to justify infanticide as well as feticide, on grounds that without linguistic abilities normally not developed before the second or third year of life, human infants do not have a self-concept. However, Tooley recognizes that it is possible a nonverbal concept of self emerges as early as a month after birth, pushing back the 'cut-off point' between potential and actual personhood to the first few postnatal weeks; but then he worries that if there *is* such a nonverbal self-concept all kinds of infra-human species devoid of language functions might also qualify as persons whose right to life we humans routinely override.

Let us see what can be salvaged here. If it were true that without a verbal conceptual scheme no self-concept is possible, would this imply that beginning persons have no right to life (assuming, again, that any entity has this)? Consider, first, that there are some otherwise normal children who were raised in isolation by uncaring parents, cut off from human language, who if not rescued by age 10 or 12 are thereafter unable to learn language, even in an artificially enriched linguistic environment. Conversely, consider that some higher primate species who never develop symbolic language in natural conditions have been trained in similarly enriched environments to do so using plastic cutouts, computer consoles, and American Sign Language. If what Tooley suggested were true, it follows that the isolated, otherwise normal human 12-year-old unable to learn to talk has no right to life, while the chimp who can sign "You take out cabbage and give me monkey chow" is a person with a right to life! Yet what morally relevant difference is there between the isolated child and the run-of-the-mill infant toddler? The fact that the former is artificially speechless and the latter naturally so cannot serve to distinguish between them. And if not, the lack of a verbal self-concept in beginning persons cannot justify denying them whatever right to life anyone has.

5. ACTUAL PERSONS

Tooley's qualms about the person-status of languageless infra-human species can now be addressed. The only solid evidence for a nonverbal self-concept comes from Gordon Gallup's [4] studies of self-recognition in a reflecting surface by higher apes, something lower apes such as monkeys cannot learn to do. Yet monkeys rely on recognition of *other* monkeys' faces to establish their place in the troop's dominance hierarchy. How can this be? After all, brain-damaged humans who lose the ability to recognize faces not only cannot identify their own but cannot recognize those of close friends or loved ones. Apparently it is because chimpanzees and other higher apes have a self-concept to begin with that they quickly learn to recognize their own faces and bodies in a mirror. Lacking this, lower apes such as the monkey can identify and react to other monkey faces appropriately, but persist in seeing the reflected face and body as that of just another conspecific of similar age, sex and size. So if it were true that regarding oneself as a continuing subject of experiences is what qualifies an organism for personhood and the right to life, on present evidence only our closest phylogenetic relatives would make the grade.

But even this seems strained. According to many contemporary philosophers, the kind of rude nonvocal but still verbal abilities demonstrated by chimpanzees after arduous human training, plus the evidence for a nonverbal self-concept already in place in such species, is a far cry from what *actual* persons like you and me are able to do. For example,

H. Frankfurt [3] has influentially espoused the view that a necessary condition of being a person is the capacity for having what he calls 'second-order
volitions', i.e., the desire not to will what one wills and will something else
instead. And this clearly requires a rich verbal conceptual scheme, for how
else is one going to think the equivalent of, "I wish I were less ambitious";
or, "If only I could love her in return"? Beings that do not have this ability
are simply characterized by Frankfurt as 'wantons', and include nonhuman
animal species, mental defectives, and the small children I called beginning
persons.

More than a decade ago, I would have welcomed Frankfurt's stipulation,
because at that time I could not see how any entity could be a moral subject
as well as a moral object, hence a moral agent and a full-blown person,
without a complex verbal conceptual scheme. But since then I have come
to distrust such maneuvers by philosophers, for the reason that they are
dangerously exclusive. Who am I to say, for example, that someone with a
lesion to Broca's area, a motor aphasic unable to think in propositional
language anymore, is therefore a mere 'wanton', a nonperson without a
right to life? Except in the narrow legal sense that such a human may not
sign a contract or witness a will because of linguistic incompetence subsequent to the brain damage, I might indeed prefer to regard such a human
as a person with a language defect, no more and no less than that. And in
that case I would have to conclude that moral agents are just a subclass
of persons.

Then what is a person? I have come to share the scepticism of D. C.
Dennett [1] over ever being able to give an exhaustive list of the necessary
and sufficient conditions of being a person; as he says, it might turn out
that the concept of a person is only a free-floating honorific that we all
happily apply to ourselves, and to others as the spirit moves us, rather as
those who are *chic* are all and only those who can get themselves considered
chic by others who consider themselves *chic*. In any case it is not my task
here to say exactly what a person is, but only to argue that a person is more
than a living human organism[2]; it is a conscious entity that builds a personal
life from agency and experience, and until and only for so long as it has a
capacity for conscious experience does the notion of a right to life, if there
is such a thing, take hold.

6. FORMER PERSONS

Probably there has been no time before this when philosophers have been more conscious of the brain dependence of the human mind. Yet in spite of this, they sometimes talk of the brain as if it were a replaceable or sub-stitutable organ a person has, on a par with the heart, a kidney, or the cornea of the eye. For example, John Perry [13] has suggested that some day it might be possible to make a duplicate 'rejuvenated' brain exactly like the original except for having healthy arteries, etc., which could then be used to replace the latter when it starts to wear out. If the copy were exact enough, he argues, all the individuating psychological characteristics of the person, including the long-term memories he has, would persist and exact similarity is as good as makes no matter to saying one and the same person has survived the operation. John Hick [7] has even extended this notion to the next world. He asks us to imagine that upon our earthly demise God will create a replica of each of us in a special Resurrection World, complete with an exactly similar brain containing the same memory traces, dispositions, etc., and holds that it would be unreasonable for these resurrectees not to regard themselves, and be regarded by others there, as continuants of the persons whose earthly pasts they recall as their own.

What such claims overlook is that for any future person to be me, any statement true of me now would have to be true of him as well, otherwise he is not me. Now it is true of me that I can really remember certain mile-stone events in my life, e.g., a delayed honeymoon on the island of Corfu. But the person with the duplicate of my brain came into existence as a subject of experiences only upon duplication, just as the replica of me in the Celestial City would come into existence upon my death, not before. But then neither the duplicatum nor the replicatum of me, given that the brain each has is what makes each a subject of experiences, could possibly have been a subject of experiences at the time of my honeymoon in Corfu, and so could not really remember the events there, but only seem to. If so, neither would be me and it would be vain for me to anticipate any experiences they are going to have as experiences I shall have. Duplication or replication of a brain cannot endow the resultant person with a retroactive personal history; not even God can change the past and tomorrow make true of it what was not true of it before. In sum, it is the spatiotemporal continuity of a particular living brain that is the anchor of personal identity through time.

If we have this straight, we may now ask when exactly does a person's life end and he or she become only a *former* person? At the beginning of this paper I suggested that on the Lucretian view personal life spans one's total conscious experience, and that this is necessarily shorter at both ends than the life of the organism supporting that conscious life. We have seen how this is probably so for the first several months of fetal development, but one might well wonder if it is true at the end of organic life in any more than a picayune sense. After all, if the organic basis for conscious life is the brain and total brain infarct subsequent to, say, cardiac standstill or lung failure causes the death of masses of central neurons by oxygen deprivation within, normally, a matter of minutes, organic death of the brain follows very quickly upon loss of consciousness. It is true that electrical activity can persist in the spinal cord for hours, and some somatic cells may take up to two days to die, such as those composing cartilage in the knee, but these lingering signs of life are no obstacle to a medical finding that the person has died.

Such is indeed normally the sequence of events, but not always. Consider the following case reported by Ingvar et al. [8].

Case 8. The patient (Th. Sv.) was a female who had been born in 1936. In July 1960, at the age of 24, she suffered severe eclampsia during pregnancy with serial epileptic attacks, followed by deep coma and transient respiratory and circulatory failure. In the acute phase, Babinski signs were present bilaterally and there was a transitory absence of pupillary, corneal and spinal reflexes. A left-sided carotid angiogram showed a slow passage of contrast medium and signs of brain edema. An EEG taken during the acute stage did not reveal any electrical cerebral activity. The EEG remained isoelectric for the rest of the survival time (seventeen years). After the first three to four months the patient's state became stable with complete absence of all higher functions.

Examination ten years after the initial anoxic episode showed the patient lying supine, motionless, and with closed eyes. Respiration was spontaneous, regular and slow with a tracheal cannula. The pulse was regular. The systolic blood pressure was 75–100 mm Hg. Severe flexion contractures had developed in all extremities. Stimulation with acoustic signals, touch or pain gave rise to primitive arousal reactions including eye-opening, rhythmic movements of the extremities, chewing and swallowing, and withdrawal reflexes. The corneal reflex was present on the left side. When testing was done on the right side, transient horizontal nystagmus movements were elicited. Pupillary reflexes were present and normal on both sides. On passive movements of the head, typical vestibulo-ocular reflexes were elicited. The spinal reflexes were symmetrical and hyperactive. Patellar clonus was present bilaterally. Divergent strabismus was found when the eyes were opened [by the examiner]. Measurement of the regional cerebral blood flow on the left side (ten years after the initial anoxic episode) showed a very low mean hemisphere flow of 9 ml/100 g/min. The distribution of the flow was also abnormal, high values being found over the brain stem. The patient's condition remained essentially unchanged for seven more years and she died seventeen years after the anoxic episode after repeated periods of pulmonary edema.

Autopsy showed a highly atrophic brain weighing only 315 grams. The hemispheres were especially atrophied and they were in general transformed into thin-walled yellow-brown bags. The brain stem and cerebellum were sclerotic and shrunken. On the basal aspect some smaller parts of preserved cortex could be seen, mainly in the region of the unci. Microscopically the cerebral cortex was almost totally destroyed with some remnants of a thin gliotic molecular layer and underneath a microcystic spongy tissue with microphages containing iron pigment. The white matter was completely demyelinated and rebuilt into gliotic scar tissue, and there were also scattered macrophages containing iron pigment. The basal ganglia were severely destroyed, whereas less advanced destruction was found in the subfrontal basal cortex, the subcallosal gyrus, the unci, the thalamus and hypothalamus, and in the subocular and entorhinal areas. In the cerebellum the Purkinje cells had almost completely disappeared and were replaced by glial cells. The granular layer was partly destroyed. The cerebellar white matter was partly demyelinated. In the brain stem some neurons had disappeared and a diffuse gliosis was found. Several cranial nerve nuclei remained spared. The long sensory and motor tracts were completely demyelinated and gliotic, whereas transverse pontine tracts remained well myelinated ([8], pp. 196–198).

This clinical picture, confirmed by the autopsy findings, goes by various titles in the literature: cerebral as opposed to whole brain death; neocortical death without brain stem death; and more recently and appropriately, as 'the apallic syndrome', because the characteristic feature is selective destruction of the paleum, the cortical mantle of grey matter covering the cerebrum or telencephalon. As it happens, the neurons composing the paleum are the most vulnerable to oxygen deprivation during transient cardiac arrest or, as in the above case, asphyxiation. Whereas with whole brain death, therefore including the brain stem that mediates cardiopulmonary functions, the patient can be maintained on a respirator only up to a week in adults and two weeks in children before cardiac standstill, the apallic patient can breathe spontaneously and demonstrate cephalic reflexes, which are also brain stem mediated, for months and even years if fed intravenously and kept free of infection, thus allowing organic recovery after the top of the brain is gone.

I said 'organic recovery' is possible with destruction of the cerebral cortex; but on the Lucretian model *personal* life thereupon comes to an end, for with the paleum gone the very capacity for conscious experience goes as well. That such was indeed the case with this patient is obvious from the time of stabilization a few months after the anoxic episode: how else can one explain the persistently flat EEG, the inability to move even the eyes voluntarily, the reduction of cerebral blood flow to less than 20% of normal, and the spastic flexion of extremities? Thus 'the *patient*' was nonsentient and non-cognitive for seventeen years, but the *person* was not, for she had died all that long ago, and what was left was a still breathing *former* person.

How can one be sure? Perhaps a homely analogy will help the medically uninitiated to understand this. Suppose we wanted to find out if anyone lives in an apparently abandoned house, on the top floor. But we dare not break into it to see, for legal and ethical reasons. So we stand outside, watching and listening. We can hear the furnace go on, but that could be due to an automatic thermostat. We also see the lights go on in the evening, but that could be the result of an automatic timer to thwart burglars. We dial the phone number and hear the instrument ringing, so the lines are still intact, but no one answers. We measure the heat flow from the furnace and find not enough is reaching that top floor to keep any occupants alive there in winter. Finally, we attach listening devices to the outer walls and videocameras to the windows, but absolutely no real activity is picked up. Surely at this juncture we would conclude it is pointless to go on fuelling the furnace and scrubbing the walls. Nobody is home upstairs.

Yet as things now stand, so long as the furnace goes on and the lights light up by themselves, we are supposed to be committed to heroic maintenance measures tying up scarce medical resources, even though there is *no one* being helped by these efforts. Lucretius would call this rank superstition and advise us to dispose of such former persons as reason dictates. After all, he would surely say, unconscious breathing and heart beating has no intrinsic value to a departed person; you could do no more harm to *that* individual, now dead, than you could do by opening a grave and stabbing a corpse. And I think he would be right.

No doubt this hard Lucretian line will appall many hearing it for the first time. I shall close by anticipating objections and trying to defuse them in advance.

7. OBJECTIONS AND REPLIES

Objection: Current legislation in the United States, and apparently Canada is following suit [10], is in accord with the 1968 Harvard Statement, which allows a determination of death subsequent to the *whole* brain dying above level C_1, as evidenced by prolonged absence of cephalic reflexes and of spontaneous heart and lung activity. What you are suggesting is presently proscribed by law.

Reply: Superstitutious attitudes often get enshrined in law. Why not change the law? It's been done before.

Objection: It is unconscionable to prepare a patient for burial who is not apneic.

Reply: Spontaneous breathing is normally promissory of a return to conscious functions; with the apallic patient it is not. You can always stop the breathing.

Objection: That's euthanasia, whether passive or active, and it's illegal.

Reply: You're still confusing the patient with the person. If euthanasia means 'mercy killing', it has no application here. How can you be *merciful* to someone already long beyond any possible suffering?

Objection: Nevertheless such actions would harden medical people. How do we know they won't just go through the wards disposing of helpless persons, such as mental defectives, the recoverably comatose, and the senile?

Reply: It is not because the apallic patient is helpless that I am recommending disposal, but because he is a dead person. The categories you mention retain a capacity for conscious experience, even if diminished, and to dispose of them would be to deprive them of the rest of their personal lives. You can still harm such people.

Objection: You take it for granted that the paleum is the seat of consciousness and a personal life. Yet Wilder Penfield [12], that great explorer of the cortex, believed to the end of his days that it was only a way-station and that the true site of personal being is central grey matter in the upper brain stem, which in the patient you referred to seems to have been well preserved. How can we be sure such patients are not secretly conscious?

Reply: On this issue Penfield was wrong. Split-brain surgery for relief of epilepsy yields independent streams of consciousness in the disconnected hemispheres, yet the brain stem is untouched.

Objection: Still, the autopsy showed a fairly well preserved hypothalamus and thalamus. Would this not indicate that the patient could feel thirst and pain?

Reply: *Who*, exactly, would be feeling pain or thirst? Someone who cannot remember, dream, think, anticipate, or come into contact with reality? But even supposing our concept of a person could be reduced to sensory islands like these, what harm would accrue to such an individual if he or she were prevented from experiencing further thirst and pain? In my own case, were this my "personal" future, I would prefer to go without it; and so too, I think, would any rational person.

Objection: The clinical picture included withdrawal reactions to noxious stimulation.

Reply: Which can be mediated by spinal arc pathways alone, as has been shown by experiments with paraplegics [5].

Objection: But if there's any uncertainty at all, why not give the patient the benefit of doubt? There have been misdiagnoses of even total brain death. It is always better to mistakenly assist a dead person than to mistakenly abandon someone who might otherwise survive.

Reply: The only misdiagnoses of total brain death I have heard of involved reduced oxygen requirements due to hypothermia or barbiturate intoxication. But of course one must be cautious. Take six months, use four-vessel angiography, the bolus technique, measurement of regional cerebral blood flow, EEG, brain scan, everything. When there is no longer room for doubt, there is no longer reason for concern.

Objection: Lucretius was an atheist. Why should a religious physician accept that personal annihilation is the result of the cessation of any particular bodily function?

Reply: You could say the same for whole brain death. What matters is not whether the soul survives the body and goes on to another world, etc., but the point at which a person's life ends in *this* world.

Objection: This is not so much an objection as a query. How is it that organic life can exceed conscious life so long, whereas a similar picture at the beginning of life is quickly fatal? I mean the anencephalic infant. Although the head is flattened, brain stem reflexes and spontaneous heart and hung activity are present, as in the apallic syndrome, yet the infant dies within weeks or at most a few months.

Reply: There are anecdotal references to one case of anencephaly where the child, under the total care of the mother, survived beyond seventeen years [9]. Nature is cruel, and a fairly long organic human life can still preclude even beginning a personal life.

Dalhousie University,
Halifax, Nova Scotia, Canada

NOTES

1 However, Engelhardt [2], whose analysis is fully supported by my own, believes that there is sufficient evidence to indicate the aborted fetus feels pain ([2], p. 334). If so, it would be a moral object and I am wrong to think otherwise. Yet being a moral object is obviously not a sufficient condition of being a person, as Tooley's example [15] of surplus newborn kittens makes clear. The reason I hesitate to ascribe a 'right to life' unreservedly even to human beings is that I cannot see how this follows from being a person. My concern is to argue against those who hold that, assuming persons do have a right to life, the early fetus has one because it is already a person.

2 I cannot exactly say what love is, but I would argue confidently nonetheless that it is more than sexual desire. For example, it includes caring about the desired person's happiness and state of mind.

BIBLIOGRAPHY

1. Dennett, D. C.: 1978, 'Conditions of Personhood', *Brainstorms*, Bradford Books, Montgomery, Vermont, Chapter 14.
2. Engelhardt, Jr., H. T.: 1976, 'The Ontology of Abortion', in S. Gorowitz (ed.), *Moral Problems in Medicine*, Prentice-Hall, Inc., Englewood Cliffs, New Jersey, pp. 318–334.
3. Frankfurt, H.: 1971, 'Freedom of the Will and the Concept of the Person', *Journal of Philosophy* 68, 5–20.
4. Gallop, G.: 1970, 'Chimpanzees: Self-Recognition', *Science* 167, 86–87.
5. Hardy, J. D.: 1953, 'Thresholds of Pain and Reflex Contractions as Related to Noxious Stimulation', *Journal of Applied Physiology* 5, 725–737.
6. Hare, R. M.: 1976, 'Survival of the Weakest', in S. Gorowitz (ed.), *Moral Problems in Medicine*, Prentice-Hall, Inc., Englewood Cliffs, New Jersey, pp. 364–369.
7. Hick, J.: 1976, *Death and the Eternal Life*, Collins, London, Chapter 14.
8. Ingvar, D. H. *et al.*: 1978, 'Survival After Severe Cerebral Anoxia with Destruction of the Cerebral Cortex: the Apallic Syndrome', in J. Korein (ed.), *Brain Death: Interrelated Medical and Social Issues, Annals of the New York Academy of Sciences* 315, 184–214.
9. Korein, J. (ed.): 1978, *Brain Death: Interrelated Medical and Social Issues, Annals of the New York Academy of Sciences* 315, 142 and 366.
10. Law Reform Commission of Canada: 1979, 'Criteria for the Determination of Death', *Working Paper* 23, 58–59.
11. Parfit, D.: 1976, 'Rights, Interests, and Possible People', in S. Gorowitz (ed.), *Moral Problems in Medicine*, Prentice-Hall, Inc., Englewood Cliffs, New Jersey, pp. 369–375.
12. Penfield, W.: 1975, *The Mystery of the Mind*, Princeton University Press, Princeton, New Jersey.
13. Perry, J.: 1978, *A Dialogue on Personal Identity and Immortality*, Hackett Publishing Company, Indianapolis.
14. Puccetti, R.: 1968, *Persons: A Study of Possible Moral Agents in the Universe*, Macmillan, London, Chapter 1.
15. Tooley, M.: 1976, 'Abortion and Infanticide', in S. Gorowitz (ed.), *Moral Problems in Medicine*, Prentice-Hall, Inc., Englewood Cliffs, New Jersey, pp. 297–317.

H. TRISTRAM ENGELHARDT, JR.

VIABILITY AND THE USE OF THE FETUS

In its landmark case of *Roe v. Wade*, the Supreme Court of the United States appealed to viability in signaling when it would be appropriate for the state of proscribe abortions for other than the preservation of the life or the health of the mother. The Court stated, "For the stage subsequent to viability the state, in promoting its interest in the potentiality of human life, may, if it chooses, regulate, and even proscribe, abortion, except where it is necessary, in appropriate medical judgment, for the preservation of the life or the health of the mother" ([7], pp. 164–165). The National Commission for the Protection of Human Subjects of Biomedical and Behavioral Research appealed as well to a distinction between viable and non-viable living fetuses in drafting its canons for regulations.[1] What I shall do in this essay is explore the sense and meaning of such appeals to viability.

I will attempt to indicate the extent to which the stage of viability could have moral implications for decisions about abortion or fetal research. That is, I shall attempt to delineate its moral and conceptual value. Having done that, I hope to be able to suggest some public policy implications of such a conceptual analysis. For example, in considering policies concerning abortion and fetal research, one needs to know whether the stage of viability, as it bears upon moral discussions, is fixed or whether it will change as technology allows us to sustain the lives of ever more immature fetuses.

Although appeal is often made to the criterion of viability, there is very little helpful analysis to suggest the origin of its moral pertinence. Justice Blackmun, in delivering the opinion of the Supreme Court in *Roe v. Wade*, noted that physicians and their scientific colleagues placed weight upon the point at which the fetus became 'viable'. He then defined viability as the stage at which the fetus would be "potentially able to live outside the mother's womb, albeit with artificial aid. Viability is usually placed at about seven months (twenty-eight weeks) but may occur earlier, even at twenty-four weeks" ([7], p. 160). I will argue that this statement is dangerously misleading in that it might suggest that the point of viability as a moral criterion could be pushed ever earlier simply by the force of scientific advances in fetal medicine. Contrary to such a suggestion, I will hold that the sense of viability pertinent to moral decisions with regard to the use of

183

William B. Bondeson et al. *(eds.), Abortion and the Status of the Fetus, 183–208.*

the fetus should not be so open to change in this fashion, but rather should be set at that point at which a near full term infant could survive without one providing what would be tantamount to a surrogate womb.

I will argue this point on the basis of two central considerations. The first is that fetuses, even viable fetuses, are not persons, and therefore need not be extended the special protection we give to persons. Secondly, in establishing restrictions with regard to easy access to abortion one must always be concerned not to circumscribe unduly the freedom of women who are actually and fully persons. In developing this argument, one must bear in mind that I am attempting to advance general secular considerations. Though I do not make appeal to religious or other special considerations, neither do I deny their validity for those who embrace them. Rather, I will be arguing that a peaceable pluralist community may not make appeal to such considerations in the development of its public policies bearing on the use of the fetus. For example, this will suggest that it would be immoral for a pluralist society to forbid by law abortion on request, in that consequentialist arguments against abortion could not outweigh the moral considerations regarding respect of the person of the woman which would count in favor of avoiding such a prohibition.

I. BEING A PERSON

Why should one be interested in deciding which of the objects of this world are persons? That will, naturally, depend upon what one means by person. Here I use 'person' to identify those entities that are self-conscious, rational, and self-determining. Such a use of 'person' is important, for it will help to determine which entities exist that can act as we, that can know they exist and act, and which can, then, reflect upon their knowledge and action and take responsibility for it. This use of person arises in discussions of the existence of other minds and can be construed as an epistemological use of the term. The exploration of such epistemological issues (e.g., on what grounds can I know that an entity is a person?) requires rendering the definition of person as a concept as precisely as possible. Such precision will be an ontological quest to be clear about a category of reality. Thus, as one begins to reflect upon the nature of persons, one will be pressed to define the concept's scope, and to explore the conditions under which it would be reasonable to hold that an entity is a person. In the end, such reflections should deliver a conceptual definition of what it is to be a person, and an operational definition that will specify maneuvers through which one could establish the existence of such entities.

One should notice that interest in defining the concept of person is not just ontological or epistemological. One is not simply concerned with categorizing the entities that furniture the world. One is interested as well in the concept of person due to its role in ethical theory. Thus, in addition, one will be interested in identifying those entities that are self-conscious, rational, and self-determining, because they will, as well, be the moral agents of the universe. They will be the entities who are responsible for their actions and who are bearers of both rights and duties.

I will begin with the assumption that our language often bewitches us in our attempts to be clear about what it is to be a person. The fact that we have but one word 'person' may suggest that we have but one concept of person. Such is likely to press us to irresolvable puzzles regarding the essential characteristics, if any, that underlie all of our various usages of 'person'. If the assumption is that there is *one* underlying meaning, the search will be in vain. Though we speak of both adults and infants as persons, it is, so I will argue, not the case that they are persons in the same sense.

If by person one means a self-conscious, rational, and self-determining entity, it is reasonable to hold that, though normal adult humans are such beings, infants are not. Or if one regards the issue from the moral point of view, infants are not moral agents, though normal adults usually are. This difference is of singular importance in judgments concerning the moral standing of human beings in different stages of the human life cycle. This is the case, for it is persons in this strict sense who constitute the *mundus intelligibilis* of Kant ([4], p. 438). It is persons who are invoked in hypothetical choice theories or hypothetical contractarian theories in order to generate views of the good and principles of justice.[2]

This central place of persons in the strict sense in moral reflections flows from the very notion of a moral community. If one views ethics as a means of resolving moral disputes in a fashion not based upon force, but rather upon peaceable negotiation, in a context where the participants are held accountable for their actions, the only original members of that community, of the moral world, will be persons in the strict sense: entities who are self-conscious, rational, and self-determining and therefore accountable for their choices, and who have interests. Insofar as there is a sense of rights and duties not reducible to interests in particular goods and values, it will be founded on the necessary condition for such a community, namely, mutual respect of the free choice of its members. Such a view of rights is the least presumptuous and therefore the least difficult to establish. It presumes only that the ethical life is based upon peaceable negotiation and the eschewal of force against the innocent. It does not presuppose that one can discover a univocal and morally obligatory view of the good life, nor grounds for imposing such a view upon unconsenting innocent persons. The proposed understanding of ethics, which offers ethics as the logic of pluralism, as the means for peaceably negotiating contrary moral intuitions, leads one to hold that most claims of rights and duties are in the end reducible to interests in goods and values usually pursued through practices created by particular communities of persons. A cardinal exception involves those rights and duties to which one is committed in virtue of committing oneself to the moral life, namely, to respecting the standing and freedom of the moral agents with whom one may negotiate. Respect of freedom, not as something to be valued, but as a side constraint, or condition for moral life, produces the deontological matrix within which teleological or consequentialist considerations, such as those bearing on the use of the fetus, must be framed.

Nothing mysterious is meant here. Rather, one is reminded that a concept of the moral community, a *mundus intelligibilis* (to employ a Kantian phrase ([4], p. 428)), a community of moral agents, is invoked as soon as one begins the endeavor of determining with others what the nature of the moral life ought to be. The only possible participants in such a discussion are moral agents, persons in the strict sense. It is for this reason that persons possess such a singular place in ethical reflections, in the moral life, and in the constitution of the moral universe. It is in terms of an appeal to such a community that general moral absolutes can be produced, such as: one should not take the lives of unconsenting innocent persons. This is not to deny that taking the life of an 'unconsenting' human for sport, if that entity is not a person in the strict sense, may still in important senses be morally offensive; it will, however, not offend against the very notion of a moral community. That is, rules with regard to the termination of human biological life, which life is not also that of a person in a strict sense, will need to be justified in terms of whether such practices will in general support the interest of persons in particular goods and values, including those of moral character. One may also wish to take into account here any pain involved in such taking of life, a consideration that is by no means restricted to human life alone. Which is to say, human biological life may be a moral object in a special sense, even when it is not a moral subject in the sense of a moral agent. But such is the case with non-human life as well. In any event, in such comparisons one will, however, have to remember that whatever pain and suffering is endured by a human fetus or infant, it is surely not as severe as the pain and suffering that normal adult mammals can experience, and is not of the same moral significance as imposing pain on an unconsenting person.[3]

Thus, if one attempts to identify entities who are persons, members of the moral community, one will be attempting to determine which objects are also self-conscious, rational, and self-determining. Not all humans will be persons in this sense. Nor will appeals to potentiality secure for potential persons the standing of actual persons. If X is a potential Y, it follows that X is not Y. Moreover, if X is only a potential Y, it follows that X does not as a consequence of that relationship have all the properties of a Y. In fact, to the contrary. Thus, if X is a potential president, it does not follow that X has presidential rights.[4] Rather, it is the case that X potentially has such rights, which is far from having those rights.

In order to avoid the confusion and mystification often associated with the use of the term 'potential', it might be wise to substitute the term 'probable'. Thus, one might speak of a zygote being a 0.4 probable person, indicating that it has a 40% chance of becoming a person. The extent to which an entity is a probable person would then play an important role in the value one attributed to it. In any event, even though human sperm, ova, zygotes, embryos, fetuses, and infants are potential persons (or probable persons), this will not confer upon them eo ipso the standing of actual persons. Since the focus here is upon fetuses, this means that there is not a general secular argument that would secure for them a greater intrinsic value than the value held by adult organisms of similar sapience and respon- siveness to their environment. That is to say, considered only in that regard, they would have a position comparable to that of lower vertebrates. However, fetuses play a role in endeavors that do have important moral standing, and therefore secular arguments may be available to give greater moral worth to the fetus in terms of these extrinsic considerations.[5]

How human fetuses will be valued will depend upon such issues as a society's interest in having more persons, or more persons of a particular sort. Thus the fact that many zygotes do not implant is likely to be cele- brated by individuals or communities impressed by the present over-popula- tion of the earth.[6] Similarly, the fact that most chromosomally defective zygotes do not survive to term is likely to be considered a fortuitous happen- ing by individuals insofar as it is less difficult and less costly to raise persons free of handicaps than those who are not so blessed. The view would be that it is better to prevent the birth of excess numbers of persons, or of handicapped persons, for once such persons come into existence, they have strong rights to forebearance and can make persuasive claims upon our beneficence. By avoiding such births, one avoids a needless moral test of one's virtues, and some of the tragedies of human life. Such avoidance (i.e., through abortion) is much more on a par with a couple deciding to postpone initiating a pregnancy until the circumstances are more fortuitous, than it is with an interference with the rights of a person. Further, to abort a fetus does not harm the person the fetus would have become, any more than those possible persons are harmed who will not be brought into existence due to the fact that the readers of this article are not mating, but are instead engaged in philosophical reflection. (I do not wish to claim that such a conjunction of activities is formally or even materially impossible, only unlikely.) Which is to say, in abortion no one (i.e., no person) is killed, though a human organism is extinguished. This may involve an evil in addition to what is involved in a choice not to reproduce, however, not the evil of murder.

This point is anticipated by St. Thomas Aquinas in his argument that early abortions do not involve the taking of the life of a person.[7] Potential persons, all else being equal, have no actual rights, though one must distinguish between the potentiality for becoming a person, and the potentialities of a person. However, the actual persons they might become will, should they come into existence, have strong rights and claims upon us, though they may still be regarded as disvalued and prevented from existence as long as they are merely potential persons. Generally, actions that will injure future actual persons are immoral, as are actions that injure present actual persons. However, when the injury to the future actual person is due to a causal chain that is a part of the gestational history of the body of that person, it is not clear that one is obliged to avoid causing that injury at the cost of avoiding that person's existence [3]. In any event, the intention to abort alters the value of the fetus. A fetus that is to be aborted may no longer have positive significance for the mother and may indeed be of negative value for her. On this basis, at least, a fetus-to-be-aborted should receive different consideration from a fetus-going-to-term. This should be the case as well with regard to the use of the fetus in research, though current federal regulation fails to acknowledge this difference ([9], p. 47733). The value of potential persons will be determined by the benefits and costs associated with their lives, or the termination of their lives under specific circumstances, where costs are understood in the broadest sense (including psychological, financial, and such social costs as impeding the realization of moral goods). The assumption of such costs will be justifiable when they are outbalanced by other psychological, financial, moral, and social goods, and insofar as the freedom of persons in the strict sense is not violated.

Thus, one could, for example, understand the moral probity of investing considerable funds per organism to ensure that all whooping crane embryos are brought to term, while not investing such energies to prevent the loss of embryos in the case of humans, reasoning that the world has far too few whooping cranes, and in general far too many human persons. Once such persons come into existence, though one might wish there had been fewer of them, one will be strictly bound by duties of forebearance not to kill them, unless they act as unjust aggressors. One is drawn to distinguish between the inherent dignity of persons, and their right not to be used as means merely, versus what value such persons might have for themselves or others. The dignity of persons expresses itself in the obligation to respect the freedom of other persons as a constraint upon one's actions. It is to be contrasted with the various ways in which individual persons may be valuable to themselves or others (e.g., market value).

Such reflections require distinctions to be drawn between 'human' and 'person'. Here I use 'human' to identify a particular variety of animals, of the genus homo in the family hominidae of the suborder anthropoidiae of the order primates of the class mammalia. It will depend on the circumstances of each case whether one will restrict the term 'human' to only some of the species within the genus homo. In any event, 'human' need not denote personal characteristics. As already indicated, there are many instances of human biological life that are not instances of human personal life. One might think here of human zygotes, fetuses, infants, and brain-dead but otherwise alive human individuals. All of these are surely instances of life and in fact of human life. They are not porcine, feline, canine, or simian. Moreover, just as not all humans are persons, not all persons need be humans, as the characters in the popular science fiction movies *Star Wars, The Empire Strikes Back*, and *E. T.* and in fact the genre of science fiction and indeed religious reflection attest. Self-conscious, rational, self-determining extraterrestrials, angels, and gods are persons, though they are not humans. Thus we arrive at the distinction I sketched in the Introduction between human biological life, which is defined in terms of certain biological characteristics, and human personal life, which identifies those instances of human biological life that are also persons.

This would appear to do violence to many of the settled ways in which

we in our culture deal with human life. We currently accord humans the
status of persons at birth and remove that status at brain death. What are
we to make of the status of infants, the severely mentally retarded, the
severely senile, and the severely brain-damaged? It would appear, all else
being equal, that killing them would be equivalent to killing an animal of
a similar level of sentience. Although this would be a serious act, it would
in itself not have the seriousness of killing, for example, an adult higher
primate. However, all else is not equal in the case of infants, the severely
mentally retarded, etc., for they play important moral roles within particular
communities of persons. I indicated in the Introduction that a plausible
reconstruction of this state of affairs is that our settled practices presuppose
more than one concept of person. The first would involve the strict sense of a
moral agent, an entity that could be a member of a moral community. It is
through appeals to such a notion that we would understand certain entities
to have strong, though abstract, natural rights to forebearance, so that it
would be an equally heinous moral act to slay for sport and without consent
an innocent human person or an innocent extra-terrestrial person. Our treatment of instances of human life that are not also persons must be explained
in terms of general practices established to secure important goods and
interests, including the development of kindly parental attitudes to children,
concern and sympathy for the weak, and protection for persons in the strict
sense when it is not clear that they are still alive. This practice of imputing
personhood thus depends upon the moral geography of a particular moral
community. For example, one may wish to treat infants as persons in order
to secure attitudes of love and attention to children;[8] in addition, one will
wish to ensure that the person the infant will become will be secure against
injuries that would antedate his or her personhood. Again, because one might
fear false positive determinations of the fact that one was no longer a person
strictly, one might, for example, treat individuals such as Karen Quinlan as
if they were persons strictly, though all the available evidence suggests the
contrary (i.e., their status is the consequence of a false negative test for
death). That is, one would establish operational criteria for deciding in a
conservative fashion what was a person strictly.

   In summary, with regard to the concept of person and the analysis of
human ontogency, one will need to distinguish between human personal
and human biological life. Further, one will have to recognize that our
moral concerns involve more than one sense of person. In addition to the
strict sense of person as a bearer of rights and duties, we will often have
good moral grounds for creating other senses, which confer upon instances

of human life certain of the rights of persons strictly, though none of the duties, due to the absence of moral agency. These other senses indicate the value of such instances of human life for a community of persons. Where precisely one draws the compass of such social senses of person will depend upon utilitarian and other consequentialist considerations. Of course, one will also have moral interests in infants as instances of biological life or indeed human biological life. But these will not be as serious as the concerns that a community expresses by conferring upon such life the rights of persons due to the special values such life has for a community of persons. We have drawn the line for such imputation of personhood along one border at birth, conferring upon instances of human life above that border rights of persons as civil rights, similar to the rights possessed by persons strictly as natural rights.

The fact that birth as a moral criterion represents a line that is created, not discovered, suggests how one must proceed in examining the significance of viability. That is, one confers upon birth a moral significance because of certain practices that sustain the achievement of certain values, goods, and interests. We must now explore the possible functions of the criterion of viability in terms of the goals such a moral criterion would serve.

II. THE MORAL SIGNIFICANCE OF VIABILITY

An initial reflection on the possible moral grounds for holding that viability is of ethical significance in the development of practices regarding the fetus is likely to offer at least four possible accounts.

(1) The point of viability is that point at which the fetus becomes a person in the strict sense of a moral agent.

(2) At the point of viability the fetus has become a sufficiently well integrated organism to experience significant pain in the process of being aborted.

(3) The point of viability identifies a stage at which the interests of the State in such goods as procuring more citizens outweigh interests in maximizing the liberty of women to decide late in their pregnancies not to carry a fetus to term. As a consequence, late gestation fetuses may be treated as if they were persons.

(4) At the point of viability, one has usually given a woman sufficient time to decide whether she wishes to carry a pregnancy to term (if health concerns should give late grounds for abortion, one would presume, as is currently the case, that a woman would with her physician have total liberty

in procuring an abortion), so that one can give predominance to such utilitarian and teleological considerations as the effect of late abortions on attitudes towards parenthood, on the emotional well-being of physicians and nurses, and on the establishment of a general high regard for the value of human life.

The arguments that have been advanced on this point suggest that the first position is untenable. There is no evidence that viable fetuses are self-conscious, rational, self-determining entities. They are not persons in this strict sense. Nor does there appear to be any evidence to support the second proposition in a convincing fashion. There do not appear to be any well-established arguments that society should be greatly concerned about pain in an organism at the level of sensitivity of a fetus, especially considering the serious issue of a woman being able to decide freely whether she would wish to be a mother. Indeed, newborn infants are considered to have such a limited capacity to appreciate pain that they are held not to suffer in a significant fashion (it would appear that there is not full connection of the frontal lobes of the brain until some time after birth), so that, for example, circumcisions are performed without anesthetic. In any event, what is central to the arguments here is that there is not the suffering that is present in the case of a person in the strict sense where pain can also be intellectually appreciated as suffering.

The third view can, I believe, be subsumed under the fourth. One is, after all, interested in balancing the concern to respect the decisions of the mother who is a person in the strict sense, with interests that others might have in establishing fetuses as persons because of possible benefits from such treatment. Given the argument already forwarded that the boundaries for the social concept of person are created, not discovered, one might very well imagine a utilitarian argument to the effect that human biological life should be accorded personal status from the moment of conception. However, the arguments against such a practice will be both deontological and utilitarian. The deontological argument will be based on regard for the freedom of the woman who is the only person in a strict sense immediately involved, and who possesses strong claims in the matter (i.e., presuming that the woman did not promise to bring the fetus to term as a part of an agreement with her husband, her lover, or parties for whom she promised to act as a surrogate mother, etc.). One will, therefore, not be able for utilitarian or other consequentialist reasons to circumscribe the woman's liberty of decision to the point of denying her sufficient time to consider an abortion and to determine, should she wish, whether the fetus is defective. In fact, the second consideration would likely be strong enough to preclude the proscription of abortion at a time that would interfere with the ability to acquire adequate information from pre-natal diagnostic maneuvers or cause her to risk her life or health. Due to these considerations, fetuses may not be treated as persons.

These last considerations would also form a part of a utilitarian argument. One would not wish to set the upper allowable limit in gestation for abortions at a point that would preclude women from aborting defective fetuses on the basis of pre-natal diagnosis, if such fetuses would as infants not be treated anyway, or would constitute a serious burden on society. Or at least, one would wish to have an exception or a loophole in the proscription of abortion after a particular point of 'viability', should those abortions be sought on the basis that a pre-natal diagnosis indicated that the fetus would be severely deformed, or to protect the life or health of the mother.

These deontological and utilitarian considerations, in practice, will make it possible for many women to have late abortions by disingenuously claiming (with the aid of some physicians) that carrying the fetus to term will damage their mental health. Still, requiring such a claim is itself of moral value. It is a way of requiring that women seeking abortions past the point of viability advance a reasonable justification in order to reaffirm the moral seriousness of late abortions (e.g., the importance of avoiding distress to others by such procedures, and of developing attitudes of respect for human life that will enhance the lives of persons). Such a requirement allows one to acknowledge the moral consequences of late abortions, while recognizing the utilitarian considerations in favor of easy access to early abortions. These will include the role of abortion in population control and in preventing the birth of unwanted children or the birth of children under circumstances in which the births themselves would be a burden to the mothers.

Thus, in the creation of a secular proscription of the abortion of fetuses late in pregnancy, one would seek a line that allowed women self-determination, the preservation of their lives and health, the effective use of pre-natal diagnosis, and the achievement of other societal goals such as the prevention of the births of unwanted children, while avoiding undue insult to practices of parenthood and of attention and kindness toward children, etc.

Current notions of viability offer an appealing point for drawing such a line, in that it is also reasonable to wish to avoid the delivery of fetuses, who would not readily survive as infants. Not only may such a circumstance thwart a woman's desire not to be a mother, but it is also quite reasonable to presume that such events are likely to be traumatic for those who view them or who come to know about them. Viability, therefore, can function as a reasonable point after which abortion should not be performed without good reasons. Of course, though an abortion after that time would offend against a moral practice and the goods it sustains, it would not involve active infanticide. Or to put the matter another way, there do not appear to be sufficient untoward consequences from later abortions to merit extending to late gestation fetuses the status of persons. The point of birth has functioned successfully as a point at which to confer personhood in a social sense. Further, the fetus is not necessarily embedded in a social matrix. Fetuses can, unlike infants, be ignored and they will tend to go to term. It is infants that must necessarily be embedded in a social context and given a social role in terms of which they receive care. For this reason, it is difficult to envisage imposing personhood upon instances of human life prior to birth; they are not necessarily placed within an active social matrix in which they themselves play an active role.[9] Finally, the fact that one would need to allow late abortions to preserve the life or health of the mother, or on grounds of fetal defectiveness, would appear to be a strong bar against conferring personhood on the fetus.

The current criterion of viability appears thus to be a reasonable social criterion for balancing the interests in favor of abortion with those in favor of fetal life.

III. WHEN IS A FETUS VIABLE?

The advantage of the criterion of birth for conferring personhood is that it is a fairly determinable event. One can determine whether a fetus has made it outside the mother and drawn a breath. Then and only then are the rights of a person conferred from inheriting estates to being granted a tax deduction. Viability is not as clear a criterion, even if one wishes to set it at a point at which at least one fetus has been known to survive. Moreover, if such an analysis of viability is embraced, one might then envisage developments in the neo-natal care of premature infants pushing the point of viability ever earlier. Indeed, one can imagine advances in *in vitro* fertilization and gestation proceeding to the point at which a zygote could be brought to term *in vitro*. At that point, all conceptuses would be viable in the sense of being at a stage at which there were known survivors. Would or ought such possible developments in science to so alter the stage of viability as to forbid absolutely all abortions (except in circumstances involving the life of health of the mother, as is currently the case)?

Such a possibility would appear to be indefensible. After all, viability functions as a useful criterion as long as it is late enough in pregnancy to allow the use of pre-natal diagnosis and to allow women time to reflect upon whether they would wish to be mothers. Even in the best of future possible worlds, there are likely to be contraceptive failures, failures to use adequate contraception, and revisions of judgment regarding motherhood once pregnancy has begun. Since fetuses born much earlier than 28 to 24 weeks' gestation are unlikely to survive long without aggressive treatment, allowing a fetus of, say, twenty weeks' gestation to die without employing aggressive treatment is unlikely to create great moral costs. Should there be such costs, however (which is more unlikely the earlier in gestation the fetus is aborted), it would then be justifiable to use abortifacient techniques that guaranteed the death of the fetus. One is concerned primarily with respecting the freedom of the mother. As a consequence, one would wish as well to forbid attempts, against the will of the mother, to sustain the life of a fetus prior to the established general upper limit for abortions. Or to put it another way, given the absence of a generally defensible secular argument that fetuses are persons, it will follow that a secular society will not have the moral authority (right) to use force to constrain a woman to become a mother. Such would be the case if biomedical science were able to push the point of viability ever earlier as a moral criterion and appeal to it as a justification for employing force in order to attempt to sustain early fetuses. In addition, such attempts would likely have other untoward consequences (e.g., the survival of unwanted or deformed fetuses).

As a consequence, one will be forced to distinguish between viability as a moral criterion and viability as a medical generalization. The latter is likely to become ever earlier as our ability to treat premature infants advances. However, the former should remain fixed at the point at which survival would not be possible without special intervention often tantamount to a surrogate womb. Indeed, the criterion should probably remain fixed at the level it was understood to be set at in 1973. One would need to be extremely cautious about placing the moral criterion any earlier, in that this might interfere with the woman's ability to use pre-natal diagnosis adequately in her decision of whether to bring a fetus to term. Such constraints would limit her freedom to control the quality of the fetuses to which she would give birth. It would in addition have some consequences of marked disutility (i.e., the birth of handicapped children in need of expensive support.[10]

One might ask whether such a policy would not lead to unequal treatment for entities that are in other respects equal. One would be ready to employ aggressive means to sustain the life of a wanted premature baby, but not that of an unwanted fetus at a comparable stage of development. There is not, however, parity between the premature infant and the possibly viable fetus. The first is already born and therefore already plays a role under the social rubric 'child'. Personhood has been conferred upon it through the passage of birth. Beyond that, the wanted premature infant accrues value due to the interest of its parents. Thus, even if a fetus were born of an abortion procedure and were viable only in the sense of having reached a point in gestation at which there were known survivors, given special medical attention, but in a period in gestation before the point of viability as the upper limit for abortion, there would not be a *prima facie* moral obligation to employ therapy beyond that usually used to support the life of a fetus at the point of viability in the sense of this upper limit for allowable abortions. Treatment would be given at that level in order to support minimally the general practice of preserving infants.

Since fetuses are neither persons nor highly developed sentient organisms, it appears unreasonable to hold that a biological criterion of viability can in some simple fashion be given moral force. As a result, if advances in biomedicine move the point of viability to an earlier stage as a medical generalization, it does not follow that viability as a moral signpost should be placed earlier. Quite to the contrary. The criterion of viability, in that it reflects a balancing of various considerations, is likely to be influenced only marginally by improvements in chances of viability through new medical interventions. Viability as a moral criterion is perhaps best defined as a point at which fetuses, should they be aborted, would die, given the level of support thought to be obligatory in the case of full-term or near full-term births. That is, it indicates a point at which a fetus brought *ex utero* could reasonably be placed in the social role of a child. In this way one could offer a useful interpretation of the Supreme Court's identification of viability as the point at which a fetus would be capable of meaningful life *ex utero* ([7], p. 163). Again, the fact that parents interested in saving their premature children might wish to invest resources in extending the role of child to very premature infants (by placing such a child in what would be tantamount to a surrogate womb, thus restricting the full realization of the child) would not detract from the legitimacy of maintaining a fairly constant criterion of viability for moral decisions at somewhere between 24 and 28 weeks.

Given the considerations to be balanced in creating such a line, it would be appropriate for legislatures, should a community of interest be strong enough, to give legal force to the criterion of viability, as long as the woman's interest in preserving her life and health, and in avoiding the birth of a defective fetus, were not compromised. Given such constraints, it would then be appropriate for a legislature to establish a criterion of viability for such purposes somewhere between 24 and 28 weeks gestation, with exception beyond that point being made for abortions sought on the basis of fetal defectiveness or because of a risk to the health or life of the mother.

It is important to note that these considerations lead us to two distinct genres of viability. The first is a set of biological generalizations of this sort: no infant of x gestational age and/or y weight has ever survived; or infants of x gestational age and/or y weight have only survived in z (some presumably small number) % of the recorded cases; or infants of x gestational age and/or y weight have survived, but only with special intervention of z sort. The second genre of viability criteria are not biological generalizations, but moral judgments made in part by taking into consideration empirical data, especially those concerning viability in the first genre of senses. They are of the sort: abortions for q reasons are not allowed after r weeks of pregnancy because of reasons s through z. One might for the sake of avoiding confusion substitute a new phrase for the term viability, when viability is used as a moral criterion. In this way one might avoid confusing viability as a biological generalization and viability as a moral criterion. One might use a phrase such as "upper limit for aborting the fetus without special justification". That phrase would identify a criterion based on a complex set of grounds, including moral judgments of the consequences of aborting fetuses after viability, in some biological sense of viability.

These conclusions with regard to abortion should be extendable to the use of fetuses in research. Women who are now able to have abortions for whatever reasons they choose prior to viability, should be able to subject their fetuses to dangerous and harmful research as long as those fetuses will be aborted prior to viability. Strong utilitarian concerns may, however, argue against funding such research, except when it is certain, or nearly certain, that such damaged fetuses will be aborted.[11] One would not want to damage future persons out of our interests in the welfare of such persons and in order to avoid the costs that would be associated with their care, in addition to respect for them as persons.

However, since the the central issues in the controversies regarding the use of the fetus turn on whether fetuses are persons in the strict sense, whether there are adequate grounds for assigning a social sense of person to fetuses, and whether special protection should be conferred upon the fetus, resolving such issues will be central to deciding whether fetuses developed by researchers will be open to their use until the point of viability. One might imagine, for example, scientists some time in the future developing fetuses *in vitro* to early stages of gestation in order to do adequate research on fetal physiology towards the goals of avoiding birth defects and increasing the health of those fetuses that are indeed brought to term. Since fetuses are not persons in a strict sense, major arguments against such a proposal will be consequentialist arguments. And, moreover, there are strong consequentialist considerations in their favor. Important scientific information is likely to be gained from such research. If there is a reasonable prospect of acquiring such information, then the moral presumption would be that scientists may generate fetuses for research, and perform harmful experiments upon them as long as they are not brought to term, do research upon nonviable fetuses *ex utero*, and expedite the death of fetuses prior to viability (again as long as the fetus is not brought to term). This presumption would be defeated only given reasonable expectations of greater costs from such practice. (One would presume that at least 'greater costs' are required in order to restrict the freedom of scientists).

However, concerns about offenses to parental feelings and sympathy for children might move society to set a lower 'viability' standard for such research, than the standard for abortion, as suggested in the National Commission report.[12] One might also wish to discourage such research from being displayed openly (thus, for example, we no longer have public executions, even in states approving of such executions). The issues at stake here can at best be indicated very generally, namely, the concern to acquire better knowledge in order to assure better health for the future persons we will bring into existence, while avoiding practices that might brutalize us as a civilization. The evidence in favor of such research being beneficial would appear much more substantial than the evidence concerning its detrimental side effects. As a result, since there do not appear to be good reasons for holding that fetuses are persons in the social sense or other clear grounds for the special protection of fetuses, one might, therefore, be able to conclude that the freedom to experiment and gain knowledge through fetal research should be on a par with interests in sexual experimentation with the right to abortion. That is, general arguments about the nature of persons as moral agents, about the imputation of a social sense of person, and for protection of the fetus suggest that there is likely to be great moral latitude in the use of early gestation fetuses in research.

IV. CONCLUSIONS

I have attempted through these reflections to analyze the conceptual pre-suppositions underlying the criterion of viability in its role as setting an upper limit for abortions (save in the case of abortions where the life and health of the mother is at stake, as is currently the case, or to avoid a defective fetus going to term, as ought to be the case). The argument I have forwarded is offered as a general secular one, appealing to considerations open to all without special appeal to religious, ideological, or metaphysical presuppositions. Again, I do not wish to suggest that such special appeals are improper. Rather, I have restricted myself to those considerations that can feasibly provide the moral cement of a pluralist society.

Ethics in this sense must function as a means of negotiating about moral intuitions without recourse to force or special metaphysical or moral insights as its very bases. It will also not have the moral force of conclusions arrived at, for example, within a religious arena. In secular terms, it will not be possible to hold that others ought to see that fetuses are persons, as it can be argued, for example, that normal adult humans are persons. Nor would strong utilitarian reasons for endowing fetuses with personhood be available as they are available for endowing infants with personhood. As a result, those who hope for more robust conclusions in defense of the fetus must restrict themselves to special domains of consideration framed by religious or particular metaphysical presuppositions. Such conclusions can, however, be persuasive only for those who agree with the special premises they pre-suppose. Those who hold such positions will need therefore to convert through witness, not coerce through force. As a consequence, the general rules of a pluralist society cannot prohibit abortions without that society becoming immoral in the strong sense of using force without moral authority and against the very fabric of a peaceable community.

To summarize, then, given this background, the criterion of viability can be used as a line expressing the upper limits for abortion in circumstances that do not involve the life or health of the mother, or the abortion of a defective fetus. In such circumstances no upper limit may be set. Moreover, the use of viability as a moral criterion does not indicate that personhood should be conferred on fetuses.[13] Rather, viability expresses the point at which in many circumstances there has been an adequate balancing of the woman's rights of self-determination with consequentialist considerations in favor of abortion or in favor of the preservation of fetal life. Therefore, one must distinguish between the criterion of viability as a moral criterion and viability as expressing a medical generalization about the likely chances of a fetus surviving. The criterion of viability should continue to function as it does now, precluding abortion after 24 to 28 weeks of gestation, save in cases involving the life or the health of the mother, and as I have argued, abortions performed to avoid bringing a defective fetus to term. In this way, one will be able to respect adequately the freedom of the women involved as well as to achieve important moral goals, including a moral regard for the fetus. Scientific progress should not move the moral criterion earlier.

Center for Ethics, Medicine, and Public Issues,
Baylor College of Medicine, Houston, Texas

NOTES

[1] The National Commission for the Protection of Human Subjects of Biomedical and behavioral Research in 1975 offered a more ample account of viability. Thus, for example, the report provided the following definitions:

" '*Viable infant*' refers to an infant likely to surive to the point of sustaining life independently, given the support of available medical technology. This judgment is made by a physician.

'*Possibly viable infant*' means the fetus *ex utero* which has not yet been determined to be viable or nonviable. This is a decision to be made by a physician. Operationally, the physician may consider that an infant with a gestational age of 20 to 24 weeks (five to six lunar months; four and one-half to five and one-half calendar months) and a weight between 500 to 600 grams may fall into this indeterminate category. These indices depend upon present technology and should be reviewed periodically." ([11], p. 5).

The Report further amplified these definitions in the following fashion:

"The concept of viability implies a predication as to whether a delivered fetus is capable of survival. A prematurely delivered fetus is viable when a minimal number of inde-pendently sustained, basic, integrative physiological functions are present. The sum of these functions must support the inference that the fetus is able to increase in tissue mass (growth) and increase the number, complexity and coordination of basic physiolog-ical functions (development) as a self-sustaining organism. This development must be independent of any connection with the mother and supported only by generally accepted medical treatments. If these coordinated functions are not present, the fetus is nonviable. This may be the case even though some signs of life are apparent.

The following functions, taken together, constitute the minimal number of basic integrative physiological functions to support an inference of viability:

(1) Perfusion of tissues with adequate oxygen and prevention of increasing accumu-lation of carbon dioxide and/or lactic and other organic acids. This function consists of the following components:

(a) inflation of the lungs with oxygen;

(b) transfer of oxygen across the alveolar membrances into the circulation and elimination of carbon dioxide from the circulation into the expired gas; and

(c) cardiac contractions of sufficient strength and regularity to distribute oxygenated blood to tissues and organs throughout the body, and to eliminate organic acids from those tissues and organs.

(2) Neurologic regulation of the components of the cardio-respiratory perfusion function, of the capacity to ingest nutrients, and of spontaneous and reflex muscle movements.

These functions in the prematurely delivered fetus cannot at present be assessed separately in a consistent, reliable and exact manner. The absence of the sum of these functions, however, can be assessed indirectly in a reasonable and reliable manner by measurement of weight and an estimation of gestational age. Thus, organisms of less than 601 grams at delivery and gestational age of 24 weeks or less are at present nonviable; signs of life such as a beating heart, spontaneous respiratory movement, pulsation of the umbilical cord and spontaneous movement of voluntary muscles are not adequate in themselves to be used to determine the existence of basic integrative functions.

A weight of 601 grams or more and gestational age over 24 weeks may indicate that the minimal basic functions necessary for independent growth and development are present. Such a prematurely delivered fetus may be considered at least possibly viable. At these weights and gestational ages, a sign of life such as a beating heart, spontaneous respiratory movement, pulsation of the umbilical cord or spontaneous movement of voluntary muscles indicate possible viability." ([11], pp. 55–57.)

As the definition of 'possibly viable infant' suggests, these definitions were held to depend directly, and erroneously, as this paper argues, upon the technologies available to sustain the life of a premature infant. This intent is clear in the proposed regulations of August 23, 1974:

"Current technology is such that a fetus, given the benefit of available medical therapy, cannot survive unless the lungs can be inflated so that respiration can take place. Without this capability, even if the heart is beating, the fetus is non-viable. In the future, if technology has advanced to the point of sustaining a fetus with non-inflatable lungs, the definition can and should be modified.

The Department has therefore chosen to specify, in the definition of viability of the fetus (46.303 (e)), that heart beat and respiration are, jointly, to be the indicator of viability." ([8], p. 30651.)

Current regulations define viable as it pertains to the fetus as the state of "being able, after either spontaneous or induced delivery, to survive (given the benefit of available medical therapy) to the point of independently maintaining heart beat and respiration" ([10], p. 12).

[2] After Rawls defines moral persons – "Moral persons are distinguished by two features: first, they are capable of having (and are assumed to have) a conception of their good (as expressed by a rational plan of life); and second, they are capable of having (and are assumed to acquire) a sense of justice, a normally effective desire to apply and to act upon the principles of justice, at least to a certain minimum degree. We use the

characterization of the persons in the original position to single out the kind of beings to whom the principles chosen apply" ([6], p. 505) — he then appends a notion of potentiality, for which he does not argue ([6], p. 505).

[3] The arguments for this viewpoint can be sketched here only in very general terms. They begin with the fact that there is no generally accepted view of the good life, nor a generally accepted theory of how to establish such a view. This circumstance provides sufficient grounds for holding (if one understands by ethics, the establishment of choices among lines of conduct by appeal to reason, not force), that there will be no strong arguments in most cases for one concrete view of the good life over others. One will, though, be able to distinguish between those concrete ways of life based on force versus those based on respect for the free choice of moral agents. One will be able to make this distinction because such respect is part of the very view of ethics as an alternative to force. Such a view of ethics is not based on a metaphysical assumption, an intuitive truth, or a self-evident axiom. Rather, insofar as one is concerned to resolve, without recourse to force, disputes concerning which lines of conduct are proper or improper, one will have bound oneself to respect freedom as a side constraint or a restraint upon one's action. Respect for the freedom of the participants in such negotiations, that is, respect for persons as moral agents, becomes a canon of morality presupposed by the practice of participating in the rational process of peaceably discussing the merits of different views of the good life with other persons. Respect for freedom as a side constraint is thus acknowledged as a necessary condition for the possibility of ethics, or the peaceable community, the community in which moral disputes are resolved without the use of unconsented-to-force against the innocent. Through this view one can establish a transcendental argument (i.e., showing the necessary conditions for the possibility of) for the notion of freedom as a side constraint as advanced by Robert Nozick [5].

Beyond that canon there is very little hope that conclusive arguments will emerge to provide conclusive rational grounds to settle moral disputes. Insofar as different persons have different psychological inclinations and abilities to experience and participate in life, they will frame different views of the good life. Some concrete views of the moral life may be eliminated and others judged to be preferable in terms of such formal criteria as maximizing the diversity, unity, and intensity of human values in concrete ways of life. However, the class of ways of life which are acceptable in terms of respecting the freedom of other persons, and in terms of these general, somewhat formal aesthetic criteria, is likely to include many incompatible, concrete life styles. It is in terms of such ways of life that one will create the boundary for the social concept of person and the moral significance of criteria for fetal viability. However, it is respect of persons as moral agents that constitutes the hard core of morality.

In these considerations, it is useful to distinguish between what one might term the hard dimension and the soft dimension of ethics or morality. The hard dimension of ethics is constituted of those elements of the moral life to which one is committed in terms of the very commitment to morality itself. This hard dimension can be further distinguished in terms of a hard core and a hard periphery.

(I. A) The hard core of ethics is the very condition for the possibility of a moral community: a community that attempts to resolve without coercion questions about the nature of the good life. This condition, mutual respect for the freedom of all moral agents, fixes the boundary between the peaceable community and that community that will allow the imposition by force of the view of some on others without their consent. It is the hard core, for it is the minimum necessary condition for the notion of ethics as an endeavor raising questions about proper moral conduct and resolving such questions without force. This view has the advantage of relying only on the general notion of the possibility of envisaging moral agents asking questions about the nature of the good within an enterprise of seeking answers through agreement, not through force, while making no presuppositions about the correctness of one particular view of the good life. As a consequence, respect for persons in the strict sense will be an element of the hard core of morality; respecting infants is not.

(I. B) The hard periphery of ethics is constituted by the various schemata for hypothetical imperatives through which one articulates a particular view of the good life. Thus, once one has decided upon the goods to be pursued in child-raising, and has determined certain psychological and other conditions of the human context, it will follow where one ought to draw the compass for the social concept of person and to establish the stage of viability as a morally significant line in the use of the fetus.

Unlike the hard dimension of ethics, which is grounded in the notion of *the* moral community and of the rational pursuit of goals, and which is therefore strongly inter-subjective in its claims, the soft dimension is grounded in concerns which frame *a* partricular moral community. While the soft dimension aspires to universality (e.g., "All should recognize that personal liberty is to be valued more highly than personal security"), its propositions cannot be established by conclusive rational argument. In fact, elements of this dimension of ethics can often be established through the medium of the arts in which the virtues of particular ways of life can be portrayed. Thus stories about heroes witness for, and convert people to, particular ways of life.

Moreover, the soft dimension of ethics provides the content of the moral life. From the hard dimension of ethics it will follow that one ought to keep one's promises, not what promises one ought to make. From the hard core of morality, it will follow that agreed to fidelity in marriage should obtain. However, apart from a particular context, one will not know whether this includes or excludes polygamy or polyandry, or certain extra-marital liaisons (or, for example, under what circumstances divorce will be morally acceptable). That is, again for example, promise keeping is grounded in the very notion of *the* moral community as an intellectual construct through which one understands the basic moral constraints upon persons. The notions of what promises ought to be made are grounded in the context of *a* particular moral community of persons who are also, for example, humans sharing a particular historical cultural viewpoint.

(II) One can distinguish between the soft core and the soft periphery in the soft dimension of ethics.

(II. A) The soft core of ethics will encompass those values and interests that most persons in most societies take to be essential to a moral life. This is likely to include valuing freedom, valuing sympathy for one's fellow persons, and concerns for fairness in the distribution of commonly held goods. Such, though, is part of the soft dimension, not the hard dimension of ethics. This is the case since appeals to ideal observers (or to groups of hypothetical contractors) who are fully informed, vividly imaginative, fully knowledgeable (or in the case of John Rawls's contractors, rendered specially ignorant), dispassionate, impartial, and seeing all from everyone's perspective, will not suffice in order to discover the lineaments of *The* Moral Life. An observer (or a set of hypothetical contractors) must have interests. It, or they, must want certain things or have interests in certain states of affairs. They have *A* moral sense. However, the difficulty will be in establishing, without a *petitio principii*, which moral sense such an observer or group of contractors ought to have. After all, moral preferences, rankings of goods and evils, appear to be functions of psychological and cultural idiosyncracies, and not matters of pure reason, deducible from a rationally discoverable concept of a rational person, or discoverable by an appeal to the notion of an impartial or rational intuiter, or to a group of rational contractors. Such is the case since rankings of goods and values reflect interests in attaining particular goods and avoiding particular evils. As a result, one would expect that the criteria for inclusion within the social concept of person will vary from culture to culture, or from society to society. Such variance can be a proper reflection of the difference in accepted rankings of goods and evils, and in dispositions towards particular human interests. Notions of what constitutes a life of maximum unity, diversity, and intensity, and of the virtues of such canons in choosing among concrete views of the good life, belong in the soft dimension.

(II. B) Insofar as such variance in the acknowledgement and ranking of goods is pronounced, the values and moral propositions involved will be part of the soft periphery of ethics. As a consequence, the character of the moral life will be as much created as discovered. Though the characteristics of persons in the strict sense (persons as moral agents) will be discoverable, those of persons in the social sense (humans upon whom the rights of persons are conferred) will be created. The status of infants and fetuses, and the moral significance of birth and viability, will be the moral creation of a particular society. Finally, the term 'rights' in the case of persons in the social sense is a marker for a set of moral concerns concretely specifiable only within a particular moral community. In this sense we are all also persons socially. That is, in virtue of the values we bear within a particular community, we possess 'rights' beyond those abstract rights that depend on our very nature as moral agents. Thus, our right not to be shot for sport without our consent or to have promises kept are hard-core rights, while noncontractual 'rights' to empathy and sympathy which fashion the concrete nature of the moral life reflect the geography of moral concerns that frames a particular moral community.

4 The example of presidential rights was explored by S. I. Benn ([1], p. 102).
5 The reader should note that I stress here *secular* argument. It is important that the reader understand that here, and in fact throughout these arguments, I am indicating what can be delivered by a secular argument without special religious appeals. This distinction is important not only because it acknowledges integrity of religious arguments for religious commentaries, but also because it sets limits on the extent to which a secular society may impose religious values upon its members. Thus, it would be a violation of the notion of the moral community for a secular society to impose by law a particular religious or metaphysical view upon its unconsenting members. Such issues are not open to general, secular resolution and therefore one cannot presume that free individuals would have delegated to the state the right to impose a particular view. And to use unconsented to force against a person would violate the very notion of a moral community. These considerations set moral limits on majoritarian democratic action.

The U.S. Constitution is flawed because it allows, by an appeal to a two-thirds majority of the House and Senate and a three-fourths majority of the States, the imposition of any law whatsoever (except for altering equal representation in the Senate by

States), ranging from the establishment of the Shiite Moslem faith or the execution of all Jews, to the proscription of abortion on request in the first two trimesters of pregnancy. On this point (among a number of others), the First Constitution of the State of Texas was superior, for it forbade any restrictions of the basic rights of citizens as enumerated in the Bill of Rights of Texas. Article 1, Section 25 of the Texas Constitution of August 28, 1845, stated that "To guard against transgression of the high powers herein delegated, we declare that everything in the 'bill of rights' is exempted out of the general powers of the government and shall forever remain inviolate". The Bill of Rights adumbrated the natural rights or non-delegated rights of persons. It could not be presumed that the citizens had ceded these rights in agreeing to participate in a majoritarian democracy. Such basic rights of self-determination and liberty remain, therefore, outside the domain of a majoritarian democracy. Thus, for example, supporting an amendment to the Constitution to proscribe early abortion would be an immoral act in that it would be incompatible with the view of a moral community based on mutual respect, not force. Such an amendment would be imposing, as the Inquisition did, one view of moral life upon unconsenting innocents, when that view was not establishable through general rational appeals, and which view would restrict the basic freedoms of moral agents. They cannot be presumed to have ceded such a right to the state. Such a restriction would lack moral authority.

This view is central to the concept of the nation state, which includes many particular communities without itself being simply another community. The nation state exists to protect the hard core of morality including particular created moral frameworks insofar as they do not do violence to the hard core of morality. Which is to say, the nation state can frame and support a general view of public welfare insofar as individuals may exempt themselves from such welfare programs, and insofar as such programs do not involve force against unconsenting innocents. A moral nation, however, may not violate the basis of the peaceable community. Further, since the nation state embraces numerous communities (e.g., Roman Catholics of Irish descent, Reform Jews, Southern Baptists, urban homosexuals, atheists, Hassidic Jews, and Amish), it may not impose the views of some dominant community on the other communities, but must respect the freedom of all its members. The result is that the nation state must in many respects be amoral. It may not constrain individuals from engaging in private activities that offend certain or most moral communities, as long as such activities do not offend hard-core Morality (e.g., the nation may not forbid abortion). The state, instead of being a community with a concrete view of the good, is the secular unity of numerous communities. It is only this view of the state that offers the prospect of the peaceable collaboration of numerous communities with disparate views of the good life, and the prospect of the respect of the freedom of individual persons.

Finally, it should be added that these arguments do not count against laws forbidding abortion, as long as they are without any sanctions. Such could be interpreted as a simple expression of the moral opinion of the majority of the citizenry.

[6] An excellent discussion of zygote loss is provided by John D. Biggers's paper submitted to the Ethics Advisory Board of the U.S. Department of Health, Education, and Welfare ([2], Essay 8).

[7] St. Thomas Aquinas held that the rational soul, which sonstitutes the person, enters the fetus only some time after conception (*Summa Theologica*, Part 1, Question 118, Article 2). St. Thomas as a result recognized that abortion before 'sense and motion'

was less of an evil than abortion thereafter (*In Aristoteles Stagiritae: Politicorum seu de Rebus Civilibus*, Book VII, Lectio xii). St. Thomas's view that early abortion did not constitute the taking of the life of a person or homicide is found also in his *Commentum in Quartum Sententiarium Magistri Petri Lombardi*, Distinctio XXXI, Expisitio Textus.

[8] It may be questioned whether infanticide would have adverse moral consequences. For example, one might suggest that the Hawaiians, who practiced infanticide, had a quite defensible way of life, while the Germans, who forbade infanticide, produced in the early 20th century the horrors of Fascism. The issues are in any even complex.

[9] My point here is that in order for infants to survive one has to decide whether or not they will be placed in a social role. That is not the case with regard to fetuses. For that reason, the point of birth is a time at which one is pressed to decide whether or not one will impute personhood.

[10] One should note that the interest to minimize as far as possible the number of fetuses that would go to term and result in the birth of handicapped persons is fully compatible with an interest in maximizing the protections and privileges of those persons who are handicapped. Once persons actually exist, they have strong actual claims upon our attention, sympathies, and actions. In fact, a concern to aid the status of the handicapped person may be positively tied to programs in pre-natal diagnosis and abortion. This may be due to a general concern to diminish suffering or to maximize the resources available for the handicapped.

[11] One would need to explore the moral significance of tort for wrongful life arguments. Torts for wrongful life arguments have held that persons have a claim to compensation for injuries that are tied to the very circumstances of their having come into existence. According to these arguments, persons could therefore sue for having been born under circumstances worse than non-existence. In order to understand the moral strength of the claim for recompense to persons who were damaged as a result of injuries that occurred to their bodies before they became persons, and which injuries could then have been avoided only if one prevented the existence of that person, one would need to decide if such an injury is a violation of a duty of forbearance or one of beneficence. That is, can one be said to have treated another in disregard of his status as a free being by allowing such an injury, or does it rather violate some canon of beneficence? If persons came at once and fully into their self-possession, one could simply ask the person involved whether existence was worse than non-existence. If the afflicted individual found life not worth living under the circumstances, one could assist him or her in suicide and offer some compensation for the sufferings prior to the suicide by supporting, after the sucidide, projects that the person found important. However, persons achieve that powers of decision only years after their birth. Therefore, a considerable amount of suffering is likely to be endured before such a decision can be made.

Another way of putting the question is, whose body is there before there is a person to have that body? And may one knowingly give a person a seriously defective body? The dictum in the recent court case of *Curlender v. Bioscience Laboratories*, 165 Cal. Rptr. 477 (Ct. App. 2d. Dist. Div. 1, 1980), holding that parents could be sued by children for having been born defective, raises these issues. For a recent analysis of tort for wrongful life suits, see [3].

[12] That is, the National Commission through its concept of viability created a limit

of 24 weeks (as opposed to the Supreme Court's 24 or 28 weeks) and through its concept of pre-viability a limit of 20 weeks' gestation for particular uses of the fetus. See Note 1.

[13] The distinctions introduced in this paper could be summarized in this fashion:

Human biological life – human life that need not involve the life of a person, e.g., zygotes and fetuses. 'Human' here indicates species membership.

human personal life – human life that also involves the life of a person. Unless specifically indicated, this refers to persons in the strict sense as in the case of normal adult humans.

persons in the strict sense – persons in the sense of moral agents: self-conscious, rational, capable of free choice and having interests. This includes not only normal adult humans, but possible extra-terrestrials with similar powers.

persons in the social sense – humans who are not persons in the strict sense, but to whom some of the special rights of persons have been imputed because of utilitarian and other consequentialist considerations, e.g., infants.

possible persons – persons that could under certain circumstances come into existence. As merely possible persons they have no actual rights.

potential persons – a shorthand expression indicating entities that are not yet persons and therefore do not have any of the rights of persons, but which have a probability of 'becoming' persons. The 'entity' (e.g., fetus has 'continuity' with the 'entity' (embodied person) who will follow it in the sense of there being some physical continuity over time; an analogous continuity exists, for example, between the body of a person before and after total brain death. One entity is followed by another entity, though there is much physical continuity. There are also special and important changes in physical structure. Thus one can distinguish between what became of a body and what became of a person.

viability as a biological generalization – a point in gestation before which, for example, no infant has been known to survive.

viability as a moral criterion – a point in gestation after which abortion may be procured only with special justification, such as consideration of the health or life of the mother, or because the fetus is probably defective. This line represents a balancing of various consequentialist concerns as well as the recognition of the requirement of respecting the freedom of the pregnant woman.

BIBLIOGRAPHY

1. Benn, S. I.: 1973, 'Abortion, Infanticide, and Respect for Persons', in Joel Feinberg (ed.), *The Problem of Abortion*, Wadsworth, Belmont, California, 92–104.
2. Biggers, J. D.: 1979, '*In Vitro* Fertilization, Embryo Culture and Embryo Transfer', in U.S. Department of Health, Education, and Welfare, Ethics Advisory Board, *HEW Support of Research Involving Human In Vitro Fertilization and Embryo Transfer: Appendix*, Department of Health, Education, and Welfare, Washington, D. C., Essay 8.
3. Holder, A.: 1981, 'Is Existence Ever an Injury? The Wrongful Life Cases', in Stuart F. Spicker, Joseph M. Healey, and H. Tristram Engelhardt, Jr. (eds.), *The Law-Medicine Relation: A Philosophical Exploration*, D. Reidel Publishing Co., Dordrecht, Holland, 225–239.

4. Kant, I.: 1911, 'Grundlegung zur Metaphysik der Sitten', *Kant's Gesammelte Schriften*, Preussische Akademie der Wissenschaft Edition, Vol. 4, De Gruyer, Berlin.
5. Nozik, R.: 1974, *Anarchy, State, and Utopia*, Basic Books, New York.
6. Rawls, J.: 1971, *A Theory of Justice*, The Belknap Press of Harvard University Press, Cambridge, Massachusetts.
7. *Roe v. Wade*, 93 S. Ct. 705 (1973).
8. U.S. Department of Health, Education, and Welfare: 1974, 'Protection of Human Subjects. Proposed Policy', *Federal Register* 39 (August 23), 30618–30656.
9. U.S. Department of Health, Education, and Welfare: 1979, 'Protection of Human Subjects of Biomedical and Behavioral Research', *Federal Register* 44 (August 14), 47732–47734.
10. U.S. Department of Health, Education, and Welfare: 1978, *PRR Reports: Code of Federal Regulations* 45 CFR 46, Washington, D. C.
11. U.S. Department of Health, Education, and Welfare, National Commission for the Protection of Human Subjects of Biomedical and Behavioral Research: 1975, *Research on the Fetus: Report and Recommendations*, Department of Health, Education, and Welfare, Washington, D.C.

ROBERT C. SOLOMON

REFLECTIONS ON THE MEANING OF (FETAL) LIFE

The peculiar fact about what we call *self-consciousness* is that, when it reflects on itself, life without it seems unimaginable: indeed, it is impossible to imagine a world without ourselves. So says just about everybody: Descartes, most famously, reflected on his consciousness of himself and made it the foundation of his philosophy, an indisputable axiom in a world of doubt. "I think, therefore I am"; it was the one sure thing. Immanuel Kant similarly reflected on his own self-consciousness and discovered that he was not only the center of the world but its source as well, and it was a small step from Kant to the philosopher J. G. Fichte who said, in effect, "I am everything".[1] In England, John Locke, too, discovered his self in self-consciousness, and when David Hume denied that he found any such self in himself, he still never challenged the stage on which this familiar egotistical game was being played, namely, the stage of self-conscious reflection. We have seen Kafka endow a dog or a burrowing creature with dignity – even a cockroach – by granting it at least fictional self-consciousness. And Hegel – the one philosopher in the modern tradition who saw rather clearly that selfhood and self-consciousness presuppose interaction with other people, still made the Fichtean move: the world is self-consciousness, and it is only that which gives life meaning and has intrinsic value.

In self-conscious reflection, to use the standard metaphor since the seventeenth century, one stands before a mirror, mirroring oneself. It is not just a reflection, but a reflection of a reflection, and a reflection of a reflection of a reflection, and so on, as often as you like. Thus the 19th-century German philosophers talked about seeing the infinite in themselves, and the content of the mirror's reflections, the context of the reflection and the placement of the mirror all became relatively negligible. We are so impressed with this metaphysical curiosity that we too turn it into everything: Professor Engelhardt [2] here resembles Kant, if not Fichte, in taking personhood to revolve around moral self-consciousness. Professor Puccetti [8] emerges with Locke; personhood is based in self-conscious memories and expectations.[2] Professor Soupart [12], on the other hand, seems implicitly to deny personhood and self-consciousness to the fetus, granting it, however, a not unhonorable role in medical science: "it undoubtedly deserves a high

William B. Bondeson et al. *(eds.), Abortion and the Status of the Fetus,* 209–226.
Copyright © 1983 *by D. Reidel Publishing Company, Dordrecht, Holland.*

degree of respect when treated as a research *object*" ([12], p. 100, *my emphasis*). Presumably if it were also a self-conscious subject, this degree of respect would not much impress us.

If there is a shared premise in these distinguished papers (with whose conclusions, I should quickly say, I am largely in agreement), it is this: it is self-consciousness, which is intrinsically valuable, that bestows personhood on what otherwise might be just another biological organism. This is not, perhaps, quite the extravagant claim made by some of our philosophical ancestors, but it is, for all practical purposes, essentially the same. Self-consciousness is the "light of the world". Our concept of a 'person' – and let's say straight out that this word is a *moral* one and not at all a 'scientific' one – thus finds a concrete criterion for its application, one which itself seems to be non-moral and wholly 'objective'. To be a person is to be self-conscious, nothing less, and not necessarily much more. To be self-conscious, or potentially so, is therefore to have certain rights, not least among them – the right to life itself, the right to *be* self-conscious.[3]

SELF-CONSCIOUSNESS AND THE SOCIAL:
THE MISSING INGREDIENT

To be self-conscious is to be a person and have rights. How can I disagree with this? Well, for one thing, it does not follow that to be a person and have rights is to be self-conscious, which I would argue allows into candidacy for personhood dogs, cats and horses, who have rights but not self-consciousness, and perhaps even 'lower' forms of life as well, including fetuses and, perhaps, some plants. There are non-humans who are ostensibly self-conscious, for example, Koko the sign-speaking gorilla of Stanford.[4] I will mention, but not pursue, the possibility that not all humans who are self-conscious deserve recognition as persons, though this is too controversial an issue to treat parenthetically. But simply smudging the line between the human and the non-human, or raising a few controversial cases in which people do not deserve treatment as persons, is not enough to show that self-consciousness is not a satisfactory criterion for personhood in general. Indeed, at most this would show that abortions should be outlawed in gorillas too if they are to be outlawed in humans, or that some fetuses (for example, potential dictators) might be rightfully aborted (though the criterion for potentiality here becomes extremely problematic, along with the much abused notion of 'innocence' as applied to fetuses). But my argument here goes beyond this opening up of the concept of a person: I want to attack the self-importance we attribute to the notion of self-consciousness itself and the general philosophical assumption that underlies this. In his book, *Die Fröhliche Wissenschaft*, Friedrich Nietzsche [6] dissents from the philosophical orthodoxy by reminding us that self-consciousness only becomes interesting when we realize how *in*essential it is to us. He says,

... we could in fact think, feel, will and recollect, we could likewise 'act' in every sense of the term, and nevertheless nothing of it at all need necessarily 'come into consciousness' (as one says metaphorically). The whole of life would be possible without its seeing itself as it were in a mirror; as in fact even at present the far greater part of our life still goes on without this mirroring – and even our thinking, feeling and volitional life as well, however painful this statement may sound to older philosophers ([6], p. 78).

What Nietzsche is saying seems almost obvious – as soon as we step outside a philosophical context, however much we sometimes prefer the company of philosophers, and whether or not this is the case – we tend to think more highly of people who are deeply reflective. But, to tell you the truth, I often prefer the company of my dog, who is hardly self-conscious, to the company of other self-conscious beings, and, indeed, I value his life more highly than many of my fellow persons. And what's more, albeit philosophically, I sometimes wish that I could be just like him. Self-consciousness isn't everything.

Why is self-consciousness so important to the abortion and right-to-life debate? I agree with the spirit of the discussions presented here in general that if there is to be any civilized debate on these crucial bioethical issues, the considerations must be non-religious, rather than the purely doctrinal question of when the soul – if there is one – enters the pre-natal body or leaves a diseased one. I also agree that the medical criterion of 'viability' raises serious dangers in the face of present technology. Already, we have dramatic cases of 'viable' creatures who count as 'persons' only by appeal to the most dubious arguments – that they once were persons or, given a womb and a good education, might yet be persons. (It is finding the education, not the womb, that seems to be the greater problem today.) Given the very real possibility that, in only a few years of further research, a fetus might be 'viable' even in the first few weeks, perhaps even as a zygote, it is desirable for reasons that Engelhardt [2] mentions – to have criteria which are *morally* determined rather than dependent upon technological advances. But a criterion for moral determination – albeit with at least some scientific backing, may not be as simple as we have made it sound. Indeed, what has emerged from these presentations is a viewpoint so reasonable that it is only at the risk of considerable confusion and misunderstanding that I want to argue that we are debating a question that has no answer.

What is missing from all of these accounts, including the traditional accounts we have inherited from Descartes, Locke, Kant and others who remain our models in this debate, is the *social* context in which personhood and rights are ascribed, and the fact that self-consciousness and individual worth become of significance only within a *social* network. Self-consciousness itself is not the criterion for personhood, but only becomes so within a certain kind of society that prides itself on reflection, in certain emotions such as shame and embarrassment as well as pride, and on the basis of an anthropologically peculiar sense of individual autonomy that misleadingly suggests that the criteria we apply to ourselves are the universal truth of personhood as such. But even in such a society, it is simply not true that self-consciousness plays the absolute role that we have suggested so often in our imminently self-conscious philosophies. Neither having a self-consciousness nor having the potential for self-consciousness is a necessary or sufficient condition for personhood and rights. Those conditions emerge only within a more general sense of social worth, in which the self-ascribed worth of self-consciousness is only of partial importance.

THE TRANSCENDENTAL PRETENSE

In an earlier work, *History and Human Nature* [11], I introduced a notion which I called 'the *transcendental pretense*'. It is, in a phrase, our tendency to project our own virtues onto the whole of the species, most of whom, not surprisingly, turn out to be not so virtuous as we are. They are less sophisticated, less efficient, less understanding — 'underdeveloped' in our most paternalistic of phrases. The imagery here is that of *potential*, as if there were some pre-ordained path of development, which *we* have all but completed, from the savagery of the state of nature to the civilized accomplishments so evident at an academic cocktail party. Thus we who write the essays and defend the rights of the fetus (or deny them) tend to employ as our criteria for personhood virtues which are distinctively our own, much as Tolstoy once described the writing of history in *War and Peace*:

... history is written by learned men and so it is natural and agreeable for them to think that the activity of their class is the basis for the movement of all humanity, just as it would be natural and agreeable for merchants, agriculturalists and soldiers to entertain such a belief (if they do not express it, it is only because merchants and soldiers do not write history) ([13]).

And so it is with metaphysics too; we define what it is to be a person in terms of our own accomplishments, and we argue for and against abortion on the grounds of the fetus's *potential* for achieving similar accomplishments, in particular, philosophical self-consciousness. But this cannot be — by the nature of the case — the argument *of the fetus*; it is *our* argument to the effect that the fetus has the potential for certain virtues of value *to us*. One question that follows is the question that Puccetti [8] put much more politely — "*so what?*" Another question, which I want to pursue here, is "of value *to whom*"? If the possibility of self-consciousness is not of any value to the fetus (any more than the logical possibility of self-consciousness is of value to the kittens in Michael Tooley's [14] much quoted example), then what kind of criterion is being invoked here? It can only be because *we* so value it. The virtue we so fundamentally treasure in ourselves (as Puccetti's pedagogical examples show so keenly) is extrapolated from our particular social context to human life as such, aside from any social context; self-consciousness itself is said to be intrinsically valuable, and this is precisely what I want to challenge here.

To assume that self-consciousness is in itself the criterion for personhood is to eliminate from proper consideration virtually every member of the animal kingdom (excepting, perhaps, a few apes and water mammals); they have rights, if at all, by virtue of our sense of compassion, our designation of them as valuable. But this is not how we see our own rights, or the rights of our potential progeny. Moreover, to assume that self-consciousness is the criterion for personhood raises horrendous problems concerning human beings who are not, in our sense, self-conscious. Some people have no autonomous sense of individual worth apart from society. They have no sense of a right to life, apart from the right given them by society. Does this make them less persons, or qualify their rights, in our eyes? Jean-Paul Sartre [10], a good humanist through and through, nevertheless raises questions about the non- (or 'proto-') humanity of the 'primitive' tribesmen studied and celebrated by his colleague Claude Levi-Strauss. Of course, it can be argued that they, like any fetus in our more 'civilized' countries, have the *potential* for becoming self-conscious, perhaps even becoming philosophers. But at this point we surely begin to suspect that the argument itself has somehow gone awry, and it is the transcendental pretense that has let it do so.

The transcendental pretense is not in itself objectionable; on an everyday basis, intellectuals tend to evaluate everyone on the basis of intelligence and athletes evaluate everyone on the basis of physical prowess and Marxists and radical feminists tend to evaluate everyone on their attitudes on 'the issues'. And our way of dealing with this slightly obnoxious tendency in ourselves is to segregate ourselves willingly, with the proviso, "you don't impose your standards on us, we won't impose ours on you (even if they are superior)". But where moral questions are concerned, this small-scale liberal social compact never works, for it is the nature of such questions that they do not simply define preferences but present universal demands. If my neighbor is partial to broiling children – even his own – I have no qualms about bringing in the law. If there is overpopulation and mass starvation in India, most of us feel the right to intervene. And this does not seem to depend, in either case, upon mutual consent. But it is the transcendental pretense that makes this possible, for it is the essence of the argument that our values regarding the right to life are not just our peculiar preferences but universal moral concerns which we have the right to enforce whenever and wherever we can.

When questions about the transcendental pretense – usually under the less philosophical title 'ethnocentrism' – are discussed, the examples usually tend to be comparisons and contrasts between ourselves and some well-documented cannibal tribes in New Guinea or some virtually extinct mountain people in Eastern Africa. That is not the strategy I want to invoke here. Consider my neighbor who broils his children; in what sense is that my business? How does that differ from my neighbor's wife, who wants to get an abortion? Suppose they believe that nothing is a person unless it is fully self-conscious with a provable I.Q. of over 150? What if my neighbors simply want to eat one of their chickens? In what case is my language justifiably the 'pro-life' language of murder, as in the case of culinary infanticide? And that language, to be sure, is not the language of Julia Child.

SELF-CONSCIOUSNESS, RATIONALITY, SELF-DEVELOPMENT AND MORALITY

The version of the transcendental pretense that concerns me here is that modern European criterion of personhood as individual self-consciousness. That is, to be a person, or a fully developed person anyway, is to have a conception of oneself, to see oneself as an individual with rights, to have plans and ambitions for oneself, whether or not oneself alone. An earlier version of the same pretense was to be found in the Christian concept of the soul – which said, in effect, that each person had a soul whether he or she knew it or not, and, in the interests of saving that soul, others had the right to intervene, even to kill. The modern version, partly because it was the invention of rather worldly, utilitarian-minded philosophers, is slightly more modest, but it too evalutes personhood on the basis of its own virtues and values — with an emphasis on *self-consciousness, rationality, self-development* and *moral responsibility*. These are, to be sure, the virtues and values according to which we evaluate ourselves and each other; but are they more than this? Do they transcend our peculiarly self-conscious and development-minded culture? Should they be the sole or at least bed rock arbiters of right to life? Does the fetus, by virtue of its *potential* for these properties, have the rights of a person? Do the lack of these properties *cancel* such rights?

Regarding Engelhardt's [2] criterion of 'rationality', I think I can get you to agree without much argument that rationality, at least, is a culturally peculiar product; Tom Robbins in *Even Cowgirls Get the Blues* [9] notes that there are hundreds of ways to live on the earth, but only one wrong way — which is called rationality. That's a bit overboard, perhaps, and not just a little faddish, but it makes the point. What we call 'rationality' is a virtue that emerged with a few Greek orators, a minority of Medieval monks and the Enlightenment; and even today, one has no trouble finding defenders of alternative views who see rationality as trouble, interfering with our naturally religious or socially obedient natures. 'Rationality' means: using common sense, cool deliberation, having faith in science, as opposed to blind obedience, belief in witchcraft and sacrificing virgins to the river gods. Now I do not subscribe to any of these alternative views, but I would not hesitate to call those who do, 'persons'.

So too with Engelhardt's [2] criterion that a person be 'self-developing'. This is a peculiarly bourgeois notion since the only sense to be given to the implicit contrast between the personal self-development that bestows individual rights and the development that one can point to in a frog or an oak tree, comes down again to self-consciousness, to plans and ambitions, rather than mere growth. Indeed, it is the growth of self-consciousness itself that many of us value most, though not exclusively. In order to have the moral thrust this criterion is supposed to have, the self so developed must be an *individual* self. But this notion of an individual self is clearly a cultural peculiarity, as this particular metaphor (which today goes by the somewhat unhappy name 'human potential movement' and which 150 years ago the poet Goethe called *Bildung*) is to be found only in a small number of cultures with which we, not surprisingly, identify. Consider, as an example, Aristotle's Greece. But it is not *self*-development that we are talking about here — even though we think we are. A human being alone, without a culture, is not a "talented but unfulfilled ape" as Clifford Geertz has often argued, but "a wholly mindless and unworkable monstrosity" ([4], p. 68). The individual self does not develop: culture develops us, and, in certain cultures, develops us as individuals. If I can mock Nietzsche this time, one might say, "man does not live for potential: only the German philosopher does". (And some of our fellows in California, of course.) What counts as 'self-development', i.e., what makes development possible, is our role in a culture. I myself have ambitions, as do we all; but let's not make the mistake of making that one of the criteria for personhood. We think of ourselves in terms of potential, but that has nothing to do with rights to life or personhood.

Finally, Engelhardt [2] argues that persons must be members of the moral community – which fetuses are presumably not – and it is membership in such a community that bestows rights. This looks attractively like my own insistence that individual worth and right to life are to be accounted for only within a community. But this is not quite the case, for what Engelhardt [2] means by 'membership' is, in my opinion, much too strong. Indeed, he argues that only moral agents have rights, which excludes not only fetuses and animals but any number of persons who, for a variety of reasons ranging from serious illness to political impotence might be excluded from consideration on these grounds. The confusion here seems to me to be between the members of a moral community in whom rules and values are embodied and the 'objects' of moral concern which, presumably, will include all members, including fetuses, and any number of other beings as well, e.g., foodstuffs, artwork, icons or the weather. Nor will it do to say that the rights of persons apply only to potential members of that community, for as Puccetti [8] has argued, there is a significant difference between potential persons potentially having rights (which is almost trivial) and potential persons having rights, which is nonsense. However not only fetuses but even cows and plants may be objects of moral concern and thereby have rights, so long as we are clear that rights are granted in being recognized. This may hold whether or not the bearer of rights in any sense is or can ever become conscious of its rights. So none of this is sufficient to defend the right to abortion on the ground that the fetus, which is not a member of the moral community, cannot be the bearer of rights. Neither is the argument that fetuses are potential members of the moral community any reason to insist that they have a right to life. To say that rights are endowed by the community is not to say that only members or potential members of that community have rights. It is only to say that, outside of a social network, the language of rights and 'right to life' does not have a meaning at all. And within an appropriate community, anything whatever might have a right to life (if it is alive, of course) so long as the community

deems it to have that right. Indeed, this almost resembles a tautology —
fetuses have the right to life if they are deemed to have a right to life. But
it is not. Like 'business is business' and 'boys will be boys', this apparent
tautology has hidden within its grammatically repetitive structure one of the
most violent moral disagreements of our times.

What is self-consciousness? Self-consciousness is too easily confused with
mere consciousness, and consciousness with mere sentience — and this is
true even of some of the great philosophers. Worms and, I surmise, fetuses
are sentient. This alone surely gives no claim to the right to life, though
perhaps we will all agree that even flies and mosquitoes should die painlessly
whenever possible. Dogs and very young children are fully conscious, but
not self-conscious; yet I think we would agree that they have a claim to rights
to life. Dogs have no particular potential for development, but this does not
seem to me to change the argument. Most children do have such potential,
but I would even argue that it is unfair and degrading to children to consider
them valuable and grant them rights on the basis of their future potential.
Children have a right to life as children, and not as potential adults.

Self-consciousness, finally, has a particularly stringent set of conditions;
not least is the ability to speak and the opportunity to learn a language, a
special kind of language which is complete with self-reference and an abstract
set of concepts which in a loose sense might be called 'metaphysical'.[5]
But however much we may identify with other speakers of such a language,
surely it is not this that endows personhood; there are cultures that have
no language of self-reference; they have no first person singular. There are
cultures in which self-reference is a grammatical contingency; there is no
self (for there is no language of the self); there is only someone speaking.
And in any case, self and self-consciousness are not inherent to the individual
alone but rather to the society. No less an outspoken individualist than
Jean-Paul Sartre has argued throughout his life that the self is ultimately
a construction, and a construction largely constituted by other people. That
we have a sense of self, and what this sense of self is, is not itself, a product
of self. Nor is it the case that the self is self-contained, or of intrinsic value
in itself. Indeed, in a culture such as Aristotle's Greece, the idea of a self
not defined in terms of its society would be all but unthinkable. The Jewish
conception of immortality is quite explicitly remembrance in the minds of
others, and the value of life as life is just this too.[6] It is self-consciousness
as *Sittlichkeit*, as organic membership in a community. And here we come
to what I see as the heart of the matter — that the artificial focus on self and
self-consciousness in what we have been saying here makes it look all too
much as if selves were valuable in themselves, when in fact, they are of value

only in and through others. Indeed, I would want to push this argument further than many of you might — to argue that the value of life itself is never first of all a matter of intrinsic worth but of value to others. Is there, then, no intrinsic value to human life? That does not follow. We are taught to value ourselves and each other as 'ends in themselves' — no small cultural accomplishment, to be sure — but the genealogy is the reverse of our usual image: intrinsic worth is a product of, not prior to, extrinsic worth. The value of a fetus, therefore, turns not on its intrinsic worth as a 'potential self-consciousness' but simply on its being valued as such. Someday it may make claims on its own behalf as a self-consciousness, but as a fetus, its worth is *entirely* in the hands of others. Its value has nothing to do with its own potential self-consciousness, except insofar as others value that potential self-consciousness. Indeed, even as adults, our worth is hardly dependent upon our own self-consciousness, no matter how conclusive that sometimes seems to us. We are what we are *to others*, little more, and nothing less.[7]

THE SOURCE OF WORTH: THE SIGNIFICANCE OF THE FETUS

In his most lampooned and lamented comment of all, John Stuart Mill famously declared in his pamphlet *Utilitarianism* that "the sole evidence that it is possible to produce that anything is desirable is that people actually do desire it" ([5], Paragraph 56). Teachers of philosophy ever since have delighted their undergraduate audiences by showing so easily how this claim falls apart with the distinction between 'desirable' as 'able to be desired' (which yields a tautology) and 'desirable' as '*ought* to be desired' (which is the morally relevant claim, but which does not follow at all). A few brave souls have defended Mill, for example, by appealing to his *System of Logic* where he spells out the connection between 'desirability' and "the excitation of the feeling of approbation", but the fallacy seems to remain intact *so long as 'people' is taken to refer to individuals rather than cultures and societies*. Individuals, of course, often want what they ought not to, but there comes a point at which it becomes absurd to distinguish what *a people* want and what they ought to want, except from some outside standpoint which can be simply dismissed as irrelevant. A society launches into a wave of religious fanaticism which disrupts institutions and very likely leads to its defeat by some political rival; *we* say (or they say, in retrospect) that they ought not to have had those desires, but only by appeal to a law of (secular) survival which is, within that religious consciousness, not an ultimate criterion, if it counts at all. More to the point, the Spartans committed infanticide regularly, and many societies besides our own continue to take advantage of the modern medical technology that makes abortions relatively safe and painless; from what standpoint are these practices to be criticized as 'not desirable', if not within the society in question and according to what "the people actually do desire"? Whose decision is it that some Spartan babies are not worth saving? Whose decision is it that a woman in our society has the right – or does not – to have an abortion and terminate the life of a fetus that is, in some sense, 'hers'? Who, in such cases, are 'the people'?

The idea that society in general will decide makes little sense in our heterogenous culture; we know what will happen – open moral warfare with victory going to the politically strongest party. We try in fact to appeal to 'the standards of the community', but what this tends to mean in practice is that conservative communities have the right to prohibit the activities of minorities, while more liberal communities will continue to be controlled by federal or state legislation.[8] Appeals to majorities in such issues in such societies are clearly beside the moral point, and the essence of the abortion issue in America is that there seems to be no common moral ground – except for the general prohibition on murder – upon which the issue can be resolved. And so the issue returns to the notion of the intrinsic worth of human life, including fetal life. If the fetus is indeed a person, is killing a fetus murder? And that is where the current dispute reaches its impasse, debating such criteria as 'self-consciousness' and appealing to such undebatable authorities as 'the word of God' or, in lieu of God, Jerry Falwell. But my proposal here is that we not only reject the criterion of self-consciousness, which has been so often used to distinguish the fetus from full-fledged personhood, but reject the notion of intrinsic worth which lies behind the 'pro-life' argument as well. And what this will do – without reconciling the differences – is to at least disarm the two sides, by showing not that there is nothing to fight about, but that the fighting has neither a point nor an end.

How did we come to recognize the supposedly intrinsic worth of human life, including perhaps, the proto-human life of the fetus? An adequate answer to that question would involve the whole history of ethics, but I think a short answer could be gleaned from Hegel's moral philosophy.[9] That answer is that, as tribal and communal society began to enlarge beyond the size in which traditional bonds could hold people together and give them a distinctive and integral place in society, people began to compensate for the loss of identity within the community with a view of *individual*

rights, a sense of abstract, intrinsic worth which had no relationship to
one's worth *to* anyone or anything. In Hegel's view, this was poor compensation for what had been lost, but in a large and impersonal society, it provided
the only protection the isolated individual could depend upon. And in our
society in particular, we have the unusual propensity to value life intrinsically,
without reference to social ties and social roles. It is this notion of intrinsic
value that initiates the abortion question about the right to life of the fetus,
for if it were not the case that persons had intrinsic rights, it is doubtful
that one could imagine a plausible argument concerning the intrinsic rights
of fetuses.[10]

In a society such as ours, where anonymity is a standard fact of life and
impersonality a daily experience, in which being a stranger in town is as
common to most of us as being 'at home', an unusually broad concept of
respect for persons is required, not because we are more 'civilized' than other
cultures, but because we have more of a problem identifying ourselves and
other people. Respect for persons as such, even when we know nothing
else about them, is the prerequisite for the very existence of a society such
as ours, not by way of a set of conventions that are usually referred to as
'the social contract' but as a straightforward *causal* pre-condition. If we did
not have respect for persons *qua* persons, our society could not survive.
And so too is the value of non-persons to be decided, by reference to their
potential roles in a society of a certain kind. Intrinsic value, in other words,
is itself a *social convention* whose purpose is to serve the good of society
as a whole. And what is to count as a person – adults, men, women, children,
children of citizens, members of a certain class – is also a matter of social
determination. The intrinsic value of an individual depends on whether he
or she (or, in the case of a fetus, perhaps, it) is embodied in a society which
is concerned with the intrinsic value of the individual.

To suggest a genealogy of morals is not yet to undermine or reject that
morality. To deny intrinsic rights to the fetus is not in itself to say anything
about the justifiability of abortions, but to understand the origins of our
notion of intrinsic worth is indeed useful in clarifying the kind of question
the abortion question ought to be.

*The worth of a fetus is the worth it has according to the people involved
with it, and who will be involved with it after birth.* There is all the difference
in the world between two unborn babies of whatever trimester, one of whom
has a mother who sees her pregnancy as an act of God and acknowledges
the fetus as a full-fledged person from the very moment she first hears the
news from her doctor, and another whose mother views her pregnancy

as an invasion of her body not unlike a tumor, to be gotten rid of as quickly as possible. The first endows the fetus with full rights, by virtue of the fact that she so views it; the latter will claim that 'one's body is one's own', and she will not listen well to those who claim that she is no longer the sole inhabitant of her body. Does her fetus have rights? I think that this is the wrong question. Contrary to the whole tradition of 'rights' talk, I want to insist that rights are not 'had', they are endowed, and sometimes claimed. The fetus cannot claim rights, so do we endow it with rights, *a priori*, regardless of who it is or will be? The fact is that we are a society torn apart on such issues, which cannot be resolved even by the calm and considered deliberations of the medical, legal, or philosophical professions. And this is not a question of freedom (of religion, for example) which might well obey the liberal proviso that each can do as he or she pleases so long as there is no interference with others' rights, for the question here is precisely whether or not there is an 'other' involved. And to this, I suggest, there is no single, transcendental answer, since there is no criterion for persons apart from the fact that others recognize them as such. And, in the case of the fetus, this is exactly the point that we cannot agree upon.

In the case of the mother who wants her child, supported hopefully by a father and an indefinitely large family and community, the question of worth does not even arise. It is taken for granted. The baby is valuable because it is *wanted*, and that value is then projected into the baby itself as 'intrinsic'. The difficult case is the one in which the baby is totally unwanted, unwanted by the mother, a matter of indifference or inconvenience to virtually everyone else. According to what I have been arguing, it might be concluded — too quickly — that there is no worth whatsoever to that unwanted fetus, but that is not true. Complicating the issue is the fact that that proto-baby is valued, albeit abstractly, by precisely those people who insist upon the intrinsic value of all human life, including fetal life. They thereby bestow some value on that unwanted child, but the consequence of that, it seems to me, is that they also thereby incur some considerable responsibility for it.[11]

The value of a fetus to society in general may well turn on straightforward economic and biological considerations. For example, a society that is dangerously underpopulated will see every fetus as not only a potential person but as a full person with all rights, especially the right to life. On the other hand, a dangerously overpopulated culture might well see the fetus as a virtual parasite, to be considered as much the same as the carrier of a disease, without rights, like a rat during the plague years. In our society, however,

222 ROBERT C. SOLOMON

certain inordinate fears aside, neither of these extreme situations is presently plausible, and the question of worth of the fetus tends to turn on a large variety of more individual factors, including religious commitments (which are beyond the scope of this essay). But if one simply considers the difference between the status of a fetus in a family that desperately loves and wants children and the status of a fetus that is the accidental by-product of a casual affair, it becomes clear that we are not at all talking about the same kind of worth. The first is worth endowed by love; the second is worth endowed only by an abstract principle. Indeed, it is one of the peculiarities of the abortion question that the issue of rights comes up only in those cases in which the fetus is threatened, and virtually never in the contrasting situation in which the fetus is already accepted with enthusiasm into a family and perhaps an entire community that are already preparing for its arrival and its future life as a member of the community. But it is in the (fallacious) extrapolation from the undeniable sense of worth in the latter case to the more unsettling and abstract questions in the first case that the *faulty notion* of the *intrinsic worth of the fetus* is born. We move from our feelings about babies of our own to an unsupported metaphysical postulation of the intrinsic worth of the individual fetuses themselves. But not only do fetuses as such lack such intrinsic worth; we do too.

ON (NOT) ANSWERING THE ABORTION QUESTION

In a community that cannot agree on the personhood of fetuses in an *a priori* way, there is no *a posteriori* criterion for doing so. But I want to correct the impression that my insistence here that there is no intrinsic worth to individuals and no intrinsic rights as such is a purely negative proposal, like Dan Dennett's suggestion that we first of all call *ourselves* 'persons', and then others "as the spirit moves us" [1]. My answer is not so cynical or merely negative: it is to say that personhood need not turn on *self-consciousness*, but that human life, fetal life, and self-consciousness are all of value insofar as they are of value to others as well as ourselves. This answer may not be popular in these days of 'pulling your own strings' and 'looking out for number 1', and some may object to the consequence that, since fetuses are not self-conscious, their value is *entirely* extrinsic and in the hands of their potential parents or guardians. But it seems to me that too much emphasis has been placed on the impossible question, whether a fetus is a person or not, apart from any consideration of the concerns and values of other people and society in general. The utilitarian tries to take this into account, in his or her considerations of how miserable everyone might become if a child is unwanted, but the problem with this account is that it tends to turn *against* the fetus in an *a priori* way, since the fetus by its very nature has a limited capacity for pleasure and pain and, in any case, the question only arises when the child is unwanted. This leads to the inevitably absurd *cul-de-sac* of arguments about the potential pleasures and pains of a merely potential and almost wholly unknown proto-person, and leaves this all-important moral question mainly a matter of imagination. On the other hand, dogmatic moral principles about the *a priori* right to life of the fetus make it sound as if considerations regarding the concerns, desires and happiness of everyone else are tangential if not morally irrelevant. And consequently, the welfare of the child-to-be is also neglected, in the name of an abstract 'right' that no longer makes any reference to human concerns and interests. The value of the fetus, and therefore the value of the child-to-be and person-to-be too, is constituted by its place in *a network of social relationships*, and if these cannot be boiled down to an *a priori* principle neither can they be dismissed as irrelevant.

What, then, are we to say about our most dangerous domestic dispute, far more disruptive than party politics or financial affairs, where at least we have some firm agreement on the goals at stake? My answer will probably not satisfy everyone − since I want to say, in effect, that there is no answer, because there is no single principle or ontology that we can agree upon in this still (thankfully) heterogeneous and pluralistic society. There will be groups and neighborhoods and perhaps whole cities and states which hold the fetus in such reverence that, to be a member of that community, is to share that sense of reverence. In that community, abortion is out of the question, but not because of law, for no law is needed. There will be groups and neighborhoods and whole cities and states in which the fetus is considered to be no more than a potential person, not yet eligible for the rights of a person. There, abortion will be considered as an operation on the woman: the fetus does not count at all. But most often, given the complexity and inter-mixing of subcultures and moral groups in our society, there will be no such clear-cut answer, since there will be no such clear-cut community. The decision will be − though not in the sense usually intended − a strictly individual or family choice. This is not because all moral choice ultimately rests with the individual so much as because it is in the individual − usually the pregnant woman − that the powerful vectors of competing moralities confront one another. Indeed, it may be a difficult choice; often it will be made by appealing to one competing group of demands rather than another. But this is not to say – as we are so prone to rationalize *after* such decisions – that the principle of the chosen group (whether 'right to life' or 'right to one's own body') should therefore be imposed on everyone else as well. One makes one's choice; one lives with it. One chooses one's community (or to stay in one's community) and one lives its mores. Religious civil war is not going to make those choices any easier.

I have been accused, as you will well imagine, of having fallen prey to that horrible thesis known to philosophers as 'moral relativism'; but why is it, I want to ask in return, that finding value in human relationships and community is considered 'relativism' (or worse, 'nihilism'), while appealing to abstract and often inhuman principles and imposing them on everyone else is considered to be 'moral'? My tone may not be humble but my thesis is: there *is* something of ultimate value, even if it is not either human life or self-consciousness *simpliciter*.

What does this mean, in terms of medical practice, in terms of the law? I am afraid it means that we should go on functioning as our country has always functioned – chaotically, and without a fixed rule of procedure. Part of that chaos has always been and will always be some self-appointed guardians of universal morality and the transcendental pretense, perennially clamoring for restrictions on the Immoral Minority; and part of that chaos will always be certain moral dilemmas facing the individual caught between two subcultures, both of which have their appeal. And, of course, we will have more conferences. But this is far preferable, I would say, than opening up one more intimate feature of American life to the underworld and governmental controls or setting us up for internal organized conflicts which might not too outrageously be compared to the Thirty Years War in Germany, which finished that country for almost two centuries. But to be without law is not to be without morality. There are *internal moral constraints*, though they are not universal, and are often at odds with each other. They will have to do.

The University of Texas at Austin

NOTES

[1] Heinrich Heine, parodying Fichte, wrote, "Himself as everything: How does Mrs. Fichte put up with it?" (*Werke I*, 358).
[2] The self-consciousness criterion for personhood today tends to take a linguistic turn:

Harry Frankfurt, for example, in a classic paper on the subject 'Freedom of the Will and the Concept of a Person' [3] takes our ability to have 'second order desires', i.e., desires concerning our desires, as the criterion for personhood, and this in turn presupposes a language in which such desires can be described and evaluated. Michael Tooley [14] in 'Abortion and Infanticide', the most controversial paper yet written on the abortion topic, argues that even kittens would be persons if they developed a language in which to be self-conscious. Indeed, the classical literature in Europe from Descartes to Sartre often finds itself tangled in the web of language and self-conscious experience, ascribing properties to the one that properly belong to the other. But this is another topic.

3 Puccetti [8] does distinguish personhood from rights claims, Engelhardt [2] does not. Soupart [12] dodges the question, though the logical connection seems to be implicit in his discussion.

4 Elizabeth Anscombe was asked what would happen to our concept of 'being human' when they teach apes to speak. She said, quite simply and prophetically, "they up the ante".

5 I will not consider here the rudimentary self-consciousness that may be possible in creatures without such a language.

6 Engelhardt has offered in discussion the example of the orthodox Jewish woman who, despite her desire for a child, is ordered by the elders of her community to have an abortion in order to save her life. The identity of the child is the identity it is given by the community, and in such a society, even a mother's love is not sufficient to override the lack of recognition of the community at large. (Of course, there is always the question of whether any community in our society is ever sufficiently closed or impervious to alternative moral interpretations.)

7 I am leaving entirely open the question of whether one of the 'others' − in fact the only 'Other' that counts − might be God. To say that the life of a person or a fetus is sacred is, in any case, quite different from the claim that life is intrinsically valuable, and since the question about whether God does or does not value each and every human life − indeed whether or not he exists − is a question which cannot be answered without religious authority, I shall say no more about it here.

8 One thinks, for example, of Pitkin County, Colorado, in which the community clearly approves of cocaine and other pratices verboten in the larger society; but there we do not see the familiar appeal to 'community standards' among federal enforcement agencies.

9 In particular, his early 'theological' essays of 1793–1799 and his Philosophy of Right of 1820, coupled with selected passages from his Phenomenology of Spirit and his lectures of 1802–1806.

10 Thus Robert Nozick, to choose but one recent example, confidently begins his Anarchy, State and Utopia, stating "individuals have rights" ([7], p. 1).

11 For those who argue against abortion, therefore, I think the obligation is quite clear − that one accepts responsibility for the welfare of the child. It is worth noting that the Catholic Church, in accordance with this principle, has long seen its particular obligation to take care of the children that would not have come into the world except by its insistence.

BIBLIOGRAPHY

1. Dennett, D. C.: 1978, *Brainstorms: Philosophical Essays on Mind and Psychology*, Bradford Bks., Vermont.
2. Engelhardt, H. T., Jr.: 1982, 'Viability and the Use of the Fetus', in this volume, pp. 182–208.
3. Frankfurt, H.: 1971, 'Freedom of the Will and the Concept of a Person', *Journal of Philosophy* **68**, 5–20.
4. Geertz, C.: 1973, *Interpretations of Cultures*, Basic Books, New York.
5. Mill, J. S.: 1971 *Utilitarianism*, edited by S. Gorowitz, Bobbs-Merrill Co., Inc., Indiana.
6. Nietzsche, F.: 1974, *The Gay Science*, translated with commentary by W. Kaufmann, Random House, New York.
7. Nozick, R.: 1975, *Anarchy, State and Utopia*, Basic Books, New York.
8. Puccetti, R.: 1982, 'The Life of a Person', in this volume, pp. 169–182.
9. Robbins, T.: 1977, *Even Cowgirls Get the Blues*, Bantam.
10. Sartre, J. -P.: 1960, *Critique de la Raison Dialectique*, French and European Pubs., New York.
11. Solomon, R.: 1979, *History and Human Nature*, Harcourt Brace Jovanovich, Inc., New York.
12. Soupart, P.: 1982, 'Present and Possible Future Research in the Use of Human Embryos', in this volume, pp. 67–104.
13. Tolstoy, L.: 1931, *War and Peace*, Modern Library, New York.
14. Tooley, M.: 1976, 'Abortion and Infanticide', in S. Gorowitz (ed.), *Moral Problems in Medicine*, Prentice-Hall, New Jersey, pp. 297–317.

SECTION IV

INTERCOURSE, WOMEN, AND
MORAL RESPONSIBILITY

HOLLY M. SMITH

INTERCOURSE AND MORAL RESPONSIBILITY
FOR THE FETUS

In her ground-breaking paper on abortion, Judith Jarvis Thomson [3] examines an argument against abortion that strikes a responsive chord with many people. As stage-setting for this argument, she makes the following two assumptions: (1) First, it is assumed that the fetus is a person, that is, has all the basic rights that normal adults do, and, in particular, the right to life. (Neither Thomson nor I believe this assumption is correct, but we may allow it for purposes of examining the argument in question.) (2) Second, it is assumed that the right to life does not entail the right to anything and everything necessary to maintain one's life. Thus, I have a right to life, but this right does not give me the right to use your kidneys if they are necessary to support my life. Similarly, a fetus's right to life does not entail the right to whatever is necessary for its support. For example, to use a case of Donald Regan's, suppose a woman carrying a two week old fetus is discovered to have a terminal disease that will kill her before the fetus reaches a state of independent viability [1]. However, advances of science have made it possible to remove such a fetus and transfer it to the womb of another woman where it would undergo normal development and be delivered as a healthy child. In this particular instance no willing surrogate mother can be found. Despite this, would we say that the fetus has the right to the use of another woman's body, just because it has a right to life – i.e., that another woman may be forcibly conscripted and compelled to serve as host to the fetus until it can survive by itself? Presumably we would not – we do not feel that the fetus's right to life gives it the right to *whatever* resources it needs to sustain that life. We may grant, then, Assumption (2).

With this background, the argument with which we are concerned enters onto the stage. It begins by pointing out that the case of a woman who becomes pregnant in the normal way seems intuitively quite different from the case of the conscriptee into pregnancy just described. We may trace this intuitive difference to the following facts. The normal pregnant woman voluntarily engaged in intercourse, knowing that doing so might result in pregnancy. If she did not want to become pregnant, she took a risk – and lost. Through her action she brought the fetus into existence, brought about its presence inside her, and brought about its dependence on her for continued

William B. Bondeson et al. *(eds.), Abortion and the Status of the Fetus*, 229–245.
Copyright © 1983 by D. Reidel Publishing Company, Dordrecht, Holland.

life. None of this is true of the conscriptee, who did nothing to bring on her artificial pregnancy, and may have done everything to avoid it. Since the normally pregnant woman is responsible in this sense for her pregnancy, and in particular for the need of the fetus to use her body if it is to survive, it may seem plausible to say that by her acts she has *given* the fetus the right to use her body – something that could not possibly be said of the conscriptee. Since she has given it the right to use her body, it would be wrong of her now to deny it that use by procuring an abortion – just as it would be wrong of me to forcibly take back my lawnmower from you after granting you the right to use it for the afternoon.

Let us call this the *Responsibility Argument* ([3], pp. 57–59). Abstractly characterized, it amounts to the claim that if (A) one person depends on the continued use of another person's body in order to survive, and (B) the second person acted in a manner that brought about this state of affairs, then (C) the second person has thereby transferred the right to the use of his or her body to the dependent person, and would be wrong to deny the dependent person that use. Additional details may of course prove relevant, for example the fact that the second person *knew* that dependence would result from his or her action. We can consider these as the occasion warrants.

Thomson contends that there are at least some cases of natural pregnancy – and perhaps a great many cases – in which the responsibility argument does *not* succeed in showing that abortion would be wrong. Many readers have found her treatment of this argument suggestive but unsatisfactory either because it is insufficiently detailed, or because the analogies she employs to show its failure are inapt. In this paper I propose to examine the Responsibility Argument in greater depth, or more accurately to *begin* that examination, since completion of the task surpasses the limits of the present occasion.

I

Before turning directly to a consideration of the Responsibility Argument, let me clarify some related issues.

First, there is a great deal of debate about the question of whether a woman's having an abortion should properly be considered as 'killing the fetus', or merely as throwing the fetus back on its own (inadequate) resources and so 'allowing the fetus to die'. Many of us have different moral responses to situations that differ only with respect to a death's being brought about by a killing or a letting die, so that it may be important to settle this issue. Which view we ought to accept may depend on the mechanics of the abortion in question. For example, we may feel that an abortion produced by suctioning out the fetus, whose body is rended limb from limb in the process, is undeniably a killing of that fetus. On the other hand, an abortion produced by merely detaching the fetus from the uterine wall and then discarding its intact body may be much less clearly a case of killing. In this later case we may feel that 'allowing the fetus to die' does not provide an adequate description of what happens, either. Perhaps it would more accurately be called 'discontinuing life support'. But even this category has two subcases that can elicit differential responses. Sometimes we discontinue support be *ceasing to supply it*, as when someone stops giving insulin injections to a comatose diabetic. At other times we discontinue support by *removing the dependent person from the supply*, as when we disconnect someone from a respirator. Many people feel the second of these is morally worse than the first, and it seems clear that abortion must fall into this category. However, there is no universal agreement that removing a person from a life-support source counts as *killing* that person. Until we have a better account of the nature of these distinctions, and why they are important (if indeed they are), I believe it is better to steer clear of them, and I shall try to do so in what follows.

Second, it may be important that in the case of abortion we are talking about a person who needs the continued use of another person's *body* in order to live. There are many cases in which one person needs continued use of the personal possession of some other person in order to live – for example, his medicine, or his shelter, or his food – but not his body *per se*. Since we tend to feel that the body deserves special moral protection beyond that needed for mere material possessions, it may be that what is necessary in order to give away the right to one's material possession, such as a medication. Hence wherever possible I try to construct parallel examples involving the use of bodies rather than other possessions.

Third, it is not clear to me (despite Thomson's first background assumption stated before) that success of the Responsibility Argument turns on the dependent party's being a *person*, i.e., a being with initial basic rights of its own, and in particular a right to life. Our concern is whether or not certain activities of the prospective mother amount to giving the fetus a right, and it may well be that one can give or transfer rights to creatures who would otherwise have none of their own. For example, if I leave a will in which I stipulate that the income from my estate is to be used for the maintenance of my twenty-six cats, it seems to me that I have *given* the cats the right to this use of that income, even though cats may have no natural rights of their own. Hence the Responsibility Argument *may* be important both for people who believe that fetuses are persons, and also for people such as myself who believe they are not.

Fourth, it needs to be pointed out that the dilemma raised by abortion is not a dilemma involving a *simple* conflict between a woman's right to bodily integrity and a fetus's right to life. Many conservative arguments against abortion assume that the dilemma is of this simple nature, assert with great plausibility that the right to life is stronger than the right to bodily integrity, and so conclude that abortion is always wrong. But to see a genuine case involving a *simple* conflict between two rights, we must look elsewhere. For a relevant example, consider Jones, the driver of a subway train. Jones' train is rounding a bend, on the other side of which the tracks fork and he must steer either right or left. To his horror, as he comes round the bend Jones sees the bodies of two unconscious persons lying on the tracks (flung there perhaps by an automobile accident), one on the left track and one on the right. He cannot stop the train in time to avoid hitting one of these persons. If he steers right, the person lying on that track will be killed. If he steers left, the other person (whose body is halfway off the track) will merely suffer bodily injury equivalent to that typically undergone by a woman during pregnancy and labor: several weeks of nausea, recurrent backaches, hemorrhoids, constipation, insomnia, loss of balance, leg cramps, extreme urgency of urination, discomfort during sexual intercourse, followed finally by a substantial period of severe abdominal pain. Whichever way he steers, Jones will breach a person's right, but if we ask which right it is better to breach in this situation, the answer is clearly that it is better to breach the second person's right to bodily integrity than the first person's right to life. Here the two rights are in simple conflict. Their relative priority, and the import of that priority for the decision that ought to be made, are clearcut. But in the case of pregnancy, the woman's right and the fetus's (supposed) right are *not* in such simple conflict – the rights are related to each other in a much more intimate fashion, and that fact prevents us from interpreting the problem according to the simple model provided by the subway train case. It is for this reason that it is so important to grasp the second assumption Thomson makes, namely the assumption that a right to life does not entail the right to anything and everything necessary to sustain that life.

II

In this paper I shall restrict myself to the following three questions:

(I)   If (A) one person depends on the continued use of another person's body in order to survive, and (B) the second person acted in a manner that brought about this state of affairs, has the second person thereby *waived* her right to the use of her body in favor of the first person?

(II)   Even if a woman has not explicitly waived her right to the use of her body in favor of the fetus, may the state legitimately *stipulate* that engaging in intercourse counts for legal purposes as waiving one's right?

(III)   If a person has waived her right to the use of her body in favor of another person in the manner described in Question (I), what is the *scope* of that waiver?

There are many ways to lose or transfer a right besides waiving it. For example, a felon *forfeits* (but does not waive) his right to vote, and his right not to be incarcerated; and I *lose* (but do not waive) my right to my land if the government claims it under eminent domain. In this paper I shall concentrate on the question of *waiver* alone. This means that our results will necessarily be limited. If we discover that few or no women *waive* the right to their body in favor of the fetus by engaging in intercourse, we will still not know whether or not they lose that right in some other fashion when they engage in intercourse. Hence we will not be able to conclude decisively that the Responsibility Argument is unsuccessful. However, our answer to the question about waiver may place us in a better position to carry forward the enquiry into other possible forms of loss.

To *waive* a right is to *voluntarily relinquish* it. Hence a pregnant woman has waived her right to the use of her body in favor of the fetus only if she has voluntarily given up that right in favor of the fetus. Thomson assumes this can never happen. She says, "I suppose we may take it as a datum that in the case of pregnancy due to rape the mother has not given the unborn person a right to the use of her body for food and shelter. Indeed, in what pregnancy could it be supposed that the mother has given the unborn person such a right? It is not as if there were unborn persons drifting about the world, to whom a woman who wants a child says 'I invite you in'" ([3], p. 57). Evidently Thomson supposes that I cannot give something (including a right) to someone — or waive my right in favor of that person — unless the person actually exists at the time of the gift or waiver. This seems wrong. Clearly, I can place a piece of jewelry in a safe deposit box as a gift for my children, or write a will leaving my estate to them, even though at the time of these acts I have no children (and am not pregnant). Of course the gift is not completed until it is received, and that requires the existence of the recipient. But I have done everything *I* am required to do in order to make a gift at the time I place the jewelry in the safe deposit box or sign my will. Hence Thomson's own reason for thinking that a woman cannot waive the right to the use of her body in favor of a presently nonexistent fetus seems spurious.

To determine whether or not a woman engaging in intercourse can, or does, thereby waive the right to her body in favor of the fetus, we must look more closely at the concept of waiving a right. What is it about an act that *accomplishes* a waiver of right, that *makes it true* that the agent voluntarily relinquishes her right? One possible account might be the following:

(i)   A person, S, voluntarily relinquishes a right to X in favor of a second person, T, just in case S voluntarily performs an act, A, and A results in T's breach of S's right.

I shall use the term 'breach' to denote an act that is contrary to a right, but shall leave it open what the moral status of that act is. Thus if I cause your death, I breach your right to life. If the breach is justified (e.g., I must kill you in self-defense), I shall say that the right is *overridden*. If the breach is unjustified (e.g., I kill you in the course of robbing you), I shall say that the right is *violated*. According to Account (i), if a woman voluntarily engages in intercourse, becomes pregnant, and so causes the fetus to breach the woman's right to the exclusive use of her body, then the woman has voluntarily relinquished her right in favor of the fetus by engaging in intercourse. It does not matter what the woman's *state of mind* was at the time of intercourse. Her ignorance that intercourse might result in pregnancy, or her desire not to become pregnant, is wholly immaterial to the question of whether she waives her right.

It is clear on very little reflection that Account (i) does not provide a plausible analysis of what it is to voluntarily relinquish a right. To voluntarily perform an act that happens to have a certain upshot is not to voluntarily cause that upshot. For example, to voluntarily pull the trigger of my shotgun is loaded. On Account (i), we would have to say that I voluntarily relinquish my right to vote in favor of my neighbor if I ridicule his favorite candidate and so induce him to slash the tires of my car and prevent me from voting on election day. Clearly my behavior does *not* constitute a *waiver* of my right to vote, even though it results in my *inability* to exercise my right.

This may suggest that in order to waive a right, one needs not only to perform certain actions voluntarily, but also to have a certain mental attitude toward the right that is affected by the performance of those actions. Thus we might be tempted by the following analysis:

(ii)   A person, S, voluntarily relinquishes a right to X in favor of a second person, T, just in case
    (a) S voluntarily performs an act, A,
    (b) A results in T's breach of S's right,
    (c) S believed A would or might have this result, and
    (d) S was willing that A have this result.

On this second view, a woman who voluntarily engages in intercourse, but does not understand the biological connection between intercourse and pregnancy, does not thereby waive her right to the use of her body in favor of the fetus. However, a woman who voluntarily engages in intercourse knowing that it may result in pregnancy, and being willing that this should happen, thereby waives her right in favor of the fetus. Such a view is significantly more plausible than the first account, and I suspect many people suppose it to be true. Indeed, something like this follows directly from the very popular view about rights advocated most prominently by Michael Tooley.[1] According to this view, one person violates another person's right to X only if the right-holder *desires* X. If the right-holder does not desire X — i.e., is willing to lose X — then no one who removes X can violate his right. In effect such a right-holder waives his right.

However attractive account (ii) may be, it still falls short of the truth. Just as losing my *car* is different from losing my *right* to my car, so *wanting to lose my car* is distinct from *wanting to lose my right to my car*. And it is the desire to lose my right, not the desire to lose my car, that seems relevant to the question of my waiving my right to my car. In other words, I must want not just that my right to the car be *breached*, but that my right to it be *lost*. I must desire a change in my moral status vis-à-vis the car, not just a change in my physical possession of the car. To see this, consider the following example. I am an under-cover policewoman who desires to apprehend and bring to justice a certain notorious purse snatcher. To this end I slowly stroll along streets he is known to frequent, positioning my purse

for easy snatchability. I succeed; he steals the purse. According to Account
(ii), my behavior and mental state constitute a waiver of my right to my
purse in his favor – in other words, he does no wrong in taking it, because
I have in effect given it to him. But clearly this is incorrect. I want him to
take it precisely because his doing so will be illegal and so enable me to
charge him with theft. He cannot defend himself in court by claiming that the
purse was already his when he relieved me of it, since I wanted him to take
it. Of course what is illegal and what is immoral are sometimes distinct,
but I think none of us suppose I have given him the *moral* right to my purse
any more than I have given him the *legal* right to it. Hence Account (ii)
must be rejected.

This suggests a third, and for our purposes, final account:

> (iii)   A person, S, voluntarily relinquishes a right to X in favor of a
> second person, T, just in case S wants
> (a) that S lose her right to X, and
> (b) that T gains the right to X.

On this view, a woman waives her right to the use of her body in favor
of a fetus just in case she explicitly wants her right to be transferred to
the fetus. Merely having intercourse, even knowing that this may result in
pregnancy and even being willing for this to happen, does not constitute
waiver of one's right to one's body in favor of the fetus. Hence the answer
to the first question I posed at the beginning of this Section is 'no': the
Responsibility Argument does not establish that a pregnant woman has
ipso facto waived, and therefore given away, the right to the use of her body.
Possibly there are *some* women who do waive their rights in the manner
required by Account (ii). But I suspect there are rather few. Hence if the
Responsibility Argument is to succeed in showing that a pregnant woman,
even a willing one, has transferred her right to the fetus, it must be through
some other form of gift than waiver, at least in the vast preponderance of
cases.

III

If I waive my right to the use of my car in favor of someone else, then he
does me no wrong – he acts within *his* rights – if he uses the car. But if
he uses my car without *knowing* that I have waived my right in his favor,
then he is blameworthy for his act, since he acts in the belief that he is
violating my right. And if society takes upon itself the task of enforcing

my rights, and it also does not know I have waived my right in his favor, then society has reason to compel him to cease using the car. Since, on Account (iii), my waiving my right is brought about by a mental state of mine, to which only I have privileged access, there is a strong probability that persons in whose favor I waive a right and society in general will rarely be able to tell whether or not I have waived that right. To avoid resulting inconvenience to the smooth regulation of interpersonal affairs, we commonly employ certain external modes of behavior as signals of our internal states. Thus I may say to someone, "I hereby waive my right to use my car in your favor", or more commonly, "You may use my car this afternoon", and such statements serve as evidence that I waive my right in his favor.

However, if these statements merely functioned as *evidence* of my waiver, other persons would still be in a difficult position, since I could always claim later that I didn't want to transfer my right, despite what I said. And no one could dispute my word. For this reason society may legitimately stipulate that certain kinds of behavior simply *count*, legally speaking, as a waiver of my right — *whatever* my accompanying mental state. Thus society might hold that anyone who has signed a consent form to a surgical operation has thereby waived his right not to be physically touched by the surgeon, provided the patient understands (or should understand) the content and the legal effect of the form. Under such a system, the patient could not subsequently sue the surgeon for assault by claiming that he *mentally* withheld consent when signing the form.

In view of this we might ask whether society could stipulate that voluntarily engaging in intercourse (at least with the knowledge that doing so may lead to pregnancy) counts, legally speaking, as waiver of one's right to the use of one's body in favor of a fetus who is conceived thereby. If such a stipulation would be legitimate, then it could be argued that a society which so stipulated could justifiably make abortion illegal for any woman who understands the biological connection between intercourse and pregnancy, and who is not pregnant as a result of rape. Such a woman would have legally waived her right in favor of the fetus, and would no longer have the right to evict the fetus as a 'trespasser'.

However, reflection suggests that it would not be legitimate for any society to make this stipulation. Not just *any* act can be designated as a legally binding sign of waiver. In particular, society cannot designate an act as a sign of waiver if failure to perform that act would be *independently costly* to the agent. Designating such an act as waiver would amount to *coercing* the agent to waive her right. For example, no society may say that failure to pay $500 to the Registrar on election day shall count as a waiver of one's right to vote. Such a scheme would impose a heavy cost on anyone who wishes to retain his right to vote, and so is coercive in effect. Presumably the right to vote is a right that society may not coerce its citizens to give up, and similarly the right to the exclusive use of one's body is a right that society may not coerce its citizens into giving up in favor of other individuals. (At least this is true except in extreme national emergencies.) On the scheme under consideration, in order for a woman to retain her right to the use of her body, she would have to abstain from intercourse, since engaging in intercourse would count as waiving this right. But abstinence from intercourse is extremely costly for most people. Indeed, it may not be wholly under voluntary control ([1], pp. 1594–1595). Hence designating sexual intercourse as a legally binding sign of waiver would amount to society's coercing women into giving up their exclusive rights to their bodies. Such coercion is surely illegitimate. We can conclude that no society may stipulate that a woman who voluntarily engages in intercourse has thereby, from a legal point of view, waived her right to the use of her body in favor of the fetus.

The foregoing argument rests on the implicit assumption that contraceptive measures are not available. As things now stand, of course, such measures *are* available, and the argument must take this into account. Could the state legitimately stipulate that sexual intercourse *without* the use of contraceptives counts as a waiver of one's rights in favor of the fetus? If the use of contraceptives were cost-free, or virtually so, then in terms of the foregoing argument it would appear that the state could make this stipulation. But in the present state of affairs, this is not the case. All contraceptives cost money. The most effective ones (the Pill and the IUD) carry substantial health risks. Other less effective contraceptives, such as diaphragms, foams, and condoms, are found by many couples to interfere with the spontaneity and pleasure of intercourse itself. Any form of contraceptive may be contrary to the religious views of some segments in the population. Thus the use of contraceptives is not cost-free for a great many people. To settle our question decisively, we would have to determine what *level* of cost may legitimately be imposed by the state on the refusal to waive one's right. But I am inclined to think that the use of contraceptives imposes a high enough cost on a large enough segment of the population so that the only acceptable uniform policy is one which does *not* stipulate that intercourse without benefit of contraceptives counts as a waiver of one's rights.

IV

I have now argued that a woman does not waive her moral right to the use of her body merely by engaging in intercourse, even if she knows that pregnancy may result, and is willing for this to happen. To waive a moral right, one must want that right to be lost, not just want it to be breached. I have also argued that no society may legitimately stipulate that engaging in voluntary intercourse counts as a legally binding waiver of one's right to the use of one's body.

It is difficult to know how many women actually waive the moral right to the use of their bodies in favor of the fetus. Possibly none do, but perhaps there are some. It is with regard to these women (assuming they exist) that we may now turn to our third question: what is the *scope* of their waiver? How *much* is such a woman obliged to do for the fetus, or to allow it to do to her body? In particular: if she discovers after conception that pregnancy threatens to end her life or seriously impair her health (although the fetus would survive), is she obliged to let the pregnancy continue? Shall we say "She waived her right in favor of the fetus, and now cannot change her mind; she must not end the pregnancy even though it threatens her life or health", just as we would say of someone sho sets up an irrevocable trust in favor of his child, and then discovers he faces financial ruin without those funds, "He gave the money to the child, and now cannot change his mind; he cannot take the money from the trust even though leaving it there threatens his financial future"?

To decide what the scope of the pregnant woman's waiver is in these circumstances, we must first distinguish four different types of case.

(A)   At the time of intercourse, the woman believed there was no genuine risk of the threat in question, and waived her right on that understanding.

(B)   At the time of intercourse, the woman did not consider the question of whether or not pregnancy might constitute a threat to her life or health, and waived her right in that mental state.

(C)   At the time of intercourse, the woman believed pregnancy might endanger her life or health, and waived her right only on condition that it does not, reserving the right to withdraw use of her body from the fetus if her life or health should be endangered.

(D)   At the time of intercourse, the woman believed pregnancy might endanger her life or health, and waived her right even in that event.

It may be difficult to imagine a woman, about to engage in intercourse, explicitly waiving her right in favor of the fetus. It may help us therefore, in considering the question before us, to consider at the same time what we would say in parallel cases where explicit waiver of right is easier to visualize. One such case would be that of a woman who formally contracts with a couple to serve as a surrogate womb for a fetus conceived by them but which they are unable to carry to term. Another such case would be that of a person who contracts to donate an organ (for example a kidney or quantity of bone marrow) to someone who needs such an organ transplant to sustain life. In both of these parallel cases the performance of the contracted action may pose an unexpected danger to the contractor's life or health. The surrogate mother is of course subject to all the physiological hazards that may imperil a natural mother, and the removal of a donor's organ may prove risky for unforeseen reasons. In such an event, what would we say — that the surrogate mother and the organ donor must fulfill their contracts nonetheless, or that they may legitimately back out? Clearly the answer to this question may depend on what understanding of the risk was entertained by the contractor, such as those detailed in the above four possibilities.

Returning to the naturally pregnant woman, it seems clear that if she may waive the right to her body at all, she may certainly waive it conditionally or in the qualified fashion described in Case (C) above. In such a case, she has certainly not granted the fetus a right to use her body in a manner that endangers her life or health. Hence she is not required by the 'terms' of her waiver to permit the pregnancy to continue when it does endanger her. Similarly, a woman who agreed to serve as surrogate womb for a fetus only on the condition that her life is not thereby endangered would not be obliged by the terms of her contract with the biological parents to allow the pregnancy to continue when a life-threatening condition arises. I think one could argue successfully that natural mothers caught in cases of types (A) and (B) also need not continue their pregnancies. But a case of type (D) is more difficult, since there the woman explicitly *does* grant the fetus the right to use her body even if its doing so endangers her life or health. Must we conclude, therefore, that such a woman cannot legitimately end her pregnancy when the contemplated threat materializes?

In answering this question, the first point we must be clear about is the fact that a waiver of one's future rights is like a promise: it establishes a *presumption* that one ought to allow the future breach to occur, but it does not show that one ought *all things considered* to allow the breach. For example, suppose a man of heroic impulses promises a distraught stranger to rescue her pet dog, even if it should cost his own life. The dog has been swept away in the icy currents of a flooding river, and the hero swims out with a thin rope to tie around the dog so that it may be pulled to shore by its owner. But as he gets farther out, he sees clearly that although he will be able to reach the dog and tie the rope around it, thus ensuring its survival, by then he will be so exhausted that he himself will be unable to swim back. The rope is not strong enough to pull him in. Certain death stares him in the face if he completes the rescue. No doubt his promise establishes a *presumption* that he ought to swim on nonetheless, but no one would say that all things considered he *must* do so − even though his own self interest is the only consideration that militates against his doing so. It is morally permissible for him to break his promise, and leave the dog to its fate. From this case we may conclude that the *mere* fact that a woman in a case of type (D) waives her right to the use of her body in favor of the fetus does not by itself show that she must, all things considered, allow the fetus to use her body in a way that imperils her life or seriously threatens her health.

But what distinguishes cases in which the person *must* all things considered allow the granted right to be breached (or must fulfill the promise) from cases in which this is *not* morally required? Perhaps the most obvious suggestion here is that what ought, all things considered, to be done depends on the *relative value* to the two concerned parties of performance versus nonperformance. In the case of the hero's promise to rescue the dog, the rescue has moderate value to the dog's owner (and considered in itself as prevention of death to an animal). But the rescue has great negative value for the hero − he will die as a result. Since the disvalue to the hero is radically greater than the value to the dog's owner, we find on balance that the hero need not fulfill his promise.

In the case of the naturally pregnant woman, the disvalue of continuing the pregnancy is extremely high − she will die, or her health will be seriously impaired. On the other hand, the disvalue to the fetus of terminating the pregnancy seems equally high − it will certainly die if aborted, whereas it would live if not. We may be inclined to say that where the stakes are equal, as they apparently are in this case, the fact of the promise (or the waiver of right) tips the balance in favor of the person to whom the promise was made or in whose favor the right was waived.

However, it is not clear that this principle is correct. Such a situation is created when one person contracts to donate an organ to another person who will die without a transplant, and it is then discovered that the donor himself would lose his life if the organ is removed. The stakes for either party are equally high in such a case, and yet I am inclined to say that the prospective donor need not carry through as promised. It may be that a certain level of self-sacrifice is not morally required, even to fulfill a promise where the stakes are equally high for the other person.

The details of such a case may make a difference. For example, suppose that when the person who requires a new organ advertised for donors, several suitable prospective donors presented themselves. Smith is chosen and signs the contract, stipulating willingness to donate the organ even if his life should be endangered thereby. It is then discovered that indeed his life will be imperiled by the donation. Meanwhile the other possible donors have unfortunately disappeared. May Smith back out of his contract in this situation? I am somewhat less inclined to say that he may than I was in the previous case that involved no other prospective donors — largely, I suspect, because Smith's agreeing to donate the organ and then backing out would leave the transplant candidate *worse off* than he would have been if Smith had never signed the contract in the first place. The transplant candidate is worse off because if Smith had never signed, another donor could easily have been found and the transplant would have gone through, whereas now no other donors are available, and if Smith backs out the transplant candidate must die. But even so I am reluctant to say that Smith is morally obliged to donate his organ at the cost of his own life.

Thus even if the stakes are equal for both parties to the dispute, it is unclear that the naturally pregnant woman in a case of type (D) is obliged, all things considered, to allow the pregnancy to continue when it is discovered that doing so will cost her her life. (And I suspect we would arrive at the same result in the case where the stakes are not so apparently equal, i.e., a case in which abortion would kill the fetus but merely prevent serious impairment of the woman's health.) However, I believe that it is incorrect to see such a case as one in which the stakes are equal for both parties. Of course it *appears* they are: both the woman and the fetus stand to live or die, depending on which decision is made. But this fact only shows the stakes to be equal if life and death are of equal value and disvalue to the two parties. And this does not seem to be so. To settle the question decisively we would have to have a compelling account of *why* (and when) life is a good and death an evil. Debate on this question goes back at least to the Epicureans, who claimed (without convincing anyone) that death could not be an evil to the person who dies [2]. I do not believe we have a fully satisfactory account of why death is an evil and life a good, but it seems to me that the centerpiece of such an account must be the thesis that life is a good, and death an evil, to a presently existing person insofar as that person presently has the desire to go on living, and has projects and plans that will be frustrated if his or her life is cut short. According to such an account, life is clearly a good and death an evil for normal adults, including most pregnant women. But the account does *not* imply that life is a good and death an evil to a fetus, or at least an early fetus. For a fetus has no cognitive desire to live (although like all organisms it may physiologically resist death), and it certainly has no plans or projects that would be frustrated if its life were cut short. Of course, if the fetus survives, there will be a person some years from now whose life is (probably) valuable to him or her. But this fact does not show that it is in the interests of the fetus *now* — the *present* person — that such a life exist. So far as I can see, it is all one to the fetus whether someone genetically identical with him will exist and be happy in the future, or someone genetically distinct from him, or no one at all. Nothing in which *he* is concerned rides on the issue. From this point of view it appears that future life is not a good to the present fetus, and death not an evil. And it follows from this that the stakes are not equal in the case we are considering: the pregnant woman has a great deal to lose by dying, but the fetus has very little. Hence the case is more like that of the hero who promises to rescue the dog than it is like the case of the organ donor whose organ is the only hope of survival for the transplant candidate. Hence even if we had said, as we did not, that the organ donor must fulfill his contract, we need not say this of the pregnant woman whose life is endangered. The harm to her in dying is far greater than the harm to the fetus in dying.

It might be protested that the case of the naturally pregnant woman is really more like that of the donor who agrees to make the donation, thereby making other prospective donors unavailable, and then wants to back out of his contract. For the woman in getting pregnant and then withdrawing the right to use her body from the fetus has made the fetus *worse off* than it would have been if she had never granted it the right in the first place — for then it would never have been conceived, and so not need to die. But this seems a mistake. It is not at all clear that the fetus is worse off by being conceived and then aborted than it would be never having lived at all ([1], p. 1599). If the abortion is early, the fetus has no sentient existence at all. If the abortion is late term, then the fetus may feel pain during the process, although that pain can hardly be compared with the sort of pain fully mature human beings feel. Perhaps a painful existence is worse than no existence at all. But then (if Freud is right) the fetus may experience pleasure during its uterine life as well, and perhaps the pleasure balances out the pain. In reality these are imponderables. The main point is that the pain to the fetus (if any) is not nearly so great a disvalue to it as losing her life is to the woman. Even if her total course of action makes the fetus marginally worse off, I do not think this is enough to show that she may not discontinue the pregnancy in order to save her life.

V

According to the Responsibility Argument, if one person depends on the continued use of another person's body in order to survive, and the second person acted in a manner that brought about this state of affairs, then the second person has thereby transferred the right to the use of her body to the dependent person, and would be wrong to deny the dependent person that use. I have argued that these circumstances fail to show that the second person has *waived* the right to the use of her body in favor of the dependent person, even if we assume the second person wanted the breach of her right to occur, and even if she knew that it would occur if she acted in the manner described. The only hope for the Responsibility Argument to succeed, then, is if it can be shown that a person who acts in this manner loses her right in some other fashion than by waiving it. I have also argued that no society can legitimately stipulate that engaging in intercourse counts as legally waiving the right to one's body in favor of the fetus, since doing so would amount to coercing women to renounce their rights. In the last section I have argued further than even if a woman explicitly waives her right in favor of a fetus on the recognition that her life could be endangered thereby, nevertheless she is not obliged, all things considered, to allow the pregnancy to continue if the threat to her life materializes. We may break a promise or fail to allow a previously granted breach of our right when we stand to lose our life, and when the stake for the other party is less extreme. And I have argued that death is less of an evil to the fetus than it is to the woman who carries the fetus.

University of Illinois at Chicago Circle

NOTE

[1] See, for example, [4]. In this and subsequent versions of his argument, Tooley qualifies his view in various ways that are immaterial to the point made in the text. He does not actually discuss the notion of *waiver*.

BIBLIOGRAPHY

1. Regan, D. H.: 1979, 'Rewriting *Roe v. Wade*', *Michigan Law Review* 77, 1569–1646.
2. Silverstein, H. S.: 1980, 'The Evil of Death', *The Journal of Philosophy* 77, 401–423.
3. Thomson, J. J.: 1971, 'A Defense of Abortion', *Philosophy and Public Affairs* 1, 47–66.
4. Tooley, M.: 1972, 'Abortion and Infanticide', *Philosophy and Public Affairs* 2, 44–45.

BIBLIOGRAPHY

CAROLINE WHITBECK

THE MORAL IMPLICATIONS OF REGARDING WOMEN AS PEOPLE: NEW PERSPECTIVES ON PREGNANCY AND PERSONHOOD *

One of the striking things about the philosophical debate on the ethics of abortion is how few women enter it. I believe that the relatively small number of women who enter the discussion is a result as well as a cause of the way in which the subject is demarcated, and the way in which it is conceptualized. Given the way in which the issue is presently framed, it is difficult for many women to find any position for which they wish to argue. I shall argue, first, that abortion is actually a fragment of several other moral issues surrounding pregnancy and childbirth so that the moral situation can be adequately understood only if this larger context is considered, and second, that the choice of the terms in which the analysis is generally carried out is mistaken. In particular, I shall argue that neglect of matters which cannot be adequately expressed in terms of 'rights' and the employment of an atomistic model of people (a model that represents moral relationships as incidental to being a person) confuses many moral issues but especially those concerning pregnancy, childbirth, and infant care. It is my purpose in this paper to argue for a reframing of the issues regarding pregnancy and childbirth. Such a reframing will yield different questions from those which have typically been raised in debates about abortion.

An important factor contributing to the inadequate formulation of the issues which I shall discuss is the neglect of interpretations of the human condition from women's perspective. (The problem is not confined to philosophy, but the neglect of women's perspective in philosophy is symptomatic of the neglect of women's experience in the culture generally.) It is not my purpose to give an extensive critique of the existing literature, but at least to identify many of the neglected issues, and to show how attention to the perspective of women will generate new approaches to these issues.

1. ON THE DENIAL THAT WOMEN ARE PEOPLE

It is striking that the culture has managed to ignore the implications of the fact that women are people. Of course, our own culture is strongly influenced by a number of scientific and religious traditions that explicitly deny that women have in full measure those characteristics that are taken to distinguish

247

William B. Bondeson et al. *(eds.), Abortion and the Status of the Fetus, 247—272.*
Copyright © 1983 *by D. Reidel Publishing Company, Dordrecht, Holland.*

man from the animals. Thus, St. Paul in his first letter to the Corinthians interprets the second of the two accounts of creation in Genesis as denying that woman is created in the image of God, as man is. Woman, Paul says, stands in relation to man as man does to Christ. Woman was created for man. Paul concedes that man cannot do without woman, however, since man is born of woman. In short, Paul represents women as failing to have the property of being made in God's image, although they are a necessary means to the existence of such beings.[1]

Aristotle in his work, *On the Generation of Animals*, tells us that the most common kind of deformity is to be born a woman and that the rational part of the soul, that which distinguishes man from the lower animals, is inoperative in woman. Because women do not have enough soul heat, women cannot cook their menstrual blood into semen, says Aristotle, and therefore, to put the matter in modern terms, women do not contribute any gametes to the formation of the embryo. According to Aristotle, not only are women not people in the sense of failing to be rational animals (recall that Aristotle regarded 'rational animal' as definition of 'man'), women are, in a sense, not even full parents of people on Aristotle's account, but only necessary as the custodians and nurturers of men's 'seed'. I have termed this, 'the flower-pot theory of generation'. Ideas found in Paul and Aristotle are to be found in the work of many other thinkers, although these quotations from Paul and Aristotle are among the most influential upon subsequent views of women [38].

These days, it is less common to assert outright that women lack some or all of the characteristics taken to distinguish people from lower animals. Many implications of the view that women are people are routinely ignored, however, and women's experience continues to be disregarded as though it were not relevant to understanding the human condition. (I venture that by this stage in the present volume, we will have had a remarkable amount of discussion of fetuses with little or no mention of pregnancy.)

The problem is not one of sloth on the part of individual scholars, but of general neglect within the culture. The neglect of discussion of the experience of pregnancy and childbirth within our culture and the neglect of women's perspective on the subject of human sexuality are subjects that I have discussed in detail elsewhere [37]. The problem can be illustrated by considering some of your own experience. How many of you have seen films or read novels about men's experience in war? How many have seen or read at least four such works? How many of you have seen films and read novels that deal with women's experience in pregnancy and childbirth? (I do not count

Lamaze and other childbirth training films any more than I count combat training films.) My contention is that of those people who have not borne children, more have identified imaginatively with Lassie than with a pregnant woman.

Women and men alike are given cultural representations of what is stereotypically men's experience, whether in war or playing football, and few if any representations of women's experience, not only for activities and roles that are regarded as subsidiary activities but even for activities and roles such as those of mothering that are regarded as essential. The implication is that although women may figure importantly *in* people's experience, as do horses and automobiles, there is nothing in *women's experience* that merits attention. Furthermore, the subjects of women's needs and women's moral integrity and bodily integrity are omitted regularly, as is the issue of matching women's responsibilities with the authority to carry them out. Often, indeed, an ethical double standard has been implicit, so that people in general are regarded as constrained morally by the requirement not to violate anyone else's rights, but the moral expectation upon women is that they be nurturant, that is, that they ought to go beyond respecting rights and meet the needs of others, perhaps any and all others. Some even push the double standard further and maintain that women do not have rights equal to those of men.

2. THE LIMITS OF THE APPLICABILITY OF THE CONCEPT OF A MORAL RIGHT

Like recent discussions of other ethical issues, much of the literature on abortion discusses its subject exclusively in terms of rights. The emphasis on rights often stems from the implicit assumption of what I shall call, a 'rights view of ethics'. According to a rights view of ethics, the concept of a moral right is the fundamental moral notion, or at least the one that is of pre-eminent significance, so that a moral issue is settled by consideration of rights. According to this view a person is assumed to be nothing more than a being having certain rights, human rights. (Indeed it has now become common for philosophers to define explicitly the concept of a person as a being possessing certain rights, particularly the right to life.[2]) Persons are viewed as social and moral atoms, actually or potentially in competition with one another. If any attention is given to human relationships, it is assumed that they exist on a contractual (or quasi-contractual) basis and that the moral requirements arising from them are limited to rights and obligations.

In contrast to obligations which generally specify what acts or conduct are morally required, permitted, or forbidden, responsibilities (in the prospective sense of 'responsibility for') specify the ends to be achieved rather than the conduct required.[3] Thus, responsibilities require an exercise of discretion on the part of their bearers. People without medical knowledge cannot bear a moral responsibility to give someone good medical care, and newborns cannot have any moral responsibilities at all.

In contrast with the rights view of ethics, what I shall call 'the responsibilities view' of ethics takes moral responsibility arising out of relationships as the fundamental moral notion, and regards people as beings who can (among other things) act for moral reasons and who come to this status through relationships with other people.[4] Such relationships are not assumed to be contractual. The relationship of a child to his or her parents is a good example of a relationship that is not contractual. In general, relationships between people place moral responsibilities on both parties. Each party is responsible for insuring some aspect of the other's welfare or, at least, for achieving some ends that contribute to the other's welfare or achievement. This holds even in asymmetrical relationships (whether personal or professional), such as the relationship between parent and child or between client and lawyer.

Rights and obligations do have a place within the responsibilities view. Human rights are claims upon society and upon other people that are necessary if a person is to be able to meet the responsibilities of her or his relationships. Although only moral agents can have moral responsibilities and thus can have moral rights, according to this view, moral agents may, and probably do, have some moral obligations toward, or responsibility for the welfare of other beings who are not moral agents, that is, beings who do not themselves have the moral status of people. For example, people may have a moral obligation to treat corpses with respect, or not to be cruel to animals.

I maintain that a rights view of ethics yields an inadequate view of the moral status of people or 'persons' and disregards the importance of the special responsibilities that go with personal and professional relationships. In some cases, notably in situations involving adults who are strangers, the situation may be described adequately in terms of rights and obligations alone. For issues relating to pregnancy, childbirth and infant care, however, where the relationships between the parties are those which are central and indeed necessary in order for one of the parties ever to become a moral agent, adequate representation of the situation requires that attention be given to responsibilities.

3. THE SCOPE AND LIMITS OF RIGHTS AS THEY BEAR UPON PREGNANCY AND ITS TERMINATION

Although the question of when it is moral to terminate a pregnancy is not answered adequately if we attend only to rights, some rights are relevant.

Let us pose a question: Supposing you were able to do so, how many of you would like to have an abortion?

Of course, women do not want abortions any more than they want to have mastectomies, even if the risks from each are minimal. (One of the most striking examples of misogyny in our society is the way in which women who resort to abortion are portrayed as Medea figures, that is as people who wish to destroy the fetuses they carry. Medea herself is a product of the masculine imagination, and is represented as having ripped her children's bodies limb from limb and strewing the parts on the ocean out of rage toward their father, Jason.) Philosophers have long struggled to formulate the distinction between what people straightforwardly want (such as equal pay for equal work) and those options that are selected only because of a still greater aversion to the only available alternatives. I shall call the latter sorts of options 'grim options'.[5]

One example of a grim option that philosophers employ is the option of being hung with a noose made with silk rope as opposed to being hung with a noose made of hemp rope. The prisoner making the choice does not want to be hung with a silk rope in the straightforward sense of want, but only chooses that over being hung with a hemp rope. Such cases are not easily subsumed under the heading of what which is wanted only as a means. Although the selected options could be represented as a means for avoiding the alternatives, grim options cases differ from usual cases in which something is wanted only as a means, in that the causal relation between the means and end is at best remote, and the end is the *avoidance* of some outcome rather than the *attainment* of one.

It would be a mistake to regard abortion as a means to the end of being childless, since most women who have abortions do bear children at some other time in their lives. A woman seeks an abortion most often not to avoid having children *per se*, but to avoid such alternatives as the risk of becoming an invalid as a result of the pregnancy; the inability to keep a major commitment to someone; the prospect of being reduced to poverty by loss of her livelihood; dependency on someone who would batter or mistreat her or her children; or the stigma of 'illegitimacy' on herself, her child and her family.[6] (Often in human history giving birth to an illegitimate child has meant the death of the mother, either by execution or through probable starvation, as well as social ostracism and probable death of the child.) In this country laws discriminating against bastards were not declared unconstitutional until the landmark Supreme Court decision in the case of *Levy v. Louisiana* [19] in 1968, and informal discrimination and/or ostracism continues. Many of the factors that impel a woman to resort to abortion would be changed with a change in social conditions. In particular, safe, effective means of contraception and sterilization and the elimination of rape would guarantee a woman's control of her fertility without resort to abortion.

Abortion is in many ways a prototype of a grim option, but this point seems to have been neglected in both the philosophical and popular literature on abortion. In addition to the two commonly discussed issues, the risks of an abortion and the killing of the fetus in abortion (the moral significance of which we are assessing), there is the unappealing prospect of having someone scraping away at one's inner core.

Thus, women do not want abortions, although under duress they may resort to them. Nonetheless, people can, and many do, want safe abortions available, just as people want safe mastectomies to be available. It is estimated that approximately 84 000 women die every year as a result of abortion ([6], p. 1), although a legal first-trimester abortion in the United States has a mortality risk no greater than that of a penicillin shot. The distinction between what one wants and what one *wants to be available* is crucial for understanding the resort to a grim option. Further, since the development of therapeutic medicine is a prime example of society's preparation for an undesired turn of events, the distinction between what one wants and what one wants to be available is a particularly important one in the philosophy of medicine.[7] The right that would correspond to this desire would be the right of entitlement to a *safe* abortion. It would correspond precisely to a putative right to other forms of surgical care such as mastectomies, appendectomies and the like. The desire for the availability of good care of this sort cannot be equated with actually wanting such operations. Indeed, there has been a good deal of lay criticism of surgeons for encouraging patients to have operations, especially appendectomies and hysterectomies, for trivial reasons. Therefore, rights to medical care are importantly unlike such other rights of entitlement as the right to a basic education, in that people prefer *not* to be in the position of actually needing to exercise these rights.

The second example of something that people might want and claim as a right is the general right of control of one's body. This is a prototype of the privacy rights that must be honored if one is to function as a person. (I generally agree with J. H. Reiman [25] and S. I. Benn [2] that rights of privacy are not derivative rights. On the contrary they are fundamental to being (or becoming) a person. Although the rules and conventions regarding privacy vary from one society to another, in *every* society privacy exists as the social practice by which individual moral right to control the matters relating to one's own person is recognized. I disagree with Reiman's use of the term 'moral ownership' in this context, since it suggests that the right connected with one's body or one's person is a species of property right. Sara Ann Ketchum [14] argues convincingly that it is not.)

The claim that abortion should be available 'on demand' may be intended as any one of several different claims. It may, and most often does, mean that it should always be legal for a woman to have an abortion without obtaining the approval of anyone else. What is in question is a negative right, a right to be free of interference when seeking an abortion. In contrast, the claim that abortion should be available on demand is often interpreted as closely linked to the claim that women are entitled to this surgical intervention regardless of ability to pay, which is a right of entitlement. Some, usually those who are in opposition to abortion on demand on one of the preceding interpretations, treat the view that abortion should be available on demand as a claim that abortion is *morally justified* under all circumstances. They then argue that one should deny availability of abortion on the grounds that it would sometimes be morally wrong to have an abortion. The view that women have a moral and legal right to obtain an abortion without the approval of others does not imply that it is always, on balance, morally justified for a given woman to exercise that right. It does at least suggest that the woman is *prima facie*, the best person to decide when abortion is morally justified.

Although the rights that I have just discussed are relevant to the moral issues involved, the moral aspects the condition or relation of pregnancy is of even greater importance, and it is that subject to which I now turn.

4. THE MORAL ASPECTS OF PREGNANCY AND THE STATUS OF THE FETUS

I have already given some examples of the blindness of our culture to the experience of pregnancy. As a consequence of this blindness, the relationship between the pregnant woman and the fetus is inadequately conceptualized, as is the ontological and moral status of the fetus. What we find in the abortion literature is a conceptualization based on the categories that are familiar to men's experience, so that being pregnant is represented on the one hand as similar to having a tumor, or on the other as being hooked up to an adult stranger who is dependent on that hookup for survival, or more remote yet, as occupying a house with another person whose presence constitutes more or less of a threat to one's life. Although philosophers have offered some ingenious arguments, the unsatisfying nature of these treatments should warn us that the conceptualizations upon which these arguments are based are mistaken.

Judith J. Thomson's [32] analogy about being hooked up to the ailing violinist is helpful in that it reveals some of the special nature of one's rights to one's own body and the problem with the view that one person could have rights to another's body.[8] Beyond shedding some light on the issue of one's rights to one's body, Thomson's paper comes close to constituting a *reductio ad absurdum* of the view that the relation of a woman to the fetus she carries is to be understood on the model of her relation to an adult stranger who wants or needs the use of her body to survive, and hence of the view that the fetus should be understood on the model of an adult stranger (so that rights are all that matter in this case). A claim more worthy of examination is the claim that human fetuses are relevantly like newborn human beings, and have the same moral status as newborns or one which is very similar, and that likewise their moral relationships are importantly similar to those of newborns.

I shall return to this claim in a moment but first wish to clarify my use of terms. By 'fetus', I mean 'fetus' in the strict biological sense, not a blastomere, an embryo, etc. Since the papers by Professors Biggers [3] and Soupart [30] discuss embryonic development, I will only make a few points about the stages in this process. After the ovum is fertilized, some authorities in medicine continue to refer to it as 'an ovum' until about four weeks after the last menstrual period or two weeks after fertilization. This way of speaking reflects the continuity of biological development before and after the addition of the sperm ([11], p. 125), and is in sharp contrast to the masculist neo-Aristotelian assumption that the male contribution of the sperm makes the crucial ontological and moral difference. (The neo-Aristotelian view is the basis of what became the claim of the biological father that his offspring were his property.) The demarcation between embryos and fetuses is not sharp. It occurs at roughly ten weeks after the last menstrual period or eight weeks after fertilization. Nonetheless, there are established criteria for distinguishing between embryos and fetuses. These are reflected in the definition which Van Nostrand's *Scientific Encyclopedia* gives for the term 'embryo'.

> The developing individual between the union of the germ cells and the completion of the organs which characterize its body when it becomes a separate organism. The term is difficult to limit because some development occurs after birth or hatching and in some species considered growth intervenes between the completion of the essential structures of the individual and its assumption of separate life. In the latter stage, the organism is called a fetus if it is a mammal ([34], p. 943).

A fetus then is a mammal with the 'essential structures', that is, the major organ systems characteristic of its species, but prior to its assumption of 'a separate life'. Differentiation of the tissues continues during fetal life and some differentiation takes place after birth as well. For example, sexual differentiation is not complete until puberty.

The reason that the biological category, fetus, looks as though it might have ethical import, is that fetuses are sentient, that is, possessing major human organ systems gives fetuses the ability to experience as opposed to merely react to their environment. Sentience provides one basis for the analogy between fetuses and newborns. Furthermore, whereas, as Professor Biggers has shown, a fertilized ovum has less than a 40% chance of developing into a newborn, fetuses have a very good chance, statistically speaking. (I do not intend to suggest that the killing of even an embryo has no moral significance. I am inclined to regard the killing of at least higher animal forms as something requiring at least *some* moral justification, and thus not something which it is morally acceptable to do on whim.)

Membership in the species *homo sapiens* is often mentioned as though it were morally significant, but it is hard to see how species identity could be significant in the absence of other similarities. Mere species identity (the fact that the cells of some being have the human chromosomal pattern) is hardly a morally relevant trait, since this is something that human people share with some human tissue cultures.[9] If life forms on other planets should turn out to act as moral agents and have other morally relevant characteristics of people, then mere species difference ought not to prejudice our treatment of them, or justify a failure to regard them as people. Similarly two non-persons who are similar in morally significant respects ought to be treated similarly, regardless of their species. Although the termination of a pregnancy even at the embryonic stage is a grim option, killing of a sentient human raises additional moral questions. Obviously there are differences between fetuses at ten weeks after the last menstrual period and those at term, not the least of which is viability, the subject discussed in Professor Engelhardt's [10] essay. I leave it open as to what, if any, moral significance these differences have.

The term 'person' has been used in many disparate technical senses, only some of which are morally significant. Because of the variety of technical uses to which the term 'person' has been put, I try to avoid using it and its plural 'persons', and make do with the term 'people' and use 'person' only when it is necessary to use a singular noun.

As I argued above, an individual acquires the moral status of a person in and through relationships with other people. Furthermore, people's behavior is understandable only by reference to their participation in human communities. Even in the unusual circumstance in which a person is living in isolation from other people, that person's behavior is strongly influenced by social understandings and practices that are acquired in relationships with other people. For example, Robinson Crusoe lived as a Britisher even when he lived alone.

I take it that being a human being and having language are jointly sufficient to indicate that one is a person. (Such people may be immature people, neurotic people, mad people, or for some other reasons, of limited competence, but that is another matter.) I choose the indicators of being human and having language because of what I know, or think I know, about the process of language learning in humans, its prerequisites and its consequences. I trust that it is clear that I am not suggesting that the properties of being human and possessing language are indicators which must necessarily be present for one to be counted as a person, much less that these indicators provide a definition of the concept. Rather, I propose to use the term 'people' in a way which retains all of the richness and fuzziness of that concept, so that we will be less likely to overlook features of people that are germane to their special moral status.

People are (among other things) moral agents, that is, beings who can act for moral reasons and whose acts can be reasonably evaluated in moral terms. The claim that fetuses are people is absurd if it is taken to imply that fetuses are, or are very much like, moral agents, that they have moral integrity, have moral responsibilities and are capable of making choices. The same is true, however, of newborns. Concern over responsibilities for the welfare of the fetus is better expressed by asking whether the fetus is similar to a newborn (in ways that are morally relevant) than by asking whether the fetus is a person.[10]

One motive for insisting that a fetus is a person has been to give grounds for saying that feticide is homicide. Replacing the question of whether the fetus is a person by the question of the extent of the similarity in moral status of fetuses and newborns, does not prejudge the question of whether feticide should count as homicide, since infanticide is generally regarded as homicide. Furthermore, it should be clear that saying that we need to examine the claim that human fetuses are like newborn human beings is not asserting that the moral status of fetuses is the same as that of newborns. In order to examine the claim, however, we would need an understanding of the ontological and moral status of newborns and, interestingly enough, we lack even this.

The absence of a developed philosophical account of the moral status of newborns is further evidence of the blindness of the culture to women's experience. The care of newborns has been left almost entirely to women, and therefore the store of knowledge that we have regarding newborns and the conceptual understanding that has been developed in the course of this practice, has been largely ignored. It is well to remember that when Freud put forward his theory of childhood sexuality, he recognized that what he was saying was already known by those who tended the nursery. Nonetheless, his ideas were counted as startling new discoveries.

If the day-to-day realities concerning toddlers and children have been omitted from the background knowledge upon which philosophers and other scholars and scientists rely, this is even more true of our knowledge concerning newborns.[11] Indeed, because the organization of modern life gives little opportunity for the transmission of the knowledge and practices of the subculture that is or was women's culture (for example, we no longer see our neighbors through labor and delivery), the disregard of newborns in the philosophical literature is now matched by an ignorance of them even on the part of a large number of women. For example, it is common for people expecting their first child and attending childbirth classes never to have seen a newborn, and thus they must be warned not to expect that their newborn will look like the chubby, social, emerging people depicted on diaper boxes and baby food jars. (I recall one father-to-be who regarded Elizabeth Janeway's description of infants as 'voracious' as a shocking and perhaps even hostile statement, whereas in fact, 'voracious' aptly describes newborns whose only coordinated movements are those of sucking and who do that with total involvement.)

Although we need an adequate account of the moral aspects of the relation of parents and their newborns to one another and to others in society, in order to assess the scope and limits of the analogy between the parent-newborn relation and the relation of the pregnant woman to the fetus she carries, I will at least point out points of negative and positive analogy between fetuses and newborns. For example, both fetuses and newborns are extremely vulnerable to permanent detriments later in life as a result of short-term deprivation or exposure to noxious influences. On the negative side, it is impossible for the pregnant woman to do something analogous to putting the newborn up for adoption.

A difference in the practice with regard to the disposal of the bodies of fetuses and newborns indicates a *perceived* difference between fetuses and newborns. Statistics on premature birth in the United States are compiled using the figure of 500 grams as the cutoff between miscarriage and premature birth. In many other countries the figure used is 1000 grams. The weight of 500 grams represents a weight which has been the lower limit for survival, that is, survival *supported and assisted by high technology*. (Therefore it is not an estimate of the lower limit for viability in Engelhardt's sense.) According to the law in many states, fetuses *ex utero* over 500 grams are considered premature newborns, and therefore birth certificates must be issued for them and they must be buried. Fetuses under 500 grams are treated as other tissue, and hospitals dispose of them accordingly. The procedures are no different at any Roman Catholic hospital with which I am familiar, that is, *no* hospital buries the bodies of fetuses less than 500 grams. As far as I have been able to ascertain, when a spontaneous abortion occurs outside of the hospital, people do not bury the body of fetuses and this is true even of those who profess to regard not only fetuses, but all products of conception, as people.

Whatever the extent of the analogy between fetuses and newborns, it must be the same for wanted and unwanted fetuses. If feticide which results from induced abortion is homicide, so is feticide that is a consequence of an accidental action on the part of the pregnant woman. If such an accident involved negligence on the part of the pregnant woman, she would then be guilty of negligent homicide. It may be clear that deciding the scope and the limits of the analogy between the relation of parents to newborns and pregnant women to fetuses is not a simple matter, and will have consequences reaching far beyond its impact on induced abortions.

5. THE TRADITION WHICH REGARDS WOMEN AND WOMEN'S BODIES AS A RESOURCE TO BE USED BY MEN

I have argued that our culture has neglected women's experience and the status of women as moral individuals with a need to maintain moral as well as bodily integrity, particularly in connection with pregnancy and childbirth. How then has the culture represented women? There is a long tradition which regards women and women's bodies as property to be bartered, bestowed, or used by men. Usually women have lacked the power to refuse to accept sexual partners, have had little or no option as to whether to prevent or seek pregnancy, or whether to carry to term or abort. That the prohibition of abortion has often coexisted with the practice of infanticide, infanticide controlled either by the father of the infant or by the state, shows that the prohibition of abortion often evidences the view that women and/or women's bodies are a resource to be controlled by men, rather than a concern about feticide. The prohibition of abortion within Nazi Germany evidences the same view. We find the legacy of this tradition still very much with us when opposition to abortion is supported with the reason that women should not be allowed to have abortions because this allows them to escape the consequences of what is seen as their probable sexual 'misconduct'.

The book of *Deuteronomy* (22: 13–21) stipulates that if any new husband accuses his bride of not having been a virgin at her marriage and her male relative cannot produce the 'tokens of her virginity' as evidence that she was, she is to be stoned to death. *Deuteronomy* (22: 22) also lists the death penalty as punishment for extramarital relations on the part of a married woman with no sanctions at all on similar activity on the part of a married man. Until the late 1960s, the legal definition of adultery in the state of Connecticut was extramarital activity involving a married woman. Extramarital sexual activity on the part of a married man was not covered by the statute. The Bible not only exempts men from similar jeopardy for extramarital sexual activity, but as the example of Abraham (*Genesis*, 12: 11–16) and Isaac (*Genesis*, 26: 7–10) show, men were excused for giving their wives for the sexual use of other men, and Lot (*Genesis*, 19: 1–8) and the Ephremite of Judges 19 (19: 22–24) are approved for offering their virgin daughters to be raped to insure that that fate does not befall their male guests. Not only is it a common assumption in our heritage that women's bodies are at the disposal first of their fathers and then of their husbands, but until recently, the prevailing view was that if women wandered out of the care of such 'protectors' they were 'asking for' trouble, and 'fair game' for rape. The threat of rape still severely restricts the mobility of women in society, notwithstanding the fact that rape frequently occurs within the victim's home.[12]

B. Nathanson and R. N. Osting in their book, *Aborting America* [21] profess that their regard for the fetus leads them to oppose all abortion, although they do have some concern about one kind of problem pregnancy. This is not the pregnancy that results from rape or that which involves the pregnant twelve-year-old. It is the pregnancy that results from adultery. Nathanson expresses sympathy with the view he attributes to George Williams of Harvard Divinity School, that in the case of pregnancy from adultery, the husband has the right to demand an abortion. This sentiment continues to evidence the view that women's bodies ought to be under the control of their husbands.

We find that the interest of the state or of those in power in controlling women's bodies, and through that controlling fertility, is equally represented in the tradition. In the *Republic* (Bk. 5, 460), Plato casually recommends infanticide for unpromising infants, and the recent history of fluctuations in the policies of Eastern European countries with regard to contraception and abortion show that the availability of both are manipulated to suit economic interests of those in power. The sentiment favoring such manipulation is also illustrated in an article by Alan L. Otten which appeared on the front page of the *Wall Street Journal* [13], in which Otten speaks of a 'people shortage', which turns out to be a shortage, not of people in general, but of 'native populations' of the countries of Northwestern Europe [23]. In this article, Otten raises the specter of shrinking markets and mentions such remedies as antiabortion laws, but does not even mention caring for children. If pronatalist policies were desired, then a rational and humane implementation would involve addressing the concern of women that they cannot adequately care for additional children, and would make provision to care for both existing and future children. This does not seem to have occurred to Otten who does not discuss either adjusting work life to accommodate the existence of children, or providing good inexpensive day care for children. Otten seems oblivious to the fact that even in industrialized countries, and in the United States in particular, *most* women seek paid employment out of economic necessity. Perhaps Otten is not interested in most women, but only wants to get the more affluent 'native population' women back to breeding.

A frequent complaint of feminists is that little priority has been given to the development of contraceptives that are both safe and effective. As it now stands, the methods of contraception that are reputed to be most effective has proved to have a greater mortality risk than does a legal first trimester abortion in the United States.[14]

In the 17th century, John Locke put forward a view that husbands do not have the power of life and death over their wives, but do have ultimate authority in decisions affecting the family's common interest, including the power to decide the control of their joint property. Since, according to 17th century English law the husband was given total control not only of his wife's property, but also of her person, and he had the right to imprison her and beat her so long as he stopped short of killing her, Mary Ann Warren argues that Locke's views were advanced for his time and should be termed 'protofeminist' [35]. Indeed, Locke's view that all men are naturally free and equal was taken up and interpreted to apply to women by early feminist writers such as Mary Wollstonecraft.

In Rousseau's *Émile* [27], we find further evidence of the way in which the tradition of regarding women and women's bodies as a resource for men continues, even in the work of those writers usually taken to have placed the greatest emphasis on individual dignity and autonomy. In this work, Rousseau sets out a plan for the education of a child from infancy to manhood. The emphasis is upon an upbringing that will place little or no restraint on the child Émile. This absence of restraint extends from the elimination of swaddling clothes to having as much playtime as the child likes. Rather than giving Émile commands, the tutor will arrange circumstances so that Émile learns the desired lessons from experience. Émile is to be taught to believe nothing except what is evident to his own reason. It is an education supposedly geared toward autonomy, but given the absence of responsibility for the welfare of others, one might ask whether the self-governance implied in autonomy would indeed be present. The suggestion that it would not finds support in the plan of education laid down for Sophie, Émile's future bride, who must, Rousseau tells us, like all girls "be trained to bear the yoke from the first so that they may not feel it, to master their own caprices and to submit themselves to the will of others" ([27], p. 332). Indeed Rousseau maintains that she should even be deliberately subjected to injustice since she is "formed to obey a creature so imperfect as man, a creature so often vicious and always faulty, she should learn early to submit to injustice and to suffer the wrong inflicted on her by her husband without complaint" ([27], p. 333). Unlike Émile, Sophie is to be taught to believe on the basis of authority, rather than to believe on the basis of reason.

In this sort of social scheme, it is easy to recognize the fantasies of an infant or toddler centering on having control of the mother who will forever act as a willing buffer between him and harsh reality. It is the realization of this fantasy for men at least, which explains the implicit double standard which I mentioned earlier, according to which men are at liberty so long as they do not unduly violate the rights of other men, but which holds that women are morally required to meet the needs of others and perhaps are denied equal rights in addition. The rights of women, and the responsibilities of others to meet the needs of women if women are to be able to meet their responsibilities, are rarely mentioned.

This asymmetry between the way in which the ethical situations of men and women are construed is found again in a recent article on abortion by Rosaline Weiss, in 'The Perils of Personhood' [35]. In her article, Weiss points out some of the weaknesses of the argument that the fetus is a person and therefore has a right to life. She suggests that the abortion issue be reexamined from the perspective of duties rather than of rights. The duties and responsibilities that she mentions, however, are exclusively duties and responsibilities that might exist on the part of the woman to promote the welfare of the fetus. It does not occur to her to ask what might be the duties and responsibilities of others toward pregnant women and new mothers. It is as though women are regarded as Earth Mothers, having access to all resources and being able to meet all the needs simultaneously, if they were only willing to do so. The literature on abortion shows that many people are readily able to image themselves in the place of fetus but not in the place of the pregnant woman,[15] but *if one is able to look at the matter from the perspective of the pregnant woman it becomes clear how much violence is done to the woman by abortion, and therefore that the woman's self interest would lead her to avoid (unwanted pregnancy and) abortion if she had other options genuinely available.*

6. SOME MORAL DILEMMAS OF PREGNANT WOMEN

Some of the moral issues that are commonly involved in decisions to seek or attempt an abortion are specific instances of dilemmas that face pregnant women generally. Over the centuries, pregnant women have taken pains to avoid those influences thought to be teratogenic, and an extensive lore purporting to identify these influences developed. The existence of this lore attests to the longstanding nature of women's concern to promote the healthy development of the fetus.

One dilemma commonly faced by a pregnant woman with existing children, is that she must weigh some benefits to those children against some risk to the fetus, usually in the nature of increased risk of abortion and of premature delivery and of the damage that commonly results from premature birth. For example, the medical center at which I worked is the only referral hospital for the State of Texas, and is located at the south-east corner of the state. Patients who cannot afford private care may need to travel 700 miles or more to obtain treatment. A woman in the late stages of pregnancy with a child who needs treatment may have to choose between the increased risk of abortion, or premature delivery which attends a long automobile trip, and having her child's ailments go untreated.

The typical woman in Asia and the Middle East who seeks an abortion (or attempts to abort herself) is an older married woman who has given birth to many children. In circumstances of poverty where the welfare, and indeed the survival of existing children, are likely to be put in question by another birth, that fact must figure in the woman's response to her pregnancy (unless she has been so conditioned to 'bear the yoke' or is so debilitated by mal-nutrition and disease that she has little or no response to what happens to her).

Even in this country, half of the women who have abortions are already mothers for whom the welfare of existing children is likely to be an important consideration. As Justice Brennan pointed out in his dissent on the Gilbert decision (the decision which struck down the EEOC guidelines calling on employers to provide maternity disability benefits), the United States is the only industrialized country in the world with no universal legal and social provisions for maternity. The woman whose children depend on her income may regard the welfare of those children (or of aged parents or others who depend upon her) as incompatible with continuing a pregnancy, even if she could bear the thought of giving up a newborn for adoption. Considering how many women are supporting children on salaries at or below the poverty line in this country, such fears are likely to be common. While children in this country do not starve to death in signficant numbers, many children live in conditions of poverty where their physical safety is always in question. Recent figures on poverty in the United States show that families consisting of women and their children are the most rapidly growing segment of the poor. A survey in the State of Illinois in 1980, for example, found that one child in six is being raised in poverty. The moral dilemmas facing a pregnant woman because of the competing responsibility for the welfare of her fetus and the welfare of existing children (or aged parents, etc.) are real and deserve systematic attention.

The woman who is pregnant by rape and is struggling to come to terms with and recover from the experience of rape, faces a special dilemma that exists in some form for all pregnant women, that of coming to terms with the experience of pregnancy. One author of a well-known pregnancy manual describes the early fetus in the following terms: "It is already alive, a human being, although its movements are still too feeble to be felt. And it has immense power. It can make a person take care of it, and adjust her whole organism to serve it" ([13], [40]). Small wonder that a woman pregnant by rape frequently experiences her pregnancy as a nine-month continuation of that rape. Not only does she, like many raped women, wake up at night screaming, but when she does, she finds that her body is still possessed by another. It is a significant omission that the philosophical literature on abortion has considered the rape issue only in connection with the question of whether the woman bears some responsibility for having become pregnant by having consented to sexual relations!

Being taken over by another being is an idea that has evoked both wonder and horror through the ages. It evokes wonder where it represents a desired union with God or some divine force (for example, being filled with the Holy Spirit, or being inspired by a Muse). It evokes horror where it represents being taken over unwillingly by some human or demonic force (for example, being possessed by a troubled spirit or the ghost of a person who has died, or by a demon, witch or sorcerer). Possession and inspiration provide the closest analogy to the ultimately unique experience of pregnancy. The difference in the experience of a wanted pregnancy and that of an unwanted pregnancy is as different as the two experiences of inspiration and possession. (Perhaps all or most experiences of inspiration have some element of possession in them and vice versa, and similarly with wanted and unwanted pregnancies.)

It should be noted that, like inspiration and possession, pregnancy whether wanted or unwanted is a psychological hazardous path. The rate of significant mental illness after delivery is high and is considerably higher than that following abortion. According to Freedman and Kaplan's *Comprehensive Textbook of Psychiatry* [22], postpartum psychoses, while uncommon, stand at the significantly high rate of one to two per thousand deliveries. (Notice that this rate is for *all* pregnancies carried to term, both wanted and unwanted.) This high rate of significant postpartum reaction is not surprising when one considers that bringing another person into full social being requires continual renegotiation of the self-other boundaries. Of course to say that some experience is risky is not to say that the risks are not worth taking, but it does suggest that those bearing the risk should decide whether to undertake it.

In parts of Africa and Latin America, the typical woman seeking an abortion is young and unmarried ([6], p. 106), and this is the profile of about half of the women seeking abortions in the United States. The young unmarried woman may face the same threat of poverty that confronts an older married woman and, like the oldest, the youngest pregnant women often face greatly increased risks to their own health from pregnancy. The unmarried woman, however, faces the additional stigma of 'illegitimacy'. The stigmatization of women who dare or are forced to bring forth children without being married, serves to control not merely a woman's sexual behavior but, perhaps more importantly, her option of creating families with or without men.

The postulation of a 'Principle of Legitimacy' as a 'universal sociological law' and as 'the most important moral and legal rule' concerning kinship was made in the 1930s by Bronslaw Malinowski. According to Laslett it has continued to dominate discussions of birth out of wedlock ever since. The version of the 'Principle of Legitimacy' which he quotes from Malinowski is:

The most important moral and legal rule concerning the physiological state of kinship is that no child should be brought into this world without a man — and one man at that — assuming the role of sociological father, that is guardian and protector, the male link between the child and the rest of the community. I think that this generalization amounts to a universal sociological law, and as such I have called it . . . The Principle of Legitimacy ([18], p. 5).

The only alternative to bringing a child into the world once pregnancy has begun is to abort it.

Today in the United States there are three million teenage girls having sexual intercourse who are not protected by any form of contraception. They are at high risk for pregnancy and cannot be assumed to have made a considered decision to undertake the responsibilities of parenthood.[16] If women's knowledge and control of their bodies were fostered generally (I have in mind here promulgation of the sort of knowledge found in the women's health movement), then decisions about contraception could be approached forthrightly. Although I do not believe that engaging in heterosexual intercourse without contraceptive protection when pregnancy is undesired is *necessarily* an unreflective or uninformed choice, the evidence is that teenagers frequently do so because of lack of information or because of social pressure.

We still live with the legacy of the view expressed by Rousseau that women should not be educated to make responsible decisions but to learn 'to bear the yoke'. While factions quarrel over *which yoke* the young teenage girl should bear, the present situation will continue. On the one hand, those who would forbid the young teenager heterosexual intercourse have often convinced her that premeditated contraceptive preparation shows that she is cheap, that is, too available. (The opposite of being 'cheap' is being 'expensive', which means that one still is a commodity but the price is higher. The way out of the commodity mentality is not to avoid 'being cheap' but to reclaim one's body, to reclaim it in the way expressed by the phrase "Our Bodies Ourselves".) On the other hand, societal arrangements that make the girl dependent on pleasing men pressure her into sexual intercourse at an early age. As long as we are content to leave girls subject to pressures, and simply try to see that 'the right' yoke is placed upon them, rather than support the development of their capacity to make decisions they can live with concerning their lives in general and sexual activity in particular, the only alternatives to increased maternity (and resulting morbidity and mortality) among teenagers, will be the grim options of legal abortion or illegal abortion.

If we take seriously women's role as decision makers and moral agents then we must give greater attention to the issue of providing accurate information to the woman facing a decision about abortion. Such information must of course include information about the embryo or fetus which will die as a result of the abortion procedure. It is unfortunate that there has not been more attention to this point on the part of feminists. Perhaps this is because the phrase 'informed consent' has been misapplied to inaccurate information designed to frighten and punish the woman seeking an abortion. Probably the most famous attempt to force misinformation upon women was the Akron ordinance which required that, among other things, a woman seeking an abortion be told that abortion was 'major surgery' (contrary to the view of the American College of Obstetrics and Gynecology) [1]. Dr. Willard Cates, Jr., Director of the Abortion Surveillance Branch of the National Center for Disease Control, Atlanta, Georgia, has recently discussed the harmful consequences of the Akron ordinance and other measures designed to restrict abortion services [4].

Perhaps some of the people interested in insuring a woman's right to a safe early abortion have failed to provide a pregnant woman full and accurate information about the embryo or fetus because they wish to spare the woman — but then the behavior is paternalistic. It fails to respect the woman's need to maintain her moral integrity, that is, to face her situation and make a decision that she can live with. (I also regard the effort as misguided in that there is considerable evidence that this sort of deception actually increases psychological damage in the long run.)

Dr. Raymond S. Duff has written extensively on the process of facing grim choices and of supporting parents in facing the grim choices which arise when a baby is born with severe deformities.[17] He emphasizes the harm done when hospital staff think they are sparing the parents by failing to give them all of the information or failing to cooperate with the uncoerced choice of parents to see or hold their deformed or dead babies. In a recent letter to the *New England Journal of Medicine* [9], Duff explicitly extends this to fetuses, recommending that the staff be prepared to accede to women's requests to be shown their aborted fetuses. I concur with Duff and argue that just as women who have *spontaneously* aborted have been left puzzled and angry by the paternalism of physicians who dismiss their loss as 'a matter of little consequence'[18], so women who resort to induced abortion have been inadequately prepared by those counselors who avoid discussing the embryo or fetus that will die as a result of the procedure.

7. CONCLUSION

I have argued that the moral issues involving decisions to resort to abortion need to be reformulated. Recent philosophical discussion of the subject, and most of the popular discussion, has systematically ignored certain important features of the moral situation, most commonly features which are more prominent in women's experience than in men's. A major point which has been neglected is that abortion is not something that anyone would straight-forwardly want, but rather is a surgical intervention which, like most surgical interventions, is resorted to only if the alternatives are even worse. It is there-fore misleading to speak of a right to abortion since this makes it sound as if abortion were something, like equal pay, that people might want. The right to control one's body is of course something that people can and do straightforwardly want. Indeed that right is a fundamental right of privacy, that is, exercising control over one's body is requisite for functioning as a person. An adequate representation of the moral situation involving abortion would need to come to terms with the fact that it is in the interests of women not to have to resort to abortion in order to control their bodies, just as it is in the interests of women to prevent breast cancer rather than treat it with mastectomies or 'lumpectomies' even if these operations constituted one hundred percent safe and effective treatments for breast cancer.

Of course being pregnant is importantly different from having a tumor, and often unwanted pregnancy would be wanted if there were a change in other conditions, for example if there were more social support for child rearing or no stigma attached to giving birth to children out of wedlock. Pregnancy has remained one of the least discussed subjects in philosophy in spite of much recent discussion of fetuses and abortion. There has been no attention given to the moral dilemmas commonly faced by pregnant women other than decisions about whether to induce abortion, even though decisions about how to choose between risks to the fetus and risks to existing children or between a risk of deformity and an increased risk of (spontaneous) abortion raise many of the same philosophical questions. These questions concern the moral status of the fetus; the nature of the relationships of pregnant women to their fetuses and of each to others in society; and the relative importance of future deformity, present or future pain, and continuance of life in assessing the well-being of the fetus. These philosophical questions might well be brought together by examining the scope and limits of the analogy between fetuses and newborns. To do this would require a developed philosophical account of newborns and modern philosophy has none to offer. Intimate relationships with newborn babies and with the practices which transform them into people in the full social sense which is so commonly a part of women's experience as mothers,[19] nurses, aunts and so forth, has been omitted from the background knowledge upon which philosophers rely in choosing their problems and framing their arguments. If we are to understand the philosophical issues concerning fetuses, pregnant women and the nature of the relationship created in pregnancy we will need to give close attention to women's experience and to the practices involved that have traditionally been regarded as women's work, especially infant and child care and nursing (in all the senses of that term). It is only then that we will be able to frame ethical issues in an adequate manner, that is, in a way which takes acount of all of the morally relevant features of the situation.[20]

Research Fellow,
Center for Policy Alternatives, M.I.T.,
Cambridge, Massachusetts

NOTES

* I owe many intellectual debts to feminist writing and writings and, more importantly, to specific examples of feminist practice. I am no longer able to keep track of them all. Certainly extended discussions with Carol P. Christ, particularly in 1971 and 1972 were of inestimable value to me in developing my own thought on women's issues. I note how congenial to the views presented here is Christ's reading of Atwood's *Surfacing* as showing that abortion "is not a matter of little consequence" ([5], p. 52). One of

the many catalysts to my thinking on the present issue was Adrienne Rich's discussion of abortion in *Of Woman Born* from which the following passage is taken:

"No free woman, with 100 percent effective, non-harmful birth control readily available, would 'choose' abortion. At present, it is certainly likely that a woman can – through many causes – become so demoralized as to use abortion as a form of violence against herself – a penance, an expiation. But this needs to be viewed against the ecology of guilt and victimization in which so many women grow up. In a society where women entered sexual intercourse willingly, where adequate contraception was a genuine social priority, there would be no 'abortion issue'. And in such a society there would be a vast diminishment of female self-hatred – a psychic source of many unwanted pregnancies.

Abortion is violence: a deep desperate violence inflicted by a woman upon, first of all, herself. It is the offspring, and will continue to be the accuser, of a more pervasive and prevalent violence, the violence of rapism" ([26], pp. 273–274).

I wish to thank James B. Speer, Jr. and Eleanor Kuykendall for their detailed criticism of this paper.

1 Paul suggests a very different view of the spiritual significance of gender in *Galatians*, 3: 28 but repeats the views he expressed in *Corinthians*, in *1st. Timothy* (2: 12–15) and *Ephesians* (5: 22–23).

2 For example, Michael Tooley in 'A Defense of Abortion and Infanticide' stipulates "In my usage the sentence 'X is a person' will be synonymous with the sentence 'X has a (serious) moral right to life'" ([33], p. 40); and Edward A. Langerak, in his article 'Abortion: Listening to the Middle', stipulates that he uses the term 'person' to refer to "those human beings that will have as strong a claim to life as a normal adult" ([17], p. 25).

3 Since the line between description of acts or actions and the ends achieved by those acts or actions is not sharp, obligations shade into responsibilities.

4 Readers may notice the similarity between ideas I express here and ideas put forward by John Ladd in his article 'Legalism and Medical Ethics' [15]. However, in the abbreviated version of this article, which appeared in the March 1979, *Journal of Medicine and Philosophy* [16], Ladd omits what, to my mind, were crucial parts of the view of an ethics of responsibility. That is, he does not bring out the importance of respect for rights in safeguarding people's moral integrity and because his work does not go into the view of the person implicit in different views of ethics, I hesitate to say how close my views are to Ladd's, although I owe much to having read his work.

5 Some philosophers have argued that a person cannot choose freely when faced with grim options. I have discussed problems with some of these arguments in 'Towards an Understanding of Motivational Disturbance and Freedom of Action' [40].

6 For a social history of illegitimacy or bastardy, see [18].

7 In 'A Theory of Health' [39], I have developed some related distinctions and shown these implications for the concepts of health and disease, and therefore for understanding the medical enterprise.

8 Ketchum's [14] argument that one's right to one's body is not a property right.

9 Those who argue that killing a fertilized ovum is just as bad, morally speaking, as killing a viable fetus do not seem to realize that the view commits them to a position that killing a viable fetus is *no worse* than killing a fertilized ovum.

[10] Birth constitutes a major change in status according to many *religious* traditions. In the New Testament, for example, birth is the principal metaphor for beginning, and generates such expressions as 'reborn in Christ', rather than, say, 'reconceived in Christ'. Of course, those who are willing to question the ethical validity of such religious sources, can still consider the possibility that the moral status of the fetus may be close to that of a newborn.

[11] The way in which philosophers employ background knowledge is aptly illustrated in Solomon's paper [29] where he refers to the experience of being a stranger in a strange city; however, it is reasonable to assume that people attending a conference like the one generating this volume will have had this experience many times in their lives. Background knowledge about newborn care is not something that philosophers, other than a few feminist philosophers, use in their arguments. For an interesting example of philosophical attention to infants and child care, see [28].

[12] This point has been thoroughly argued by Susan Peterson in 'Rape and Coercion: The State as a Male Protection Racket' [24].

[13] I am indebted to Barbara Tilley for bringing this article to my attention.

[14] An extensive bibliography on the hazards of various forms of birth control, together with a multifaceted discussion of the subject, is contained in [12]. See also [43].

[15] As Mary Daly observes, the analogy between the fetus in the womb and the space traveler in a capsule is a recurrent theme, and she maintains that the popularity of the identification of fetus with space travelers explains some of the popular fascination with, and generous findings of space exploration [8].

[16] The many different reasons that women have for not using contraception are discussed in [20].

[17] By 'severe deformities' one generally means deformities that produce severe retardation, and/or pain throughout life and not 'merely' crippling or disfigurement.

[18] Victoria Spelman informs me that there is a book forthcoming on the subject of a woman's experience of spontaneous abortion, which takes as its ironic title, *A Matter of Little Consequence.*

[19] Notice that Carol Christ uses the same form of words, and denies that abortion is a 'matter of little consequence' for the woman involved. See * Note. For 1974, the percentage of women in the United States bearing children some time in their lives stood at 91% as compared with 73% in 1910 [31].

[20] After the paper was written I became familiar with Carol Gilligan's psychological studies that lend empirical support to the thesis that the responsibilities view is more adequate for expressing women's moral concerns. See *In a Different Voice*, Cambridge: Harvard University Press, 1982.

BIBLIOGRAPHY

1. *Akron Center for Reproductive Health, Inc. v. City of Akron*, 651 F. 2d 1198 (C.A. 6 Ohio, June 12, 1981; re hearings denied, July 10, 1981 and July 22, 1981).
2. Benn, S. I.: 1975, 'Privacy, Freedom and Respect for Persons', in R. Wasserstrom (ed.), *Today's Moral Problems*, Macmillan, New York, pp. 1–20.
3. Biggers, J. D.: 1983, 'Generation of the Human Life Cycle', in this volume, pp. 31–53.

4. Cates, W., Jr.: 1980, 'Restricting Abortion Services: Harm and Misfortune', *Medical News* **26**, 3.
5. Christ, C. P.: 1980, *Diving Deep and Surfacing*, Beacon Press, Cambridge, Massachusetts.
6. 'Complications of Abortion in Developing Countries', Population Reports, Series F, No. 7, Population Information Program, The Johns Hopkins University, Baltimore, Maryland, July 1980.
7. Connery, J. R.: 1978, 'Abortion: Roman Catholic Perspectives', in W. Reich (ed.), *Encyclopedia of Bioethics*, Vol. 1, MacMillan and the Free Press, New York, pp. 9–13.
8. Daly, M.: 1978, *Gyn/Ecology: Metaethics of Radical Feminism*, Beacon Press, Cambridge, Massachusetts.
9. Duff, R. S.: 1980, 'Care in Childbirth and Beyond', *New England Journal of Medicine* **302**, 685–686.
10. Engelhardt, H. T., Jr.: 1982, 'Viability and the Use of the Fetus', in this volume, pp. 183–208.
11. Hellman, L. M. and J. Pritchard (eds.): 1971, *Williams Obstetrics*, Appleton Century Crofts, New York.
12. Holmes, H. *et al.* (eds.): 1981, *Birth Control and Controlling Birth*, Humana Press, New Jersey.
13. Ingelman-Fundberg, A.: 1975, *A Guide for the Mother To Be*, Humana Press, New Jersey.
14. Ketchum, S. A.: 1980, 'The Moral Status of the Bodies of Persons', unpublished manuscript.
15. Ladd, J.: 1978, 'Legalism and Medical Ethics', in J. W. Davis, B. Hoffmaster, and S. Shorten (eds.), *Contemporary Issues in Biomedical Ethics*, Humana Press, New Jersey, pp. 1–33.
16. Ladd, J.: 1979, 'Legalism and Medical Ethics', *Journal of Medicine and Philosophy* **4**, 70–80.
17. Langerak, E. A.: 1979, 'Abortion: Listening to the Middle', *Hastings Center Report* **9**, 24–48.
18. Laslett, K., K. Oatween, and R. M. Smith (eds.): 1980, *Bastardy and Its Comparative History*, Harvard University Press, Cambridge, Massachusetts.
19. *Levy v. Louisiana*, 391 U.S. 68 (1968).
20. Luker, K.: 1978, *Taking Chances*, University of California Press, Berkeley, California.
21. Nathanson, B. N. and R. N. Ostling: 1979, *Aborting America*, Doubleday, New York.
22. Normand, W. C.: 1967, 'Postpartum Disorders', in A. M. Freedman and H. I. Kaplan (eds.), *Comprehensive Textbook of Psychiatry*, Williams and Wilkins, Baltimore, Maryland, pp. 1161–1163.
23. Otten, A. L.: 1979, 'People Shortage: A Growing Problem', *Wall Street Journal* **64** (38), p. 1.
24. Peterson, S.: 1977, 'Rape and Coercion: The State as a Male Protection Racket', in M. Vetterlin-Braggin (ed.), *Feminism and Philosophy*, Littlefield Adams and Co., New Jersey, pp. 54–61.
25. Reiman, J. H.: 1976, 'Privacy, Intimacy and Personhood', *Philosophy and Public Affairs* **6**, 26–44.

26. Rich, A.: 1976, *Of Woman Born: Motherhood as Experience and Institution*, W. W. Norton and Co., New York.

27. Rousseau, J. J.: 1963, *Émile*, trans. by B. Foxley and J. M. Denton, Heineman, London.

28. Ruddick, S.: 1980, 'Maternal Thinking', *Feminist Studies* 6, 87–96.

29. Solomon, R.: 1981, 'Reflections on the Meaning of (Fetal) Life', in this volume, pp. 209–226.

30. Soupart, P.: 1981, 'Present and Possible Future Research in the Use of Human Embryos', in this volume, pp. 67–104.

31. Stellman, J. M.: 1978, *Women's Work, Women's Health: Myths and Realities*, Pantheon, New York.

32. Thomson, J. J.: 1973, 'Rights and Death', *Philosophy and Public Affairs* 2, 146–159.

33. Tooley, M.: 1972, 'A Defense of Abortion and Infanticide', *Philosophy and Public Affairs* 2, 37–65.

34. Van Nostrand, R.: 1976, *Scientific Encyclopedia*, The Free Press, New York.

35. Warren, M. A.: 1980, *The Nature of Woman, An Encyclopedia and Guide to the Literature*, Edgewood Press, Michigan.

36. Weiss, R.: 1978, 'The Perils of Personhood', *Ethics* 89, 66–75.

37. Whitbeck, C.: 1975, 'The Maternal Instinct', *The Philosophical Forum* 6, 265–273.

38. Whitbeck, C.: 1976, 'Theories of Sex Difference', in C. C. Gould and M. W. Wartofsky (eds.), *Women and Philosophy: Towards a Philosophy of Liberation*, G. P. Putnam's and Sons, New York, pp. 54–80.

39. Whitbeck, C.: 1981, 'A Theory of Health', in A. Caplan, H. T. Engelhardt, and J. McCartney (eds.), *Concepts of Health and Disease*, Addison-Wesley, Reading, Massachusetts, pp. 611–626.

40. Whitbeck, C.: 1977, 'Towards an Understanding of Motivational Disturbance and Freedom of Action', in H. T. Engelhardt, Jr. and S. F. Spicker (eds.), *Mental Health: Philosophical Perspectives*, D. Reidel Publ. Co., Dordrecht, Holland, pp. 221–231.

41. Whitbeck, C.: 1978, 'What Are We Teaching When We Teach Human Sexuality?', *Connecticut Medicine* 42, 657–661.

42. Wirsen, B., C. Wirsen, and A. McMillan (eds.): 1966, *Obstetrician*, Dell Publishing Co., New York, p. 80.

43. 'Women and Health', *Public Health Reports*, Superintendent of Documents, U.S. Government Printing Office, Washington, D.C. (September–October, 1980), p. 27.

MARGERY W. SHAW

THE DESTINY OF THE FETUS

Several comments made by Holly Smith [15] can be addressed in the legal context.

First, she talks about a *gift* made by a woman of the use of her body for survival of her fetus. In the law, a gift is usually considered irrevocable once the gift has been delivered. But an accidentally transferred possession does not constitute a gift. A gift must be understood to be made in the mind of the donor and the act must be made with a written or oral statement, or be implied by the act of giving. A woman who accidentally becomes pregnant, rather than purposefully so, does not necessarily promise her life support system to her developing embryo or fetus. We can hardly argue that the fetus has mentally anticipated the use of the woman's body, thus making the gift irrevocable.

Smith also addresses the issue of the right of the fetus to use the woman's body in terms which remind one of the law of torts. A tort is a harmful act done by one individual to another. Setting aside the basic issue of a tort being committed on an unborn fetus (prenatal tort) which Leonard Glantz [8] discusses in his essay, we could analogize the decision of a woman to have an abortion under two broad classes of torts — intentional and non-intentional acts.

An intentional tort, such as assault and battery, is an act of unconsented touching. It is the civil law equivalent of a criminal act. Since the U.S. Supreme Court has decided that abortion in the early stages of pregnancy is not a crime, it is difficult to see how it would be deemed an intentional tort. A non-intentional tort, or negligence, is not so closely tied to criminal law. The elements of negligence, all of which must be met, are the following:

(1)   the woman must owe a duty to her fetus.
(2)   the duty must be breached,
(3)   an injury must occur,
(4)   the injury must be proximately caused by the breach, and
(5)   the injury must have been foreseeable.

If the first element of negligence could be shown, i.e., that the woman owes a duty toward her fetus, then all of the other elements flow easily. But it

273

William B. Bondeson et al *(eds.), Abortion and the Status of the Fetus*, 273–279.
Copyright © 1983 *by D. Reidel Publishing Company, Dordrecht, Holland.*

is just that issue, a duty and responsibility toward the fetus, which is at
the vortex of the abortion debate and has been settled in *Roe v. Wade* [13]
such that the woman's right to the privacy of her own bodily decisions is
paramount to any right-to-life of the fetus, at least during early pregnancy.
There, the negligence argument fails. However, I shall argue later that a
woman may, in fact, incur negligence toward her fetus *if* she makes the
decision to bring that fetus to term.

I certainly agree with Caroline Whitbeck's position [18] that the condition and experiences and desires of the pregnant woman in her abortion
decision are overlooked during heated debates on the rights of the fetus and
the duties of the mother toward her fetus. I am sure Whitbeck would agree
with me that most women have both conscious and unconscious concerns
about the normalcy of the fetus while they are in the pregnant state. This
probably explains why they easily accept offers of preconception and prenatal genetic testing and even accept the alternative of aborting a wanted
fetus if it is discovered to be genetically defective.

This statement leads me to explore with you my own perspective on
pregnancy and abortion in a genetic context.

First, I will comment on some biological definitions of life, the legal
definition of personhood, and the courts' attitudes toward reproduction.
Then I will discuss the legal duties of physicians and parents toward fetuses.
Finally, I will address society's responsibilities to future generations.

The life forms of sexually reproducing organisms can be described as a
continuous cycle (see Figure 1). For purposes of convenience we divide

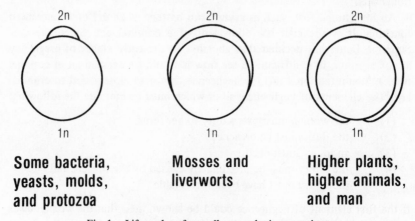

Fig. 1.   Life cycles of sexually-reproducing organisms.

this cycle into haploid and diploid stages. In fungi, such as *Neurospora*, the haploid stage predominates while the diploid stage lasts only for one cell cycle. The fertilized cell or zygote immediately undergoes meiosis to produce haploid cells which become the vegetative mold. In contrast, in the higher plants, invertebrates, and vertebrates, including Homo sapiens, the organism is made up of diploid cells. The haploid stage is confined to the sex cells or gametes.

This illustration helps us to visualize the arbitrariness or biological definitions of life. No biologist would dispute that the zygote is alive but we must also concede that the gametes are alive, and that the somatic cells that make up our tissues and organs are also alive. In the case of Homo sapiens, the gametes and the somatic cells contain only human genes, just as the zygote. For those who would argue that the human zygote is a human being or a person, they must also consider that any cell of the body which is capable of dividing has the potential of developing into a complete human being if scientists learn the techniques of cloning. This has been accomplished in a single cell from the carrot root tip and is theoretically possible for a human liver cell, bone marrow cell, or intestinal epithelial cell.

Moral and ethical arguments surrounding the sanctity of human life do not address living cells, including eggs and sperm, although debates about contraception have a hidden agenda which elevate gametes above liver cells or blood cells. Instead, discussion centers around the totality of cells that make up the differentiated organism called Man. But again, the boundaries are not clear. It is not morally wrong to remove an appendix or a cataract although some may argue that it is sinful to remove a uterus in order to foreclose reproductive capacity. I would claim that the whole human body is not considered precious or sacred but that the debate concentrates primarily on the central nervous system and reproductive system. These are the organ systems which distinguish Man from lower organisms. The gametes are the potential life source of future generations of our species and the brain, especially the cerebral cortex, gives us our cognitive and sapient qualities.

Attempts have been made to list the attributes of humanness. One such list provided by Joseph Fletcher, is made up of various aspects of cortical function [7], and is shown in Table I.

All of the criteria on this list need not be present in order for cortical function to exist but permanent absence of all of them would certainly cause us to question the existence of a human being with personhood qualities.

Fletcher argues that brain death should be defined as cortical death and not death of the whole brain and brain stem [6]. If cortical function is

TABLE I

1. Minimal intelligence;	9. Communication;
2. Self-awareness;	10. Control of existence;
3. Self-control;	11. Curiosity;
4. A sense of time;	12. Change and changeability;
5. A sense of the future;	13. Balance of rationality and feeling;
6. A sense of the past;	14. Idiosyncrasy;
7. The capacity to relate to others;	15. Neo-cortical function.
8. Concern for others;	

accepted as the primary criterion for humanness and the end of human life (not the end of biological life) is its cessation, then the beginning of human life must be its onset. The problem that philosophers and theologians face in defining personhood is that in this continuum of development and senescence of human cortical function no specific line can be drawn which clearly delineates a specific point in time between person and non-person.

American constitutional law, as enunciated by our courts, has found a simple and neat, albeit arbitrary, solution to part of this dilemma. By fiat, the word 'person' is legally defined as the individual who is born alive and becomes a member of the human community. Fetuses and stillborns are not counted as citizens in the census; they are not given income tax exemptions; they have no estates. Fetuses are considered by the law as 'potential persons' who are legally protected from harm that would cause them pain and suffering *if* they are born alive. Livebirth is a specific moment in time which can be witnessed and recorded. The time of fertilization or implantation or quickening or viability cannot be precisely determined.

The abortion debate, reduced to its lowest common denominator, is centered around the question of *who* shall decide which fetuses shall be welcomed into society. Those who support the right to life say the decision-maker is God or Nature; those who support freedom of choice say it is the mother. The U.S. Supreme Court has held that the decision during early pregnancy rests entirely with the mother in consultation with her physician [13]. Not even the husband can veto his wife's right to an abortion [11]. Rather than speaking of the rights of a fetus to be born alive, I would prefer to consider the duties and obligations of those who decide that a fetus shall be allowed to be born. Historically, the size of the human population has been controlled by both natural and man-made events such as famine, pestilence and war. We now have the power to exercise or limit our procreative options both before and after conception. I would argue that both parents should have a limited right to conceive and the mother should have a limited right to continue her pregnancy. I would further argue that these limited rights carry with them a heavy burden of responsibility to ensure, insofar as possible, that the fetus who is destined to become a member of society is given an optimal chance of being born physically and mentally sound, and will be nurtured and cherished after it is born.

Several legal decisions point to a trend in this direction. In 1884, Justice Oliver Wendell Holmes, in a case of prenatal injury, stated that there is "a conditional, prospective liability to one not yet in being" [4]. The condition is livebirth; the prospective liability is one that ripens when the one not-yet-in-being becomes a being. The courts have given people the right not to conceive ([5], [9]), and the right to abort [13]. The judge in a New Jersey case stated the limited right to reproduce succinctly: "Justice requires that the principle be recognized that a child has a legal right to begin life with a sound mind and body" [16].

Physicians have been held responsible for unwanted children after failed sterilization ([3], [12]). They have also been found liable for not determining genetic risks and not providing genetic tests, counseling, and prenatal diagnosis if a foreseeably defective child is born. The majority of cases have held that the physician owes a duty to the parents and he is answerable to them in damages for economic loss and emotional pain and suffering if he is negligent [20].

Several cases have addressed the issue of whether the physician's duty of care also flows to the child. Most suits by the child have not met with success, citing reasons of public policy, the impossibility of measuring damages when a life with defects must be compared against no life at all, and the logical absurdity that a child does not have standing to sue because if no wrongful act had occurred he would not be here to complain ([1], [14], [17], [19]).

A 1980 decision by an appellate court in California suggests a departure from this legal analysis [2]. In that case the child plaintiff had Tay-Sachs disease because the laboratories that performed carrier testing on the parents falsely reported that they were non-carriers. The court upheld the child's cause of action for physical pain and suffering and shortened life expectancy but also allowed punitive damages against the laboratories if fraud, oppression, or malice could be shown. The complaint alleged that the laboratories had been notified prior to the testing of the parents that their tests were inaccurate and could lead to disastrous results.

Not only did the court recognize the child's claim, but the judge who wrote the opinion added a remarkable comment *in dictum*:

If a case arose where, despite due care by the medical profession in transmitting the necessary warnings, parents made a conscious choice to proceed with a pregnancy, with full knowledge that a seriously impaired infant would be born, that conscious choice would provide an intervening act of proximate cause to preclude liability insofar as defendants other than the parents were concerned. Under such circumstances, we see no sound public policy which would protect those parents from being answerable for the pain, suffering and misery which they have wrought upon their offspring ([2], pp. 31–32).

If this point of view regarding parental responsibility becomes generally accepted, there are certain consequences which may be predicted. First, parents may not have a right to conceive an unwanted child if it would be destined to suffer from parental neglect. Second, it may be recognized as a legal wrong to knowingly beget defective children. Father Haring, a Catholic theologian, has argued that it is morally wrong to do so [10]. Third, if conception does occur, there may not be an unfettered right to bring a defective fetus to term, as enunciated by the California court. Fourth, if the mother abandons her right to abort a presumably healthy fetus then she incurs a conditional, prospective liability if she abuses her fetus and if the fetus is injured as a result of her acts. Newborns can suffer from fetal alcohol syndrome, drug addiction, birth defects from known teratogens or mental retardation if the mother has PKU. Any of these could be caused by the mother's failure to act responsibly during pregnancy, and could become cognizable at law by extension of child abuse statutes.

I would also urge that society's agenda should include not only protection of the fetus but also protection of the genetic pool which resides in our gonads. Reproductive hazards in the workplace and radiation and chemical toxins in the environment can damage the genes and chromosomes by increased mutations. In our short life span, we, the present generation, are entrusted with the care of all the genes for all of the generations of Homo sapiens yet to be born. All of those future generations have no other source to obtain their genes than the pool which we now hold. Surely we would wish to guard, cherish and protect from harm this precious gene pool until we bequeath it to our offspring.

The University of Texas Health Science Center at Houston

BIBLIOGRAPHY

1. Capron, A. M.: 1979, 'Tort Liability in Genetic Counseling', *Columbia Law Review* **79**, 618–685.
2. *Curlender v. Bio-Science Labs. and Automated Lab. Sciences*, 165 Cal. Rptr. 477 (1980).
3. *Custodio v. Bauer*, 251 Cal. App. 2d 303, 59 Cal. Rrpt. 463 (1967).
4. *Dietrich v. Inhabitants of Northampton*, 138 Mass. 14 (1884).
5. *Eisenstadt v. Baird*, 405 U.S. 438 (1972).
6. Fletcher, J.: 1974, 'Four Indicators of Humanhood', *Hastings Center Report* **4**, 4–6.
7. Fletcher, J.: 1979, *Humanhood: Essays in Biomedical Ethics*, Prometheus Press, Buffalo, New York.
8. Glantz, L.: 1983, 'Is the Fetus a Person? A Lawyer's View', in this volume, pp. 107–117.
9. *Griswold v. Connecticut*, 381 U.S. 479 (1965).
10. Haring, B.: 1976, 'It's Wrong to Knowingly Beget Defective Children', *U.S. Catholic* **41**, 12–17.
11. *Planned Parenthood of Missouri v. Danforth*, 428 U.S. 52 (1976).
12. Robertson, G. B.: 1978, 'Civil Liability Arising from "Wrongful Birth" Following Sterilization Operation', *American Journal of Law and Medicine* **4**, 152–165.
13. *Roe v. Wade*, 410 U.S. 113 (1973).
14. Shaw, M. W.: 1980, 'The Potential Plaintiff: Preconception and Prenatal Torts', in A. Milunsky and G. Annas (eds.), *Genetics and the Law II*, Plenum Press, New York, pp. 225–235.
15. Smith, H.: 1983, 'Intercourse and Moral Responsibility for the Fetus', in this vol., pp. 229–245.
16. *Smith v. Brennan*, 31 N.J. 353, 157 A 2d 497 (1960).
17. Tedeshi, I.: 1966, 'On Tort Liability for "Wrongful Life" ', *Israel Law Review* **1**, 513–538.
18. Whitbeck, C.: 1983, 'The Moral Implications of Regarding Women as People: New Perspective on Pregnancy and Personhood', in this vol., pp. 247–272.
19. Wright, E. E.: 1978, 'Father and Mother Know Best: Defining the Liability of Physicians for Inadequate Genetic Counseling', *Yale Law Journal* **87**, 488–513.
20. Wright, E. E. and M. W. Shaw: 1981, 'Legal Liability in Genetic Counseling', in J. L. Simpson (ed.), *Annual Review of Obstetrics and Gynecology*, Harper and Row, Hagerstown, pp. 81–103.

SECTION V

CLASSICAL AND RELIGIOUS ROOTS OF CURRENT
CONTROVERSY

RICHARD HARROW FEEN

ABORTION AND EXPOSURE IN ANCIENT GREECE: ASSESSING THE STATUS OF THE FETUS AND 'NEWBORN' FROM CLASSICAL SOURCES *

I. INTRODUCTION

The practice of abortion and exposure was a reality of everyday life in ancient Greece. Only rarely would the state or family intervene with the father's act of disposing of his offspring, be it the fetus or newborn child. This is not to say, however, that nascent life was totally without 'rights' (as we know them) in the Greek world, only that these were quite limited in scope. In assessing the status of the fetus and the newborn child, we are unfortunately handicapped by a lack of sufficient evidence. This should not deter us, though, from attempting to construct an intelligent argument as to what the status of the fetus and the newborn was in relation to the legal and social order. It is the purpose of this paper then, to deal historically with what we today would call the 'personhood' question. Overall, I will discuss the practice of exposure and abortion in ancient Greece, giving special attention to such issues as whether fetal life was considered human life, what rôle the Hippocratic Oath played, if any, in Greek medical practice, and whether the newborn infant was dependent upon the father's recognition to acquire 'standing' within the community. Thus I will approach the status of offspring (unborn and newborn) in ancient Greece from both a legal and philo-medical perspective.[1] It is hoped that as a result, the reader will better appreciate the complexity of dealing with such issues from classical sources, in addition to becoming cautious in transposing contemporary concepts and beliefs to the historical evidence.

II. THE 'GOOD' OF CHILDREN

It seems apparent that any inquiry into the practice of abortion and exposure should begin with the rôle of children in Greek society. As could be expected, the ancient Greek *oikos* (household) more than welcomed the arrival of offspring. After all, a house without children was visibly dying, unable to renew itself through another generation. Economic considerations also dictated the size of the Greek family, and it should be noted that the agricultural productivity of the average Greek homestead was quite limited. In

283

William B. Bondeson et al. *(eds.), Abortion and the Status of the Fetus, 283–300.*
Copyright © 1983 by D. Reidel Publishing Company, Dordrecht, Holland.

any case, at least one son or a son and a daughter were considered most desirable. The son was thought of as perpetuating the family and would defend its existence both on the battlefield and in the assembly. Daughters, on the other hand, though considered more of a liability in that their dowries had to be provided and their chastity preserved so as not to damage the family's reputation, were still essential, it being each family's obligation to provide the community with wives. According to Demosthenes, "For this is what living with a woman as one's wife means: to have children by her and to introduce the sons to the members of the clan and of the deme, and to betroth the daughters to husbands as one's own" (*Orations* 59.122). Overall, the importance of children should not be underestimated, for they not only provided for the family's support, but they continued ancestral worship and served to retain all acquired property. For without an heir, a man's holdings and religious obligations would be absorbed at once by the closest relation, regardless of the existing personal animosity or friendship. No doubt, there was no greater tragedy than to have one's property squandered and one's tomb and memory neglected.

The Greek legislators, as one would imagine, were particularly sensitive to the father's desire for his family's preservation and this is the principal reason for the abundance of legislation dealing with the guardianship as well as marriage of an heiress. In fact, the primary purpose of adoption was to provide a legal route for an heirless family to preserve itself, and not merely to provide parental care for a child who would otherwise lack it. Moreover, it was this concern for a clear line of descendants that required that adultery be severely punished, being a public as well as a private offense. As Lysias noted, "The adulterer gains access to all a man's possessions, and casts doubt upon his children's heritage" (*Orations* 1.33).

As for the state's rôle in the 'procreative process', it was careful, through the above legislation, to insure that family households remained viable. After all, it was the rôle of the *oikoi* to provide for the support of the entire community, in terms of both human and material resources. However, specific policies to facilitate marriage and legal offspring differed among the Greek city-states. Sparta, if we are to believe the ancient writers, had definite pronatal inclinations. According to Plutarch, bachelors were highly discriminated against, as it was considered a duty to provide the state with an assured source of military manpower. Aristotle notes that the Spartans enacted laws that would relieve a man of his military obligations if he had three sons, and of taxation if he had four (*Politics*, 2.9.18). The Spartans even went so far as to legitimize bigamy so as to maximize the number of children in the community (Xenophon, *Const. Lac.* 1). In Athens, on the other hand, and one assumes in a majority of other states, such social engineering schemes were basically unknown. Marital relations remained largely a matter of free choice, though we do occasionally hear of financial and other penalties being exacted from individuals who lacked both wives and children.[2] Only under extreme conditions, as existed during the Peloponnesian Wars, did Athens actually attempt to stimulate the birth rate. The Athenians, according to Diogenes Laertius, "because of the scarcity of men, wished to increase the population, and passed a vote that a man might marry one Athenian woman and have children by another" (*Lives*, 2.26). The reason for this apparent violation of Athenian custom and sensitivities to overpopulation, lay in the fact that the Wars had severely reduced the citizen rôles, thereby constraining Athens' politico-social institutions. In any event, under normal circumstances, the state left the choice to marry and have children to its citizens. One can see then how contemporary notions that the ancient Greeks, as with all past civilizations, stressed the virtue of a large expanding population and passed legislation to that end, are incorrect, being founded upon those instances in which a society had experienced a dramatic demographic catastrophe.

III. THE PRACTICE OF EXPOSURE

As the Greek state as a rule did not enforce any duty upon a man to have children, so the law did not interfere with the father's authority over his child, particularly the newborn. While there has been some debate as to whether the parental power of the Greek father was analogous to the Roman *patria potestas*, it is generally agreed upon that at its birth the Greek child was so completely in its father's power that it rested with him whether or not the child should be admitted into the family ([11], p. 70). He openly signified his intention to do so during a ceremony, the *amphidromia*, which took place usually during the first week after the child's birth, at which point the child was named before the assembled members of the family and proclaimed to be a legitimate offspring. However, the father had no duty to take this step. He could, on the other hand, by himself or through his agent (i.e., a slave), have the newborn child 'exposed', that is to say, abandoned wherever he pleased without worrying whether anyone would pick it up or whether it would simply perish. And though the finder of an exposed child might at his discretion treat it as a slave or a free person, he acquired no rights over it and he could not even adopt it, since adoption of a minor was a joint transaction between the adopter and the adopted child's father or his representative. Moreover, if recognized by the parents, the child had by law to be given back to them, thereby making the exposed child precarious property. As Alick Harrison points out, "The act of exposure was legally negative in character. The legal tie between the exposed child, whether it was a legitimate son or daughter or a slave, and the father or master who exposed it, remained and could be revived" ([11], p. 71).

An explanation for the exposure of legitimate children can be traced to economic considerations of the *oikos*, and at least in Athens, the absence of primogeniture.[3] Thus, a precarious balance existed between the demands for a sufficient number of children to continue the family line and the need to protect that same family from the dangers of being over-burdened by too many mouths to feed and having its property divided to the point of non-viability. Most likely it was for this reason that Hesiod advised, "There should be an only son to feed his father's house, for so wealth will increase in the house" (*Works and Days*, 375)[4]. Thus, if a father had a choice, he may have shared Hesiod's view that one son is enough, and preferred the risk of losing his only son to the danger of having to divide the family plot if more than one survived infancy. As previously noted, the liabilities associated with a daughter (i.e., dowry and chastity) would have diminished a family's predisposition to raise it, thereby making females more vulnerable than males to the act of exposure. No doubt deformed children were, as a rule, exposed. According to Plutarch, in Sparta this was done, "in the conviction that the life of that which nature had not well equipped at the very beginning through health and strength was of no advantage either to itself or to the state" (*Lives*, 16.2)[5]. It would, however, be safe to say, as does W. K. Lacey, that "the largest number and the highest proportion of exposed infants will have been those produced by unions formed out of wedlock, the bastards of slave girls, courtesans, and prostitutes of all classes" ([15], p. 210). Thus, the exposure of illegitimate children was probably viewed as an acceptable alternative to the social stigma and legal complications that would be attendant upon survival in the family.

It should be emphasized that there exists no reason to doubt that the Greek father had this absolute discretion of exposure and that this right was more than a clearly formal one. Even though no direct evidence exists of this practice in then current law codes (except for reference to a mother's right to expose her child on the condition that her divorced husband did not recognize the child), indirect confirmation of the act can be found in literature, mythology, and even in the correspondences of the time.[6] In the

Greek plays, be it a comedy of Aristophanes or a tragedy of Euripides, we often see the exposure of a child by the father, this being presented as nothing out of the ordinary. In addition, we find frequent references to the use of exposure in Greek mythology among both gods and heroes; from Zeus to Oedipus, many were exposed at their birth, and in the case of mortals, left to die by their fathers. Although the exposure motif in mythology and literature is combined as a rule with the theme of the father's fear of his son or the ruler's fear of a successor, it does demonstrate that exposure was the method in Greece for disposing of unwanted children. Lastly, in a letter, though from Hellenistic rather than classical times, a husband advises his wife, "I urge and entreat you to be careful of the child ... if it is male, let it be, if it is a female, expose it" ([10], p. 244). As the scholars dealing with this controversy have concluded, exposure was a common phenomenon and employed at the father's discretion ([3], [5], [22]). This confirmation notwithstanding, it still seems odd that the father's right to dispose of a newborn child does not form part of any of the women's tirades against men as seen in the literary sources, such as Euripides' *Medea* or Aristophanes' *Lysistrata*.

The indication given by all available evidence, is that exposure was not considered a criminal act in ancient Greece. However, was this always the case? Generally speaking, we can say that if the father had recognized the child as his, then it was considered to be a member of the family and protected by the laws of the *polis*. For once considered a member of the *oikos*, and thus the *polis*, the child became the subject of rights, though the sanctions against a breech of these rights might have been weak. Therefore, if a father exposed his child after the *amphidromia*, the possibility does exist that he was liable to the charge of homicide (i.e., murder) if the child had not been 'taken up'. However, though homicide was the most serious offense that could be committed in the *polis*, public officials could not initiate prosecution, as this duty was laid solely upon the victim's family. In short, the child's relatives would have to bring action in the court ([4], [16]). It should be noted, that once acknowledged, a son could bring an action (though this would have to be instigated by relations, if he were under age) to compel his father to enroll him as his son in his clan and on his coming of age, in the *polis*.

The question arises, what were the implications of a father actively killing his child before he acknowledged it as his own, which can be distinguished from exposure in that the latter is an act of omission rather than commission? To be sure, the child is a human being. Thus, should the father take its life by strangulation or stabbing, he could then trigger the state's involvement under the crime of *hybris* (abuse of personal power) or *miasma* (pollution).[7] Homicide in this case could not be invoked unless the child's relations brought suit. Seeing that the father had not officially recognized the child previous to his bloody deed, the child was without a family to prosecute its claim in court which was essential if a charge of homicide was to be brought before the magistrates in the first place. However, any citizen within the community could prosecute the father on a variety of lesser offenses. For instance, the crime of pollution could be leveled against the child's father if he did not seek purification rites, as it was considered customary (*nomos*) for a citizen to take religious action to purify himself (and hereby avoid infecting the *polis*) after the killing of a human being.[8] In addition, there was the crime of *hybris*, in which one did harm to another through the abuse of personal power. In short, it involved any kind of misbehavior whatsoever towards another, regardless of the status of the person harmed. As Demosthenes declared:

> So for *hybris* too the legislator allowed *graphai* to everyone who wishes. He considered that a man who attempts to act with *hybris* wrongs the state, not just the victim ... and since he found the act inexpedient, he did not allow it to be permitted either against a slave, or anyone else at all (*Orations* 21.45).[9]

Overall, it seems that the laws of *hybris* and pollution would offer little protection to the 'unrecognized' child, as the father had only to be concerned with a minor civil breach by his action.

In regard to the state's prohibitions against exposure, most likely only those states, like Sparta, which placed strict limitations on parental power and which sought to increase the citizen population, would involve themselves with such legislation. In Sparta, according to Plutarch, "offspring were not reared at the will of the father, but were taken and carried by him to a place called Lesche where the elders of the tribe officially examined the infant, and if it was well-built and sturdy, they order the father to rear it" (*Lives*, 16.1). Over time, exposure was recognized as a 'social evil', its discontinuance being seen as essential for the survival of Greece, since by the Hellenistic era, the uncontrolled use of exposure was thought to be partly responsible for the country's depopulation. Polybius lamented that in his day, "all Greece was visited by a dearth of children" as the "men becoming perverted to a passion for show and money ... if they did marry, refused to rear the children that were born". On how Greece was to be relieved from such a curse, Polybius noted, "by the men themselves if possible changing their objects of ambition, or, if that cannot be done, by passing laws for preservation of infants" (*Histories*, 37.9). In Thebes, it should be noted, there actually existed a law to protect infants, though of a late data. As Aelian recorded:

No Theban man should be allowed to expose a child ... But if the father of the child should be extremely poverty stricken, the law orders that he immediately after the child's birth (be it male or female) carry it to the magistrate together with its swaddling clothes, and they shall sell the child received to the person giving a low price for it ... that he should bring up the child in good faith ... and receive his services as payment for the upbringing (*Varia Historia*, 27).

This law, however, was exceptional even for its day. In general, during the Classical period, only rarely would the Greek father be compelled by the state not to expose his child.

IV. THE PRACTICE OF ABORTION

Although exposure was considered an acceptable method of disposing of unwanted children, that did not preclude other means to that end, such as abortion. In Aristotle's discussion in the *Politics* of whether the ideal state should enact legislation to prevent the exposure of children, "merely in order to keep the population down", he advised, "the proper thing to do is to limit the size of each family, and if children are then conceived in excess of the limit so fixed, to have miscarriage induced before sense and life have begun in the embryo" (*Politics*, 7.16.15).[10] In coming to terms with abortion in ancient Greece, one should realize that it was practised quite extensively and that the techniques used were quite advanced for the day. Keith Hopkins, in his investigation of popular ancient medical texts, reported that a vast majority of them gave specific instruction on how to produce miscarriages [12]. In fact, abortifacients appeared more frequently than either aids to conception or contraception. Also, Marcel Moissides, in an extensive study, describes in detail the various instruments and procedures found among Greek medical treatises for producing an abortion [18]. According to Moissides, if the Greeks wished to bring about a miscarriage, they had the option of turning to either intra-uterine injections, through the use of a douche with a type of saline solution; gynecological operations, involving perforation of the membrane by pointed instruments; pessaries, designed like a tampon soaked in some allegedly effective drug with a string attached for easy removal; vaginal suppositories, presented as a means of inducing menstrual flow; or a host of medications, to be administered either orally in potions or internally by fumigations or poultices. Thus, 'manoeuvres méchaniques' and 'substances abortives' were available to Aristotle, and no doubt, he, being the son of a doctor and familiar with scientific writings, was more than aware of the different methods and had them in mind when he suggested abortion as a means to limit family size.

The evidence provided would seem to indicate that abortion was not a rare procedure in ancient Greece. As for the use of abortion, no doubt the reasons were as varied as the people who employed it or recommended its use. Philosophers such as Plato and Aristotle saw it as a means of family planning, while prostitutes and courtesans viewed it as a convenient aid to their livelihood.[11] In the Hippocratic Corpus, there are numerous references to the use of abortion by such women. As we read, "Public prostitutes, if they have many sexual experiences, know if they have conceived after going to a man; they kill the embryo within them, and when it is dead it falls out like a piece of flesh" (*On Flesh*, 19). Physicians especially recognized the therapeutic value of abortion. With difficult pregnancies, writes one physician, "it would be better to destroy the fetus (to induce abortion) rather than to cut it out later (embryotomy)" (Aetios, *Medicine*, 18). Overall, the average citizen of the *polis* would most likely have regarded the use of abortion as but one means of preserving the *oikos* from impoverishment, though the medical risks involved would not have made it a primary method of birth control.

As abortion was a common practice in the Greek world, what of its 'criminality'? In short, would abortion ever have been judged to be a crime, and if so, which party was held to be wronged by the act? Was it the fetus, the father, his *oikos*, or possibly the state? In general, as a father could expose his newborn child with impunity, it would seem that the same would hold true for his authorization to abort the child before it was born. Moreover, since the *polis*, as we have seen, was not in most instances concerned with propounding a pro-natalist policy to the point of interfering with the father's prior right in *oikos* matters, any litigation involving abortion would have been left to the affected household. Therefore, the father or relative would have to bring suit in an abortion case. The question then, is what kind of situation need develop to provoke a family member to bring legal action in regard to abortion?

The answer to this problem depends partly on a comment made by Sopater, who remarked that Lysias, in his discourse 'On Abortion', was involved in a trial, "in which Antigene accuses his own wife of homicide, the woman having voluntarily aborted, and he says that she had, by aborting, impeded his being called the father of a son" ([19], p. 87). Given that a charge of homicide was applied to abortion, it would seem that the crime centered on the deliberate taking of a human life, i.e., a child's life, and one which the father sought to protect and acknowledge as his own once born. However, as we shall later see, there was plainly no consensus in ancient Greece on the standing of fetal life. Therefore the overall impression given of Antigene's accusations, is not that the fetus's 'right to life' was violated by the abortion, but rather the father's right to his child, or more importantly, an heir. For as Antigene pleaded, by deliberate miscarriage, his wife "impeded his being called the father of a son". If this is correct, then it was the father, not the fetus, who was held to be the injured party, particularly his right to enhance himself with an heir. In regard to the charge of homicide, certainly the father would have used any available tactic to bolster his claim to his off-spring and secure his prerogative in such family matters, which clearly was violated by his wife's action. A woman had absolutely no authority to dispose of the fetus without the husband's approval; this being equally true in the case of a newborn child.

Even though there does not exist a corpus of Greek legal cases from which one might draw reference when discussing the question of the criminality of abortion, there is nevertheless decisive existing evidence on this issue in Roman law. It is significant that a vast majority of these abortion cases revolve around women who deliberately deprive their husbands of children and therefore were subject to legal sanctions. The crime of abortion was, in the courts, not the destruction of the fetus *per se*, but the fetus *qua* heir to the father. As Marcianus the jurist reported in the *Digest*, "A woman who purposely produces an abortion on herself should be sentenced to temporary exile, by the governor; for it may be considered dishonorable for a woman to deprive her husband of children with impunity" (*Digest*, 47.4.1). Also, in the fifth century A.D. legal codes of the Emperor Leo, it was written, "It is unreasonable and absolutely wicked for a woman who displays such decided hatred towards a husband as to destroy in her womb the germ of his posterity (without taking into consideration the violation of Nature's law) still to have the right to cohabit with him (*Constitutions*, 31). Cicero even mentions a trial where a woman was brought before the court for 'cheating' the father through an abortion. To quote:

I remember a case which occurred when I was in Asia: how a certain woman of Miletus, who had accepted a bribe from the alternative heirs and procured her own abortion by drugs, was condemned to death: and rightly, for she had cheated the father of his hopes, his name of continuity, his family of its support, his house of an heir, and the state of a citizen-to-be (*Pro Cluntio*, 11.32).

Other examples of where the father was dead and where it might have been very much in the interest of the embryo's next of kin to procure an abortion, appear frequently in the literature, for example, in Plutarch's story of Lycurgus (*Lives*, 3.1).[12] No doubt it was on the basis of this fear, that Soranos, the great Roman gynecologist, wrote in regard to midwives, that, "She must not be greedy for money, lest she give an abortion wickedly for payment" (*Gynecology*, 1.2.4). The impression given then is that a woman and her accomplices were indeed liable for procuring an abortion without the husband's permission. Thus, it is the violation of the father's right to his child that would classify abortion as a 'crime'.

In ancient Greece, one could assume that the legal situation surrounding the criminality of abortion was similar to that in Rome. Basically, that if a relation or father brought suit, the case would have centered on the family's, or more specifically the father's, deprivation of an heir. His wife, her physician, or even other family members conspiring to deny him his right to a child, could therefore be held accountable, provided that suitable evidence existed to justify the complaint. No doubt if the father died subsequent to the abortion, a prosecutor's argument would have attempted to prove that the action of the aborters had 'killed' the father's *iokos*, by depriving him of an heir. This would have been an even stronger line of argument if the prosecutor could prove that the party responsible for the abortion stood to gain by this development. Given the extreme importance that the Greek community placed on *oikoi* survival, this accusation would definitely have prejudiced the jury against those involved in the abortion. In regard to a homicide charge, again this would have been a questionable (and less sensational) route to take, since the issue would have devolved into the 'human' status of the fetus, on which there was no majority opinion. One of the reasons, in fact, for our confusion in dealing with abortion in ancient Greece, can be traced to the Greeks' overall notion of life, particularly fetal life, as it was so totally alien to our own. Therefore, it is best that we now turn to the ancient philo-medical evidence at our disposal on the question of whether fetal life was considered to be human life.

V. THE QUESTION OF FETAL 'LIFE'

In dealing with the question of whether and to what extent fetuses were considered to be human beings in ancient Greece, one must rely more on philosophy than on either biology or related sciences. For in the classical world, as in Medieval times, the concept of life revolved around the principle of soul. In short, metaphysical speculation, rather than biological processes, ruled the debate. To any Greek, that which was said to have life must indeed have soul. As Aristotle summed up the situation, "The soul is the source or cause of the living body" (*On Soul*, 415b). This being the case, the key to establishing the status of the fetus lay in tracing Greek concepts of ensoulment (i.e., animation). However, even here, the issue is not as clear cut as it seems, for the Greeks were not of the opinion that there was any one designated soul. They held that there were many varieties of soul, nutritive and sensitive, for instance, found not only among plants and animals but in the developing fetus as well. One group was of the opinion that the fetus underwent an entire metamorphosis of souls, from plant to animal soul before it attained the rational, i.e., human, soul. Thus, when a Greek claims the fetus is 'alive', that should not be interpreted to mean that he viewed it as an alive human being; if anything, he probably considered it to be more in the realm of vegetative life than human life.

In turning to Aristotle's theory on ensoulment, the problem is further complicated in that Aristotle and those of his school held that the semen as well as the menses (which was viewed as the unformed embryo) already contained soul, thereby concluding that there was life in the womb even before conception (*Generation of Animals*, 736a).[13] However, though he believed the menses (*catamenia*) to be imbued with soul, it was the most primitive of souls, the nutritive or vegetative, i.e., that found in plants. Thus, if the unformed embryo lying within the womb was to develop into a human being, it was necessary that the semen transmit to it both sensitive soul (i.e., that found in animals and which provided the power of movement) and rational soul (i.e., that which provided thought and reason and which was found only in man). According to Aristotle, once the semen and menses unite, the sensitive and rational soul, which existed potentially in the semen, became 'actualized' (*energeia*) within the embryo at different stages in its development (*Generation of Animals*, 736a–b).[14] Now, as to when the fetus became specifically endowed with rational soul, this we are not told, though Aristotle does raise this very issue of "when and how and whence is a share in reason acquired." (*Generation of Animals*, 736a). Possibly, the reason why he did not hazard a guess was that the line of demarcation itself was unclear. As he noted, "Nature proceeds little by little from things lifeless to animal life in such a way that it is impossible to determine the exact line of demarcation" (*History of Animals*, 588b).

Some contemporary scholars have suggested that in regard to Aristotle's theory, it was at the first instance of fetal motion (forty days for a male fetus, ninety days for a female, being also the time of fetal formation) that rational soul became actualized.[15] They based their claim upon Aristotle's comment in the *Politics* where he advises that abortion should be accomplished before "sense and life had begun in the embryo"; 'sense' being synonomous with movement and 'life' with ensoulment. However, it would be an error to associate rational soul with fetal movement, for no doubt it was at this particular point of fetal formation and movement that the transition from vegetative to sensitive soul had become finalized, with the 'life' Aristotle was referring to being only that of animal life. In all his scientific treatises, movement is only associated with sensitive soul, as rational soul required thought processes which gave no outward signs of recognition. In addition, when Aristotle refers to 'life', he is designating any ensouled entity, from plant to man, and therefore is not specifically referring to human life. Therefore, when Aristotle does not recommend abortion after 'sense' and 'life' have begun, it is quite doubtful that he viewed the fetus as a human being; most likely he viewed it as potential human life. In short, at this stage in its development, the fetus had rational soul potentially but not actually. Thus, if he sought to protect its existence from abortion, it was because of what it might become rather than what it had become.

As one can imagine, theories relating to the entrance of the soul into the womb were as varied as the different classifications of soul. Perhaps the best commentary written on this controversy surrounding ensoulment comes from the philosopher Porphyry, who addressed this issue in the late third century A. D. As he wrote to a friend:

The doctrine relating to the entry of souls into bodies in view of the production of a living being has filled us with an extreme uncertainty . . . . Well then, supposing one has shown that the embryo is neither a living thing in reality . . . nor a living thing in potentiality [i.e., having the soul within, awaiting 'activation'], then it becomes easy . . . to establish the entry of the soul and the precise moment of that entry: namely that which must happen after the child is born outside the womb. On the other hand, if the embryo is potentially a living thing, in the sense that it has received the soul, or, moreover, if it is a living thing in actuality, it is difficult to determine the moment of entry, and it is not at least without a great deal of mistrust that one will accept this moment . . . so that should the occasion arise, one should note with precision what it was. For one may well define it as that moment when the sperm has been injected into the womb, as if the sperm could not be retained in the womb and become fertile unless the soul having come from the outside had been realized . . . . Or one may place the moment of the entry of the soul at the first formation of the embryo . . . or one may assign the entry to the moment at which the embryo has begun to move (*To Gauros*, 1–2).

Though the language used by Porphyry is somewhat confusing, his basic argument remains clear: that it is very difficult to assess when the soul enters the embryo. As he points out, one can either delay the entry of the soul until birth (thereby making it easy to determine when it becomes a living being), or one can place its entry into the womb either at conception, the time of fetal formation, or at the first fetal movement.

Although it is rather unclear which doctrine the ancient Greeks held to be the most plausible, all indicators do seem to point out that the majority opinion was that soul, particularly human soul, was introduced at birth, with the infant's first breath. That the word soul in Greek, *psychē*, should be derived from *psycho*, to breathe, should come as no surprise. According to Aristotle, the Orphics believed that, "soul comes in from the whole when breathing takes place, being borne in upon the winds", while the early Stoics held that the soul existed potentially within the body, waiting for the first infant's breath to actualize it through a cooling (i.e., tempering) process (Aristotle, *On Soul*, 410b; Plutarch, *Stoic Self Contra*, 1052). The Stoic doctrine concerning soul, in fact, formed the basis of Roman law on the legal standing of the fetus; basically, that it was not a human being, "it being accounted as part of the mother's belly, like as we see the fruit of trees is esteemed part of the trees until it be full ripe" (Plutarch, *De Plactis*, 15).

With so many opinions and beliefs on the status of fetal life, one can understand why the Greek courts, at least as far as the evidence indicates, did not take any particular position in regard to this issue. Porphyry's statement that the question of ensoulment "has filled us with an extreme uncertainty" surely applied to Greece some seven centuries earlier. No doubt though, in the courts, with emotions running high after the destruction of an heir, there were attempts to apply to feticide a charge of homicide; in short, to establish the human standing of the fetus. However, here the burden of proof would most likely rest with the prosecutor, and his ability to give convincing arguments in relation to fetal development and ensoulment. Moreover, one can be sure that in some minor religious communities, especially 'mystery' cults, which preached a sanctity of life (all life) philosophy, abortion was prohibited. But even in this case the evidence again is not particularly impressive. From the sanctuary of one such cult in Lydia (North Africa), we have an inscription which reads:

Coming to this sanctuary, men and women, free and slave, they must be made to swear in the name of all the gods ... not to employ nor advise others to become accomplices in the employment of filters, abortives, contraceptives, or any other means of infanticide ([19], p. 193).

This inscription is very unusual, as it views any act preventing conception as a form of infanticide, but then again, it seems we are dealing here with a religious cult concerned with fertility.

VI. THE HIPPOCRATIC OATH

This pledge against abortion with the invocation of a variety of gods, needless to say, reminds one of the Hippocratic Oath. Was this too then, one may ask, a product of a religious, rather than a medical association? According to Ludwig Edelstein, this is exactly the case, it being written for members of the Pythagorean sect who sought to enter the medical profession, a profession, one may add, totally devoid of any ethical or moral code, relying upon the individual conscience of the practitioner of the healing arts [8]. Although there has been plenty of controversy surrounding the Oath — the first reference we have to it is not until the first century A. D. — this much is certain: Greek physicians as a whole, did not believe in or follow many of its injunctions. In analyzing the Hippocratic Oath, we see that although it was formally included in the Hippocratic Corpus, its ethical prohibitions involving the use of poisons, abortives, and surgery were not in the least consistent with what we find in the other treatises, or with the realities of medical practice as revealed in the ancient literature. In the Hippocratic writings, we are given instructions on how to produce deadly pharmaceuticals for purposes of euthanasia, to conduct surgery, and as noted earlier, to perform abortions. Moreover, in novels and philosophical tracts, it appears that it was not at all unusual for a physician to violate any of the above tenets. It would seem therefore that the ethical principles in the Oath were atypical of the medical profession and the moral values of ancient society as a whole. In short, one could conclude, as did Darrel Amundsen, that the Hippocratic Oath was an esoteric document, quite isolated in its ethical code ([1], p. 26). According to Edelstein, these beliefs were reflective of the Pythagoreans, as they alone held the embryo to be animate from the moment of conception, viewed suicide as a sin against God, who had allocated to man his position in life, and believed least of all in using the knife and in cauterizing in medical practice. To Edelstein then, the Oath was truly a Pythagorean manifesto, to be used only by members of the cult ([8], p. 18).

As one can imagine, there are various problems with Edelstein's interpretation of the Oath, the least of which is the absence of any known guild of Pythagorean physicians. However, Edelstein may not be too far off in his analysis, for we see in the Oath various elements of a religious, if not 'cultish' nature and origin. When the physician, after forswearing the use of poison and abortive remedies, adds "in purity and in holiness I will guard my life and my art", we must agree with Edelstein in saying that the demand for holiness can hardly be understood as resulting from practical thinking or technical responsibility. Holiness belongs, he points out, "to another realm of values and is indicative of standards of a different, more elevated character" ([8], p. 12). Overall, we have here the terminology of a religious, rather than a medical, order. In particular, we see elements in the Oath which are reminiscent of mystery cult practices ([14], p. 91). For instance, the strong obligation on the young physician to regard his medical teacher as a parent is characteristic of the mysteries, for the novice often had a 'father' who introduced him into the secrecies of the cult and to whom he owed various duties. Moreover, in the Oath, we have the common exclusiveness of a mystery cult, as the initiate swears only to give medical instruction to his sons, those of his teacher, and to the other pupils who have taken the Oath. In addition, prohibitions against suicide and abortion were especially strong among the mystery religions ([7]. p. 130). It was held that the *aoroi* (infants who died) and *biothanati* (those who died violent deaths) were doomed to an especially gloomy existence in the underworld, as their deaths were held to be unnatural, for they had not fulfilled the allotted normal lifespan ([5], p. 110). Plato, Virgil, and Plutarch, to name only a few, all mentioned in their discussions of Hades, "the weeping souls of infants bereft of sweet life and torn from the breast, whom the ill-omened day swept off and whelmed in bitter death" (Virgil, *Aeneid*, 5.426; Plato, *Republic*, 10.614; Plutarch, *Sign of Socrates*, 590). The possibility exists then that the mysteries and the various religious cults brought to the medical profession an ethical code and set of moral obligations, which it so sorely lacked at this period in time. In any case, the Hippocratic Oath is not the standard by which to judge the actions of the Greek medical profession; after all, philanthropy had yet to be associated with medicine [9].

It should be noted, that by the first century A.D., with medicine becoming increasingly identified with humanistic principles, physicians actually became concerned with the ethical stipulations of the Hippocratiic Oath, particularly the prohibition on abortion. The Roman medical moralist Scribonius Largus, from whom we first hear of the Oath, wrote:

Hippocrates, founder of our profession, instituted the beginnings of the discipline from an oath, where by it was considered sacred for any doctor neither to give nor to show to the one pregnant any medicine by which the conceived could be destroyed, thereby going a long way toward preparing the mind of the learner for the love of humanity ([13], p. 39).

Later, Soranos mentioned that among his colleagues,

One party banishes abortives, citing the testimony of Hippocrates who says: "I will give to no one an abortive"; moreover, because it is the specific task of medicine to guard and preserve what has been engendered by nature. The other party prescribes abortives, but with discrimination, that is, they do not prescribe them when a person wishes to destroy the embryo because of adultery or out of consideration for youthful beauty; but only to prevent subsequent danger in parturition (*Gynecology*, 1.19.60).

Although these remarks were not representative of the entire medical community, they do demonstrate that the practice of abortion was constantly being questioned by various physicians.

VII. CONCLUSION

That I should conclude this paper with the growing influence of the new 'morality' on the medical profession is no accident. For the special emphasis that the mysteries and Christianity placed on the sanctity of life brought the popular acceptance of abortion and exposure under attack. The Christian Fathers were particularly sensitive to these 'pagan' practices and sought to protect equally the fetus and newborn infant from deliberate destruction. Often the Christian writers applied the term of homicide and parricide (the unlawful killing of a close relative), to those who would destroy the 'fruit of the womb' ([5], p. 43). Thus during the latter years of the Roman Empire we see a strong willingness to treat the fetus as a human being; though many within the Christian world made a distinction between the 'humanness' of the formed and unformed, as well as animated and unanimated, fetus. In any case this much is certain, the early Church came to conclude that the fetus and infant had a value separate and independent from the parents, and that they were possessed of rights equal to those people already living within the community. Of course, it would be many centuries before Christian beliefs affected legislation to that end. In fact what we see today is the continued legislative effort by religious groups to define the fetus as a human being and to restrict the parents' authority to dispose of the newborn (e.g., by refusing medical care for a stricken child). Thus the 'personhood debate', which has its roots in the classical world, has yet to be resolved to the satisfaction of everyone.

Boston, Massachusetts

NOTES

* I wish to acknowledge the assistance of Jay Pollard and Susan Ackerman.

1 For a different view on the morality of abortion and exposure in Greece, see de Boer [2].

2 It was said in Athens that a man without legitimate children was forbidden by law to be an orator or general ([17], p. 86).

3 In Athens, all legitimate sons inherited the land in equal share. Thus, over generations the family estates fractionalized to such a degree as to leave each heir with barely a living area.

4 Hesiod also noted "more hands mean more work and more increase" (*Work and Days*, 375).

5 In the *Politics* of Aristotle, one reads, "There should certainly be a law to prevent the rearing of deformed children" (*Politics*, 7.16.14).

6 Inscribed in the Law Code of Gortyn, "If a wife who is separated by divorce should bear a child, they are to bring it to the husband at his house . . . and if he should not receive it, the child shall be in the mother's power to rear or expose" ([23], p. 41).

7 *Hybris* meant more to the Greeks than just 'arrogance' ([17], p. 129).

8 It would be necessary in this case to seek the consultation of the 'expounders' (*exegetai*) of the sacred law [20].

9 *Graphai* was a written public claim. Surely the killing of a newborn would fall under the abuse of parental authority and thereby involved a change of *hybris*.

10 The most complete book on abortion in the ancient world is Nardi [19].

11 Although Plato does not specifically mention abortion, he does allude to it. See Plato, *Republic*, 5.461.

12 As we read in the story of Lycurgus, "until his brother's wife was known to be with child, he was king . . . . However, the woman made secret overtures to him, proposing to destroy her unborn babe on condition that he would marry her when he was king" (Plutarch, *Lives*, 3.1).

13 "For nobody would say that the unfertilized embryo is soulless . . . since both the semen and the embryo of an animal have every bit as much life as a plant." (Aristotle, *Generation of Animals*, 736a.)

14 Aristotle explains that just as the formation of an animal precedes the formation of any particular species of animal (i.e., as the class is assumed before that of the genus, and the genus before the species), so the sensitive soul is acquired before the rational soul.

15 According to Connery, "to Aristotle, the fetus became a full human being when it was formed because at that time the human soul was infused" ([6], p. 18).

BIBLIOGRAPHY

1. Amundsen, D.: 1978, 'The Physician's Obligation to Prolong Life: A Medical Duty Without Classical Roots', *Hastings Center Report* 8, 23–30.
2. Boer, W. de: 1979, *Private Morality in Greece and Rome*, E. J. Brill, Leiden.
3. Bolkestein, H.: 1922, 'The Exposure of Children in Athens', *Classical Philosophy* 17, 222–239.
4. Bonner, R.: 1938, *The Administration of Justice from Homer to Aristotle*, Vol. II, University of Chicago Press, Chicago.
5. Cameron, A.: 1932, 'The Exposure of Children and Greek Ethics', *Classical Review* 46, 104–114.
6. Connery, J.: 1977, *Abortion: The Development of the Roman Catholic Perspective*, Loyola University Press, Chicago.
7. Cumont, F.: 1959, *After Life in Roman Paganism*, Dover, New York.
8. Edelstein, L.: 1943, 'The Hippocratic Oath', *Supplement to the Bulletin of the History of Medicine* I, pp. 1–64.
9. Edelstein, L.: 1967, 'The Professional Ethics of the Greek Physician', in Owsei Temkin (ed.), *Ancient Medicine: Selected Papers of Ludwig Edelstein*, Johns Hopkins Press, Baltimore, pp. 319–348.
10. Grenfell, B. P.: 1904, *The Oxyphynchus Papyri*, Vol. I, Oxford University Press, London.
11. Harrison, A.: 1968, *The Laws of Athens*, Clarendon Press, Oxford.
12. Hopkins, K.: 1965, 'Contraception in the Roman Empire', *Comparative Studies in Society and History* 8, 124–151.
13. Jones, W. H.: 1924, *The Doctor's Oath*, Cambridge University Press, Cambridge.
14. Kudlien, F.: 1970, 'Medical Ethics and Popular Ethics in Greece and Rome', *Clio Medica* 5, 91–121.
15. Lacey, W. K.: 1968, *The Family in Classical Greece*, Thames and Hudson, London.
16. MacDowell, D.: 1963, *Athenian Homicide Law*, Manchester University Press, Manchester.
17. MacDowell, D.: 1978, *The Law in Classical Athens*, Cornell University Press, Ithaca.
18. Moissides, M.: 1922, 'Contribution à L'Etude de L'Avortement dans L'Antiquité Grècque', *Janus* 26, 29–38.
19. Nardi, E.: 1971, *Procurato Aborto nel Mondo Greco Romano*, Giuffre, Milano.
20. Oliver, J.: 1950, *The Athenian Expounders of the Sacred and Ancestral Law*, Johns Hopkins Press, Baltimore.
21. Pomeroy, S.: 1975, *Women in Classical Antiquity*, Schocken, New York.
22. Van Hook, L. R.: 1920, 'The Exposure of Children at Athens', *Transactions of the American Philological Association* 51, 134–145.
23. Willets, R. F.: 1967, 'The Law Code of Gortyn', *Kadmos* Suppl. 1, 230–233.

ALBERT S. MORACZEWSKI

HUMAN PERSONHOOD: A STUDY IN PERSON-ALIZED BIOLOGY

I. INTRODUCTION

What does one do with a problem that will not go away? Such is the question of the moral status of the fetus: is it a person in the sense that it has the full set of rights associated with a member of the human community? As Mary Anne Warren has rightly pointed out, " . . . it is not possible to produce a satisfactory defense of a woman's rights to obtain an abortion without showing that a fetus is not a human being, in the morally relevant sense of that term" [33]. Consequently, it is imperative that the moral status be determined. While Warren argues in Section II of her paper that the fetus is not a person as it "satisfies none of the basic criteria of personhood" ([33], p. 47), I will argue to the contrary, namely, that the fetus is a person because it possesses the essential requirements for inclusion in the class of persons. Towards this end I will:

(1)   sketch out what I believe to be the essential elements of person-hood;
(2)   show that the human fetus indeed meets these criteria;
(3)   respond to the common objections made to the position I am defending.

II. THE CONCEPT OF PERSONHOOD

The frequent confounding of the psychological self (psychological aspects of personhood), and the legal self (rights and duties conferred by law) with a more fundamental reality — the ontological self (person *simpliciter*) — which is, in fact, presupposed by the other two, underscores the importance of clearing up conceptually what is meant by 'person'.

If we proceed from the outset with the notions that we cannot directly know the self, that our awareness of self is only indirect through the acts we perform, then we seem to rule out any real possibility of knowing what the person really is, or even if such exists. To discuss this last epistemological question is beyond the purpose of this essay. The position I am espousing has

William B. Bondeson et al. *(eds.), Abortion and the Status of the Fetus*, 301–311.
Copyright © 1983 *by D. Reidel Publishing Company, Dordrecht, Holland.*

been well argued by Roderick M. Chisholm in his book, *Person and Object* [7], especially in the chapter entitled, 'The Direct Awareness of Self'. He concludes: "For in being aware of ourselves as experiencing, we are, *ipso facto*, aware of the self or person − of the self or person, as being affected in a certain way" ([7], p. 51).

One view of the person holds what is basically a reflection of a Cartesian dualism in which the person (or self) is the spirit or mind present in the body much as a driver is present in an automobile. One of the leading contemporary exponents of that position is the neurophysiologist, Sir John Eccles, long interested in the mind-brain problem. Two of his more recent writings reflect rather well his developed thought: *The Self and Its Brain* (co-authored with Karl R. Popper) [26] and *The Human Mystery* [9]. His is a "philosophy of a strong dualistic interactionism" ([9], p. 34). For him the self is the mind as a *thing* distinct from the brain (and the remainder of the body) yet strongly interacting with it.

At the other extreme is the position which holds that there is no such entity as a person, merely a sort of continuing series of conscious states that are linked together only because they follow each other in a temporal succession. Basically this is the position of Hume and those philosophers who hold that self or person is not an ontological reality but *only* a continuity of conscious states. A recent work edited by Amelie Oskenberg Rorty, *The Identities of Persons* [28], brings together a number of essays by an array of respected philosophers, a number of whom seem to weave variations on Lockean or Humean themes.

My own view of personhood can perhaps be well summarized by a felicitous phrase employed in a recent work in bioethics: human personhood is "embodied intelligent freedom" [1]. Accordingly, the existing person is a material being *radically* capable of rational thought and of electing among alternatives without an inherent universal coercion. To have a *radical* capability means that the power in question need not be actually exercised here and now, such as with a person asleep, or yet developed such as in a young child.

Hence, the human person in this view is something biological, material, and yet at the same time something which transcends biology. Being biological is a necessary condition for, and component of, the human person but it is not sufficient. Human biology is closely similar to that of the higher primates. Indeed, in many regards the entire living world has much affinity to human biology. We can conclude that personhood transcends the merely biological because of the many things that humans can do which other animals, including the higher primates, are not able to do, even in a rudimentary fashion. Humans are radically technological, record their history, conjecture about the future, and recognize good and evil. Experiments with communication among the great apes have claimed their abilities to be similar to human communication [12], but other studies have shown that these are essentially different ([19], [21], [30]). The uniqueness of human language together with the above-mentioned activities argue for some factor, some principle, which clearly distinguishes human persons from any of the great apes no matter how closely these latter can *mimic* some forms of human behavior.

This other factor must be non-material, because the capacity to form abstract concepts — for example, of truth, justice, infinity, wave-particles, or an abstract idea of a class of material objects without identification uniquely with one member — bespeaks a source which is itself non-material. Whatever we term this factor — psyche, spirit soul, life principle — is not important here. What is important is the recognition that the human person has both material and non-material principles; it is not a pure spirit. Rather it is an *embodied* spirit. Paul Ramsey somewhere describes the relationship in these terms: the body is the physical manifestation of the soul, and the soul is the spiritual expression of the body. Consequently, I would argue, the human person is a composite but intrinsically unified being which results from an ontological fusion of two *principles*: body and spirit.

But note the important distinction between the term 'body' as used to refer to the *material principle*, and as used to refer to this 'living' human body. In the latter sense, to say *living* body is redundant for a human *body* can only be living. The dead 'body' is better termed 'cadaver'. In this description, the life principle is the *formal* principle. Clearly, neither material or formal principle is tangible or visible. What is touched, seen and exists is their conjoined product: the individual living person.

Personhood then, may be viewed as the animated human body itself (understanding the term 'body' as described above). When a living human body ceases to be animated, it ceases to live; we say, "Sam Jones is dead". If, indeed, the person is somehow identified with the living human body, then its origins could well be considered to be co-terminous with that of the living body.

To be a human person, then, requires first of all that an individual has the appropriate biological makeup, namely, a human genome. Secondly, the individual must be a true organism with the radical capability — given the appropriate environmental support and the absence of disease or trauma — of being or developing into an adult human being which manifests clearly those characteristics which people commonly associate with human person: rationality, self-awareness, the power to love and to relate, etc. This radical capability is not something which is gradually acquired over time. Rather, it is inherent from the beginning and its presence is known because the human organism will normally develop into an adult human and never into an individual of another species. Unlike knowledge or physical strength which are acquired, a human being is a person *ab initio* and remains such through the vicissitudes of life, disease, trauma, and senility until the death of the individual.

III. THE HUMAN FETUS AS PERSON

A decade ago, Callahan ([6], p. 378) conveniently divided responses to the question regarding the pertinent criteria for the determination of the presence of human life into three groups: genetic, developmental, and social. The first group stipulates that by their genes you shall know them; hence, if an organism is not truly a human being in the first instance (i.e., the zygote stage) it can never become a human being. The developmental approach postulates that at some subsequent critical stage the human *organism* becomes sufficiently developed so as to be indeed a human *being*. The social approach requires that an individual be accepted by a human community and be able to relate with other human beings.

Space does not permit discussion of each group since the focus of this paper will be on the genetic approach. A somewhat fuller treatment of these groups will be found in Pastrana [25], McCarthy and Moraczewski [22], and Atkinson and Moraczewski [2]. Briefly, the principal objections I would have to the developmental approach is that a choice of a particular critical developmental stage, e.g., implantation, quickening, sensitivity to pain, or self-consciousness, for example, are all to some extent arbitrary. The social approach is even more open to the objection of arbitrariness. It is the human community of adults which decides on the basis of psychological, social or moral criteria which human beings it will accept into its midst. This approach is well reflected in United States law which states that "a person is such, not because he is human, but because of rights and duties ascribed to him" [5]. The same source notes that a child *in utero* is not a person.

Both the developmental and social approaches are in my mind objectionable because "there is *nothing within the logic of either approach* that forecloses having one's neighbor or oneself declared a nonperson and thus outside the pale of the human community. Both approaches hold that there exists a 'magic circle' within, but not coextensive with, the species *Homo sapiens*. There is not basis in either approach for demonstrating that any given member of the wider class *must* be placed within the 'magic circle'" ([2], p. 71).

My own position is within the genetic approach. In brief, the human fetus is a person from the moment of the individual's first cell, the zygote, which results from the fertilization of the egg by the sperm: the pronuclei of each gamete unite to form the new nucleus, complete with a unique set of genetic information necessary for the consequent growth, differentiation and development of the new individual. It is at this point when a new living human individual appears that *this* unique human *person* begins even if it shares *human life* with other members of the species and life with all other living beings.

Several objections have frequently been forwarded as making the position that the human person begins at fertilization untenable. The principal objections seem to be the following:

(1)   embryo wastage – the allegedly high loss of human embryos would mean that large numbers of human persons die before any meaningful life;

(2)   twinning and recombination – apparently incompatible with the essential unity and incommunicability of the human person;

(3)   impossibility of meeting criteria for personhood especially in very young human fetus, and at best the fetus is a potential person.

These objections, while challenging, I believe, can be reasonably answered.

IV. RESPONSE TO OBJECTIONS

Embryo Wastage

Frequently stated in discussions regarding the beginning of human life is that there is a huge embryo wastage, that 50% or more of the embryos conceived are for the most part silently aborted. Karl Rahner, among others, has considered this datum as seriously questioning the correctness of the claim that personhood begins at fertilization [27]. To claim such is to admit that many human lives never get born, a seeming immense 'waste' of human lives.

In response two points can be made, albeit briefly.

(1) The origin of this claim is the work of Hertig *et al.*, in which they

studied 34 human ova from 211 patients with uterine and tubal pathology, who had had hysterectomies ([14] and [15]), a study which has been criticized by Hilgers [16]. Since then, only a few studies have been proposed as confirming this claim ([3], p. 47; [4], p. 11; and [29], p. 84).

(2) Even *if* there were some significant embryonic loss, say, 10–20%, there has been an even higher loss of born infants for a major part of human history. For example, fairly good vital statistics are available for the U.S. In the 1800s the rate of deaths of infants under one year of age was 15–20%; in 1875, for example, it was 226.6 deaths per 1000 children under age ([17], p. 63). In 18th century England, to cite another example, Bills of Mortality show that in 1762 one region reported 15 351 births and 8372 burials of infants less than 2 years of age ([30], p. 455). For each year over a 10-year span, the corresponding figures were similar. One contemporary physician (William Bucham) is cited as saying that "one half of the human race ... die in infancy" ([30], p. 413). I would find it difficult to argue that because of all these 'wasted human lives', these were not human persons!

Twinning

Identical twins apparently arise from a single fertilized egg although they might arise from fertilization of the ovum and its polar body ([16], p. 149). Hence, it means that at some time after fertilization the single embryo splits apart to form two individuals. According to current understanding twinning apparently can take place at different stages up to and including the early post implantation (within the second week of gestation) as suggested by the fact that about one percent of all twins are monoamniotic ([17], p. 167). If there were a single person to begin with, how can two arise?

An intrinsically integrated organism which of itself has the appropriate human genetic and cellular mechanisms for full development and which apart from genetic disorders, disease or accident would actually do so, is a human person. The qualifier 'of itself' is added to exclude haploid cells such as the egg and sperm, and diploid cells which would require de-differentiation (as in somatic cell cloning) in order to develop from a single cell stage to an otherwise normal multicellular human organism.

The fact that the developing embryo (from the 2-cell stage to early im-planted blastocyst) seemingly can divide into two individuals rather than remaining as one individual suggests that there is some defect in the functional unity of the initial embryo. Ordinarily, as the embryo develops, certain cells shut of their full potentiality for independent development. By the time the blastocyst is formed, on about day 4 ([24], p. 3), the cells have already differentiated to an inner cell mass (which will become the embryo proper and the chorion) and the outer cells which, in part, will form the placenta. This means that these outer cells are *no longer part of the embryo*. It is the *inner* cell mass which is critical here for our position on the personhood of the fetus.

Let me draw out what seems to be an implication of these data. As the zygote divides into two cells and then four, and so on, already some of the cells are destined to be the inner cell mass while the others will be the outer cells and eventually the placenta (in part) and the amnion. The recent work of Illmensee and Hoppe [18] with the mouse in which they successfully cloned three mice is significant here because of their discovery that only nucleus from the cells of the inner cell mass could be used for the purposes of cloning, an indication that only these cells retained the power to become the embryo. Since the normal development of the embryo requires that from the beginning some cells continue on to become the true embryo while the others are 'discarded' to become the fetal membranes and placenta, there appears no intrinsic reason why in certain situations a cell from the inner cell mass or its predecessor could not be separated. Because this cell is still undifferentiated (as we know from the aforementioned cloning experiments) and is endowed with the appropriate human genetic and cellular mechanisms, it becomes a new individual human being.

Further, I do not see such a process as being incompatible with the incommunicability of the human person ([25], pp. 280–282). Organ transplants from living donors such as in kidney donation do not mean the incommunicability of the donor's personhood has been violated. In the case of the very young embryo the state of the cell being 'donated' and the environment in which it occurs permits a new human individual to be constituted.

Recombination

Studies with mice, for example, have beyond doubt showed that two or more embryos can be fused at an early stage, e.g., 8-cell, and result in an individual which can grow to maturity [3]. However, for this to take place the protective cover, zona pellucida, which is normally shed just before implantation, has to be removed by chemical or enzymatic means [23]. Although there is some doubt that recombination occurs in humans ([16], p. 150), it would be difficult to explain on other grounds what seems to have been a clear case of human recombination involving the fusion of a male embryo which does not resemble, even in the slightest way, a human person.

In light of these and similar objections, how can the very young human embryo — and even the fetus and newborn — be considered truly a person? My conviction is that the response focuses on the concepts of potency and act. For many it would be acceptable to say that the fetus is a *potential* person, that the individual is first a human being, then subsequently becomes a human *person* [10].

A source of confusion here is that the notion of potentiality is not being applied in the same manner to the fetus. Some will say the fetus is a potential person but not actually one here and now. Others will say the fetus is potentially an adult person meaning that it is already a person but not yet an adult. In the latter case, *being* and *doing* are being separated, for while they are interrelated they are not interconvertible. An individual can be a person but without being capable, here and now, of exercising certain activities which pertain to human personhood *except* to be growing gradually towards the stage when the desired capabilities can be increasingly exercised.

At conception, the individual is an *actual* person even though he or she is potentially an *adult* person and the *manifestation* of personhood's characteristic behavior has yet to be actualized and expressed. The most important fact is that the human zygote is here and now an existing and *actual* person, integrated and *inner*-directed to the full realization of his or her personhood. The actualization of that personhood takes place smoothly through a developmental spectrum involving an network of factors. Initially the factors are largely intrinsic to the initial single-cell zygote. Over time, under the influence of genetically controlled biochemical and physiological factors, the fetus gradually develops into the recognizable human being. To some extent the human embryo is also dependent upon the environment to provide nourishment and warmth, and to remove the waste products of normal metabolism.

Both the human embryo within the uterus develops the way he/she does, and the human child develops to full adulthood, because of some intrinsic factor, the presence or absence of which determines the final product. A female chimp, Lucy, for example, that was raised shortly after birth in a human family alongside a human child of approximately the same age for a period of ten years, did not become a human being nor really behave as one [32]. After an initial rapid development of a few years, during which time the chimp, in some respects, outdid the human child, the human child began to develop more rapidly and continuously, whereas the development and learning of the chimp infant leveled off, reaching a plateau with little change and improvement in skills except perhaps for those associated with muscular strength. Such evidence argues for the possession by the human child of an intrinsic capacity (or, potentiality), e.g., for rational thought, syntactical language, which the ape does not possess, since both were exposed to essentially the same environment and only the human child manifested the capacity to develop rationality-based skills.

The critical point is that the human child had something *real* — a capacity, a potentiality — the presence or absence of which makes a difference. That something real is the *potentiality*, existentially rooted in his or her *actual personhood*, to develop the ability to communicate in syntactical language and to exercise other skills which are dependent on the ability to form abstract concepts. Evidence obtained from the study of feral children (children who were raised from early infancy by wild animals, e.g., by wolves, monkeys) and from better documented cases of children raised in an environment of extreme sensory deprivation (especially deprivation of adult human companionship) argues for the vital importance of contact with adult persons [11]. *Personal interaction*, too, is apparently essential for the *development* of personhood, not for its basic existence. Actualized persons are required to bring forth certain of the potentialities of the existing person, although there is some indication that a programmed computer may be an adequate substitute. The newborn human is already an existing person but needs other more developed persons to make manifest, to make actual, certain of those characteristics we identify with personhood: relational ability, awareness of self as self, etc.

V. CONCLUSION

Consequently, it is my conviction that the human person, while not fully definable (because of its special nature), is nonetheless recognizable and perceivable in its existence. Its coming-to-be is concurrent with the existence of the zygote when the material is properly disposed for future development. By a gradual process of biological, psychological and social development, personhood becomes more and more manifest, but that development and its direction are only possible because there is already present within the organism a person-rooted drive to full human life, which is realized through genetic information, cellular metabolism and neurobiological developments of the human organism/being.

Pope John XXIII Medical-Moral Research and Education Center,
St. Louis, Missouri

BIBLIOGRAPHY

1. Ashley, B. and K. O'Rourke: 1978, *Health Care Ethics*, The Catholic Hospital Association, St. Louis,
2. Atkinson, G. M. and A. S. Moraczewski (eds.): 1980, *Genetic Counseling, the Church and the Law*, The Pope John XXIII Medical-Moral Research and Education Center, St. Louis.
3. Biggers, J. D.: 1983, 'Generation of the Human Life Cycle', in this vol., pp. 31–53.
4. Biggers, J. D.: 1979, '*In Vitro* Fertilization, Embryo Culture and Embryo Transfer in Humans', in U.S. Department of Health, Education, and Welfare, Ethics Advisory Board, *HEW Support of Research Involving Human In Vitro Fertilization and Embryo Transfer: Appendix*, Department of Health, Education, and Welfare, Washington, D.C., Essay 8.
5. *Blacks Law Dictionary*, West Publishing Co., St. Paul, Minn., 1968.
6. Callahan, D.: 1970, *Abortion: Law, Choice and Morality*, The MacMillan Company, New York.
7. Chisholm, R. M.: 1976, *Person and Object*, Open Court Publishing Co., Illinois.
8. Dewald, G., C. Haymond, J. L. Spurbeck, and S. B. Moore: 1980, 'Origin of Chi 46, XX/46, XY Chimerism in a Human True Hermaphrodite', *Science* **207**, 321–323.
9. Eccles, J. C.: 1979, *The Human Mystery*, Springer International, New York and Berlin.
10. Engelhardt, H. T., Jr.: 1977, 'Some Persons are Humans, Some Humans are Persons, and the World is What We Persons Make of It', in S. F. Spicker and H. T. Engelhardt, Jr. (eds.), *Philosophical Medical Ethics: Its Nature and Significance*, D. Reidel Publishing Company, Dordrecht, Holland, pp. 183–194.
11. Freedman, D. A. and S. L. Brown: 1968, 'On the Role of Coenesthetic Stimulation in the Development of Psychic Structure', *The Psychoanalytic Quarterly* **37**, 418–438.
12. Gardner, R. A. and B. T. Gardener: 1978, 'Comparative Psychology and Language Acquisition', *The Annals of the New York Academy of Sciences* **309**, 33–41.
13. Hafez, E. S. E.: 1973, 'Reproductive Life Cycle', in E. S. E. Hafez and T. N. Evans (eds.), *Human Reproduction*, Harper and Row Publishers, Hagerstown, Maryland, pp. 42–59.
14. Hertig, A. T., J. Rock, and E. C. Adams: 1956, 'A Description of 34 Human Ova Within the First 17 Days of Development', *American Journal of Anatomy* **98**, 453–493.
15. Hertig, A. T., J. Rock, E. C. Adams, and M. C. Menkin: 1959, 'Thirty-Four Fertilized Ova, Good, Bad and Indifferent, Recovered from 210 Women of Known Fertility', *Pediatrics* **23**, 202–211.
16. Hilgers, T. W.: 1977, 'Human Reproduction: Three Issues for the Moral Theologian', *Theological Studies* **38**, 136–152.
17. *Historical Statistics of the United States, Colonial Time to 1970*, U.S. Department of Commerce, Bureau of the Census, Washington, D.C., 1973.
18. Illmensee, K. and P. Hoppe: 1981, 'Cell', *Newsweek* (January 16), 65–66.
19. Katz, J. J.: 1976, 'A Hypothesis About the Uniqueness of Natural Language', in C. Harned *et al.* (eds.), *Annals of the New York Academy of Sciences* **280**, 33–41.

20. Markert, C. L. and R. M. Petters: 1978, 'Manufactured Hexaparental Mice Show that Adults are Derived from Three Embryonic Cells', *Science* **202**, 56–58.
21. Marx, J. L.: 1980, 'Ape-Language Controversy Flares Up', *Science* **207**, 1330–1333.
22. McCarthy, D. G. and A. S. Moraczewski (eds.): 1976, *An Ethical Evaluation of Fetal Experimentation: An Interdisciplinary Study*, The Pope John XXIII Medical-Moral Research and Education Center, St. Louis.
23. Mintz, B.: 1972, 'Implantation-Initiating Factor from Mouse Uterus', in K. S. Morgissi and E. S. E. Hafez (eds.), *Biology of Mammalian Fertilization and Implantation*, Charles C. Thomas, Publisher, Springfield, Illinois, pp. 343–356.
24. O'Rahilly, R.: 1973, *Developmental Stages in Human Embryos*, Part A, Carnegie Institute of Washington, Washington, D.C.
25. Pastrana, G.: 1977, 'Personhood and the Beginning of Life', *The Thomist* **41**, 247–294.
26. Popper, K. R. and J. C. Eccles: 1977, *The Self and the Brain*, Springer International, New York and Berlin.
27. Rahner, K.: 1972, 'The Problem of Genetic Manipulation', *Theological Investigations* **9**, 226–235.
28. Rorty, A. O. (ed.): 1976, *The Identities of Persons*, University of California Press, Berkeley.
29. Soupart, P.: 1983, 'Present and Possible Future Research in the Use of Human Embryos', in this volume, pp. 67–104.
30. Still, G. F.: 1931, *The History of Pediatrics*, Oxford University Press, London.
31. Temerlin, M. D.: 1975, 'My Daughter Lucy', *Psychology Today* **203**, 59–103.
32. Terrace, H. S., L. A. Petitto, R. J. Sanders, and T. G. Bever: 1979, 'Can an Ape Create a Sentence?', *Science* **206**, 891–902.
33. Warren, M. A.: 1973, 'On the Moral and Legal Status of Abortion', *The Monist* **57**, 43–61.

JAMES J. McCARTNEY

SOME ROMAN CATHOLIC CONCEPTS OF PERSON AND THEIR IMPLICATIONS FOR THE ONTOLOGICAL STATUS OF THE UNBORN

Many people believe that the Roman Catholic Church's opposition to abortion stems from its conviction that a new human person exists from the first moment of conception and that this newly formed person has as much a right to exist as anyone else. It is clear that this is not now, nor ever has been, official Church teaching on the matter [2]. Susan Teft Nicholson points out that, besides its ethic proscribing killing, "Roman Church leadership has sought to maintain, in one form or another, a link between sexual activity and procreation", and thus it follows that "even if the fetus were not a human being, Catholics would still view abortion as evil" ([10], p. 3). An even more clear statement of this view is provided by the Sacred Congregation for the Doctrine of the Faith of the Roman Catholic Church which, while maintaining that "respect for human life is called for from the time that generation begins", nevertheless, "expressly leaves aside the question of the moment when the spiritual soul is infused" ([16], pp. 139–140). While Church teachers do feel that there are many good reasons for holding that the existence of the soul is at least probable from the first moment of existence, its official position as proclaimed by the Congregation is that human biological life has value and must be protected whether it is considered to have a spiritual soul or not. One of the justifications adduced for this position is the conviction that "if one is to understand that men and women are 'free' to seek sexual pleasure to the point of satiety, without taking into account any law or the essential orientation of sexual life to its fruits of fertility, then this idea has nothing Christian in it" ([16], pp. 141–142). Thus, given the Congregation's view on the purpose of the sexual faculty, whose procreative dimension ought never be directly interfered with, even by artificial contraception, Church teaching would still remain intact even if it could be clearly demonstrated that the 'fertilized ovum could not be the subject and bearer of rights. What would be less persuasive in this situation is the public policy argument, especially in a pluralistic society, that human biological life deserves protection by the state from fertilization onward. This position would be counterintuitive, since we do not feel any moral or legal compulsion to protect human somatic cells growing in tissue culture. What becomes very important in the public policy arena is to

313

William B. Bondeson et al. *(eds.), Abortion and the Status of the Fetus*, 313–323.
Copyright © 1983 by D. Reidel Publishing Company, Dordrecht, Holland.

determine that a person, an individual with rights, is a constitutive dimension of this fertilized cell or mass of cells.

Moving away from official Church teaching, I will now consider the views of various Catholic philosophers and theologians on the concept of person and the implications these concepts have for the ontological status of the unborn.

First of all, Robert Barry claims that "the pro-life movement bases its contention that abortion is murder on the supposition that the developing stages of human life are persons who merit the rights and protections of the Fourteenth Amendment ([1], p. 64). He suggests, and in fact argues, that "the person must be understood as an identifiable individual who is not only the subject and causal agent of certain material predicates, but is also the subject and causal agent of certain human states of mind and consciousness" ([1], p. 64). He believes that "personhood can be justifiably attributed to the developing stages of life that indicate the presence of a subject and causal agent of human states of mind" ([1], p. 64). Since the purpose of his article is "to outline the conditions that permit proper identification of individuals as persons" ([1], p. 69), he first points out the character of publicly identifiable individuals as developed by P. F. Strawson [18]. Then he shows how we describe observed individuals through our senses and perceptions. He considers the unique individuality of persons and concludes with a section on the rights of persons to existence.

For Barry, the person is a 'compound individual' because it is the subject of both corporeal traits and predicates, as well as 'personal' characteristics, which include conceptual thought, syntactical and propositional speech, intentional expression, non-public observability of its states, and a non-transferable character of these states.

He considers developing human life to be individualized on the basis of the 'unique genetic structure' of the zygote. Further, he claims that "in contrast to cells which are not derived from the zygote, this cell (i.e., the zygote) initiates the development of a primitive neurological structure shortly after it is formed". This, incidentally, is an imprecise, if not incorrect, interpretation of early embryonic development.

Barry then investigates the grounds for assigning personhood to the developing stages of life and makes the claim that there are five characteristics manifested by these stages which warrant the predication of personhood. These developing stages of life are:

(1)   subjects of developing human states of mind and consciousness;

(2)   subjects of developing human actions;

(3)   causal agents of these developing states and actions;

(4)   causal subjects of these states, and the only material individuals who can be said to 'own' these states; and

(5)   the only animate individuals who can permit identification and description of these states of mind and consciousness.

He declares that

... it is not proper to deny personhood to the developing stages of life because their capacities are not fully developed and actualized .... Personhood is attributed to animate individuals which have the capacity for conceptual thought, intentional expression, and syntactical and propositional speech, and not to those individuals who employ these forms of action ([1], pp. 77–78).

He concludes the article by arguing that

... persons have an unconditional right to life (unless the right is forsaken by a person becoming an immediate, immanent, and proximate threat to the existence and health of another person), and this is one of the elements of their distinctiveness ([1], p. 79).

James Diamond, M.D., approaches this issue somewhat differently [5]. First he presents a summary of the embryological data with heavy emphasis on the role of the 'primary organizer' which Spemann and other embryologists had emphasized a few decades ago. From this biological data combined with a supposedly Thomistic understanding of ensoulment, he concludes that

... no soul need be posited in a sperm, ovum, zygote, or unattached blastocyst; any more than the presence of a soul need be posited in any other human cell or cell cluster after it has been totally separated from an ensouled parent organism and left to survive on its residual quanta of fuels and physicochemical energies .... I can think of no reason in the purely biological order to sustain the argument that animation is possible to consider at fertilization .... The best one can do is to adduce evidence showing why animation ought not to be considered prior to the point where twinning is no longer possible in the biological order and let it go at that .... In all scientific candor, I suggest that the overwhelming weight of biological data tilts the objective scientist toward that inexactly definable time period of 2 to 3 weeks after fertilization as the time or point in process when biological hominization occurs ([5], p. 319).

This approach and an article in a similiar vein by André Hellegers, M.D. [8], have influenced the thinking of some widely known Roman Catholic moral theologians. Charles E. Curran, for example, argues that human life is not present until individuality is established, which he believes does not occur until the 14th day when biological twinning is no longer a possibility [4]. Similarly, Bernard Haering, relying also on Boethius' classic definition of the human person as "an individual substance of rational nature", concludes that "the argument that the morula cannot yet be a person or an individual with all the rights of the members of the human species seems to me to be convincing as long as we follow our traditional concept of personhood" ([7], pp. 126–127). Richard McCormick also states that he finds the statement of Curran's position in this matter very close to his own [9]. Additionally, Piet Schoonenberg maintains that as long as the possibility of twinning exists,

... the philosophical definition of the individual, which explains it as 'undivided in itself' (*indivisum in se*), is not yet realized, at least not as strictly as the individuality of the human person demands. If the fecundated ovum can split into two beings which turn out to be two persons, it is difficult to admit that it was itself a person, hence fully human ([17], pp. 49–50).

After presenting a very thorough review of many of the positions relevant to an understanding of the ontological status of early life in the human species, Gabriel Pastrana attempts to develop a biological basis for a philosophical analysis of human life and personhood. He proposes that

... when the product of conception going through those first stages of organization and differentiation has reached that point where its differentiability is determined to perform the specific functions of a biologically individual human being, this coincides with its disposition to receive the substantial form that qualifies it both specifically and numerically as an individual human being ([11], p. 282).

He believes that the biological evidence indicates that this cannot happen before the 14th day. Once this biological individual human being is formed, it should be considered a human person with "a new essence, the individual human substance composed of a sufficiently disposed material element (as shown by the biological evidence) and a substantial form; ... " ([11], p. 291). He contends that

... the new individual human substance subsists, i.e., exists in and by itself; it becomes incommunicable, so that no other form can substantially affect it without destroying it; it is distinct and specifically determined by the uniquely human rational formality, and it is open to new actualization according to the limits and possibilities of its essence. As such it is specifically distinct from other subsistent substances, whether spiritual or composite, and numerically different from other subsistent substances of the human species ([11], pp. 291–292).

Thus, the

> ... person from its very moment of existence is autonomous, incommunicable, and
> distinct; when the individual human substance at that early stage of conception is
> actualized by its own act of being it passes from non-being to existence, to being and
> existing in and by itself; it receives *esse simpliciter* ([11], p. 294).

After discussing the history of Catholic theological thinking on the matters
of ensoulment, Joseph F. Donceel presents a very thorough analysis of the
hylomorphic conception of humans, that "which Thomas took over from
Aristotle". He contrasts this approach with Platonic and Cartesian dualism
and contends that many who pay lip service to Thomistic philosophy in
this matter "are, in fact, Cartesian dualists" ([6], p. 80).

   According to hylomorphic theory, form and matter are strictly com-
plementary. Thus, "as the soul stands higher in the hierarchy of beings, the
matter which receives it, which is determined by it, must be more highly
organized". Since this is so, Donceel argues that "there can be an actual
human soul only in a body endowed with the organs required for the spiritual
activities of man". Thus, "hylomorphism cannot admit that the fertilized
ovum, the morula, the blastula, the early embryo, is animated by an intellectual human soul". He believes that only when the brain, and especially
the cortex, have developed, is the matter of the body sufficiently organized
to receive a spiritual soul.

   He thinks that the main source of confusion in this regard has been the
perception of the soul as the efficient cause of the body when in fact it
should be seen as the formal cause, which does not in itself produce anything,
but which is revealed in the actions of the subject it informs. He shows that
Thomas himself has not made this mistake, even if many of his followers
have:

> ... For one thing to be another's substantial form, two conditions are required. One
> of them is that the form be the principle of substantial being to the thing of which it
> is the form: and I speak not of the effective but the formal principle, whereby a thing
> is, and is called a *being*. Hence follows the second condition, namely that the form and
> matter combine together in one being, which is not the case with the effective principle
> together with that to which it gives being (St. Thomas Aquinas, *Summa Contra Gentiles*,
> 2, 68).

Donceel is convinced that as contemporary Thomists abandon the Cartesian
contamination of Renaissance Scholasticism, they will more clearly see that
hominization delayed until formation of the brain is much more congruent
with hylomorphic theory as understood by Thomas than any other approach.

Karl Rahner, impressed with the statistic that at least 50% of all fertilized ova never implant, contends that the presupposition of Catholic theology, that at the moment of union of the male and female cells a human being with personal rights comes into existence, is no longer held with certainty, but is exposed to positive doubt [15]. Joseph Culliton is persuaded that Rahner could very easily accept Donceel's position as to the structures necessary before hominization can take place [3]. However, Culliton also argues that Rahner's concept of the process of hominization as detailed in his book *Hominization* [14] would commit him to a view much like that held by the Congregation for the Doctrine of the Faith:

The most important fact, and that on which ethical consideration must be based, is that successively within this one continuous process there is vegetative human life, then sensitive and nutritive human life, and finally rational human life. The continuity is of more significance than the diversity because a human organism and human life exist before and after each transformation. Neither of these critical points initiates a wholly new life or a new process. Therefore, when one understands the procreative process as one continuous process effected by divine and human causalities from start to finish, one must recognize both the continuity of the whole process and the equal dignity of the human organism at each of its stages of development ([3], pp. 209–210).

Thus, Culliton contends that the dignity of the human organism rests not so much on its ontological status as hominized but on the fact that God and the parents are working from fertilization onwards through natural causes to bring this status about.

Several Catholic authors are not so much interested in biological indicators of ontological status but consider indicators of relationality and self-consciousness equally important in determining the rights and dignity of nascent human life. Charles Curran indicates that there are several French theologians who argue for more personalistic criteria for the beginning of human life [4]. These authors indicate that there is "need for an acceptance by the parents and to some extent by society itself" ([4], p. 175), if the existence of human life is to be maintained. Under this approach, the fetus is not a child until the decision of the parents "anticipates the human form to come and names it as a subject" ([4], p. 176).

The final Catholic author I would like to consider is Karol Wojtyła, Pope John Paul II. Most of Wojtyła's philosophical writing has centered around the concept of personhood and thus it would be appropriate at this time to consider Wojtyła's insights, since he will very greatly influence the development of Church teaching on this matter in the future.

Most of Wojtyła's considerations of personhood focus upon the notion

of autonomous human action and its resulting structures of self-determination, transcendence, integration, and participation ([19], [22], and [23]).
However, as important as human action is in plumbing the full depths of
the human experience, Wojtyła contends that we also have to consider, in
order to make our account of human personhood complete, all the human
dynamisms by which and through which humans both constitute their world
and are constituted by it. Thus,

. . . the objectification of the fact of 'man-acts' requires an equally objective presentation
of integral human dynamism. For this experiential fact occurs not in isolation but in
the context of the entire human dynamism and in organic relation to it ([19], p. 60).

Wojtyła argues that one of the most basic experiences that we have is the
awareness of the difference between consciously acting and having something
happen to us from within, even though we do not necessarily experience
the latter in its fullness (i.e., there are many dynamisms that never or rarely
come to conscious awareness, e.g. vegetative processes, dreams, and other
subconscious phenomena). He concludes that

. . . having the experience of the two, objectively different structures – of the 'man-acts'
and the 'something-happens-in-him' – together with their differentiation in the field of
experience, provides the evidence, on the one hand, of the essential contiguity of man's
consciousness with his being; on the other hand, the differentiation of experience gives
each of these structures that innerness and subjectiveness which in general we owe to
consciousness ([19], pp. 61–62).

However, these two opposing structures, as different as they are, do not split
the human subject from its basic ontological unity. "Though activeness and
passiveness differentiate the dynamism they do not deprive it of the unity
issuing out of the same dynamic subject; . . . " ([19], p. 64).

Thus, the human being is perceived and experienced by Wojtyła as a
dynamic unity, a dynamic subject, and all efficacy (Wojtyła's word for
human acting) as well as all that happens within "combine together as if
they issued from a common root" ([19], p. 72).

Wojtyła argues that it is precisely because the human subject is at the same
time a *being* that every acting and happening can be rooted in it:

. . . For if the 'something' did not exist, then it could not be the origin and subject of
the dynamism which proceeds from its being, of the acting and the happening. If man
were not to exist, then he would not actually act nor would anything actually happen
in him . . . . The entire dynamism of man's functioning which consists in the acting of,
and happening in, the dynamic subject simultaneously proceeds from (but also enacts)
the initial dynamism due to which a being exists at all ([19], p. 73).

But this being is not merely individual, it is personal. And Wojtyła understands personal as having a completeness "that is unique in a very special sense rather than concrete" ([19], p. 74). This is aptly expressed in English by referring to a person as a 'somebody' rather than as a 'something'. Thus,

... the person, the human being as the person – seen in its ontological basic structure – is the subject of both existence and acting, though it is important to note that the existence proper to him is *personal* and not merely individual – unlike that of an ontologically founded merely individual type of being. Consequently, the action – whereby is meant all the dynamism of man including his acting as well as what happens in him – is also personal ([19], p. 74).

The ontological unity of the human person provides the synthetic ground for those dynamic structures that are differentiated by experience:

... The two structures, that in which man acts, and that in which something happens in man, cut across the phenomenological field of experience, but they join and unite in the metaphysical field. Their synthesis is the man-person, and we discover the ultimate subject of the synthesis in its ontological groundwork ([19], pp. 84–85).

Wojtyła, then, refers to the personal subject as the 'structural nucleus' which is both the basis and source of "not only the dynamism of what happens in man, but also the total dynamism of acting with the conscious efficacy which is constitutive of it" ([19], p. 86). Thus the person is the dynamic subject and causal relation of both actions and activations even though the type of causation in each case is perceived as different.

The experience of the unity and identity of the ego is objectively precedent to and also more fundamental than the experiential separation of acting from happening .... The integration does not abolish the differences in the manner the very structural core of a being is dynamized, but simply prevents any tendency to treat person and nature as two separate and independent subjects of acting .... Nature integrated in the unity of the specific structural nucleus, which is man, would then refer to and indicate a different causal basis of the subject than the person ([19], pp. 81–82).

Wojtyła sees nature as the 'ground of causation' which dynamizes the human individual ultimately in human actions – the most revealing manifestations of personhood. He describes this natural unfolding of personhood as the 'potentiality of the man-subject'. He argues that experience itself makes us aware that both the dynamics of action and activation issue from within, that is, both of these dynamisms are potentially contained within the subject from the beginning. Thus,

... the subject is always one and the same; it is the subject that is all a person, a 'somebody', and does not cease to be a person in the whole sphere of the causations of nature which, as already noted, differs from the causation of the person ([19], p. 90).

With this philosophical stance as a background, I will now turn to Wojtyła's convictions about personhood as it applies to fetal life. In a homily given on the Smithsonian Mall in Washington, D.C., Wojtyła proclaimed that human life is sacred because it is created in the image and likeness of God, and that human life should be protected from conception onwards "in regard to the majesty of the Creator, who is the first giver of this life", and also because life is "the expression and the fruit of love" ([21], p. 277). Each of these claims, it appears to me, are based upon different grounds. The last claim, being both normative and experiential, is based both on ethical and empirical grounds. The second claim is specifically religious, and would only have validity for those who share Wojtyła's own religious presuppositions and would surely not be compelling as the basis of a claim of human personal rights, including the right to life. It is only the first claim, even though clothed in religious language, which is based on metaphysical grounds. Wojtyła would claim that human life is created in the image and likeness of God precisely because of his conviction that it is personal. As he states elsewhere,

... Man is a person 'by nature', by which he is entitled to the subjectivity proper to a person. The fact that in some cases the human subject or metaphysical subjectivity does not manifest the characteristics of personal subjectivity (as in the case of psychosomatic or purely psychical deficiencies in which the normal human self fails to develop or becomes deformed) does not authorize doubt concerning the foundations of this subjectivity, since they are inherent in the essentially human subject ([22], p. 277).

Although I believe that Wojtyła would say, on both religious grounds and grounds which relate to his understanding of human sexuality, that the reproductive process ought never to be interfered with (his position on this being very close to that of the Sacred Congregation for the Doctrine of the Faith discussed above), he is more ambiguous as to when he believes personhood actually begins.

Wojtyła says that "man is somebody from the very moment of his coming into existence" ([19], p. 180), and that "in the metaphysical sense he has from the beginning been somebody" ([23], p. 41). The problem is that he never defines this 'beginning' or 'coming into existence' in any kind of chronological way. He does make reference to a personal right to life "at the moment in which he is first conceived in his mother's womb" ([21], p. 277), and even identifies this as the time when ensoulment takes place:

... Nonetheless, at the moment at which a new human is conceived, a new spirit is conceived at the same time, substantially united to the body of the embryo which begins to exist in the womb of its mother ([20], p. 45, translation mine).

Some might be tempted to say that Wojtyła is claiming in these statements that human personal life begins from fertilization onwards, but I believe he is being intentionally vague. For in the same work in which he talks about ensoulment as described above, he presents an appendix which clearly shows him to be aware of the fact that fertilization takes place, not in the mother's womb, but in the Fallopian tubes. In addition, in both cases cited above, Wojtyła speaks of conception rather than fertilization, conception being a term that can signify the implantation of the blastocyst in the womb as well as the process of fertilization itself. I believe that Wojtyła is allowing himself the philosophical leeway not to claim personhood until individuation is established biologically, since he relies so heavily on the notion of 'metaphysical subjectivity' as the criterion for calling a being a 'somebody' rather than a 'something'.

I would therefore contend that Wojtyła's position on the beginning of personhood is similar to that of Diamond and Pastrana, because to call an entity a 'someone' for Wojtyła means that the being in question must be the personal subject of experiences, even if these are only of the 'what-happens-in-man' variety (i.e., activations).

Since the spiritual soul neither makes persons divisible into parts nor allows them to be assumed into some higher synthesis, it must be held that these potentialities (evident in the case of identical twins and chimerism) precede ensoulment (the coming into existence of a person), but ultimately provide a level of biological organization that makes ensoulment possible. Because Wojtyła does not see personhood as rooted in consciousness, he would not need to wait until brain structure has developed before affirming personhood as Donceel has argued we should do. Once a 'metaphysical subject', i.e., an individuated organism, has the capacity of 'something-happens-in-me' type of experiences, not on a conscious level but on the level of becoming, it is enough for Wojtyła to establish personhood, at least on the metaphysical level.

I have now considered several official and speculative Roman Catholic views on the concept of person and the implications these concepts have for the ontological status of the unborn. I hope that their presentation will continute to stimulate the dialogue already begun among many different schools of thought on this most vexing issue.

Biscayne College,
Miami, Florida

BIBLIOGRAPHY

1. Barry, R., O. P.: 1978, 'Personhood: The Conditions of Identification and Description', *Linacre Quarterly* **45**, 64–81.
2. Connery, J., S. J.: 1977, *Abortion: The Development of the Roman Catholic Perspective*, Loyola University Press, Chicago.
3. Culliton, J. T.: 1978, 'Rahner on the Origin of the Soul: Some Implications Regarding Abortion', *Thought* **53**, 203–214.
4. Curran, C. E.: 1973, 'Abortion: Law and Morality in Contemporary Catholic Theology', *The Jurist* **33**, 162–182.
5. Diamond, J. J.: 1975, 'Abortion, Animation, and Biological Hominization', *Theological Studies* **36**, 305–324.
6. Donceel, J. F.: 1970, 'Immediate Animation and Delayed Hominization', *Theological Studies* **31**, 76–105.
7. Haering, B.: 1976, 'New Dimensions of Parenthood', *Theological Studies* **37**, 120–132.
8. Hellegers, A.: 1970, 'Fetal Development', *Theological Studies* **31**, 3–9.
9. McCormick, R.: 1974, 'Notes on Moral Theology: The Abortion Dossier', *Theological Studies* **35**, 312–359.
10. Nicholson, S. T.: 1978, *JRE Studies in Religious Ethics II: Abortion and the Roman Catholic Church*, Religious Ethics Inc., Knoxville.
11. Pastrana, G.: 1977, 'Personhood at the Beginning of Human Life', *Thomist* **41**, 247–294.
12. Pohier, J. M.: 1972, 'Reflexions théologiques sur la position de l'église catholique', *Lumière et Vie* **XXI**, n. 109 (août-octobre), p. 84.
13. Quelquejeu, B.: 1972, 'La volonté de procréer', *Lumière et Vie* **XXI**, note 9 (août-octobre), p. 67.
14. Rahner, K.: 1968, *Hominization: The Evolutionary Origin of Man as a Theological Problem*, Herder and Herder, New York.
15. Rahner, K.: 1975, 'The Problem of Genetic Manipulation', *Theological Investigations* **9**, 225–252.
16. Sacred Congregation for the Doctrine of the Faith: 1975, 'Declaration on Procured Abortion', *Linacre Quarterly* **2**, 132–147.
17. Schoonenberg, P.: 1964, *God's World in the Making*, Duquesne University Press, Pittsburgh.
18. Strawson, P. F.: 1959, *Individuals: An Essay in Descriptive Metaphysics*, Methuen, London.
19. Wojtyła, K.: 1979, *The Acting Person*, D. Reidel Publ. Co., Dordrecht, Holland.
20. Wojtyła, K.: 1978, *Amore e Responsabilità*, Marietti, Turin.
21. Wojtyła, K.: 1979, 'Homily at Mass on Washington Mall, Oct. 7, 1979', in *John Paul II, "Pilgrimage of Faith"*, The Seabury Press, New York, pp. 276–278.
22. Wojtyła, K.: 1979, 'The Person: Subject and Community', *The Review of Metaphysics* **33**, 293–285.
23. Wojtyła, K.: 1975, 'The Structure of Self-Determination as the Core of the Theory of the Person', *Tommasso d'Aquino nel suo settimo centenario, Atti del Congresso Internazionale* **7**, 37–44.

MARY ANN GARDELL

MORAL PLURALISM IN ABORTION

The essays in this volume attempt to secure an understanding of the status of the fetus and the ethical issues at stake in the development of practices regarding the fetus. On first inspection, the conclusions drawn by many of the authors may seem disparate and incommensurate. This pluralism of conclusions, theoretical frameworks, historical traditions, and methodologies in the discussion of the status of the fetus and morality of abortion is not only the concern in this essay, it is in fact the condition in which moral philosophy finds itself when confronted with any of the numerous moral dilemmas of the twentieth century. Moral pluralism is the condition of human existence in the absence of a generally convincing Divine Revelation or the imposition by force of an orthodoxy of belief. The abortion debate thus reveals the character of the moral conflicts arising in Post-Christian, politically free, industrial societies. One need not expect that an assessment of this moral pluralism will conclude on a pessimistic note. Rather, and in line with Engelhardt's [2] suggestion, I will argue that the state of moral pluralism characterizing the abortion debate reflects an acceptance of both the limitations of human reason, and of the obligation to respect the autonomy of competent individuals. Considering the precedence of centuries of the imposition of moral orthodoxies by force, this acceptance is no small accomplishment. In fact, it is a point to be celebrated.

To appreciate the pluralism of beliefs at stake regarding abortion, one might begin with the observation that Fathers McCartney [7] and Moraczewski [8] hold distinct views about the fetus and its importance in the development of practices regarding the fetus. Though these two Catholic theologians share a methodological tradition (e.g., a somewhat common understanding of theology), and in fact a religious tradition (Roman Catholicism), they draw divergent conclusions: while McCartney holds that the human conceptus acquires personhood sometime *after* conception ([7], p. 322), Moraczewski is convinced that the human conceptus "is an existing and actual person, integrated and *inner*-directed to the full realization of his or her personhood" ([8], p. 308) from the moment of conception. Evidence from the historico-theological rootage of Roman Catholicism accounts for the competing views. Consider the argument developed by St. Thomas Aquinas (1225–1274) in

William B. Bondeson et al. *(eds.), Abortion and the Status of the Fetus*, 325–331.

Summa Theologica (Part 1, Ques. 118, Art. 2), which can be interpreted as
an influence on the position espoused by McCartney. The infusion of the
vegetative or plant soul is followed by the sentient or animal soul; both
precede God's endowing the spiritual or human soul. It is at this point in
human ontological development that the spiritual soul is infused and the
unique, never-to-be-repeated individual being may be said to exist. This view
of the evolutionary ontogeny of humans was to find its full development after
Darwin in the late nineteenth century (e.g., as expressed in Ernst Haeckel's
(1834–1919) understanding of embryology ([4], [5])), and even later in the
twentieth century by members of the Church (e.g., Pierre Teilhard de Chardin
[15]). Moraczeswki in contrast draws upon non-developmental metaphysical
views of human ontogeny in order to assert the appearance of persons
instantaneously and coincident with the formation of the first biological
individuality. One finds then a conflict derived from differences in metaphysical viewpoints, though both agree with respect to the ontological claim
that there is an immortal soul endowed by God, the Creator. Here, authors
who presuppose a uniformity of belief turn out to support a pluralism of
convictions.

   In contrast, the authors who recognize the inevitability of pluralism of
beliefs, come to remarkably similar conclusions. The essays in this volume
by the biomedical scientists and lawyers, for example, provide a study of
reflections by individuals working with different methodologies who yet
arrive at similiar views of the task at hand with respect to abortion. Professor
Biggers [1], for instance, suggests that developmental physiology provides
the empirical content necessary to answer what he sees as a fundamental
question of immediate concern in the abortion debate, namely, when does
life begin? He sees the answer to be one of clarification on both the ontological and normative levels of analysis. Ontologically speaking, life has been
continuous in evolution from its beginning billions of years ago. This is not
to say that all life at whatever stage of evolutionary ontogeny holds equal
moral status. Rather, the pending issue in contemporary moral debates on
abortion is a normative one, namely, when to treat human life, e.g., egg,
sperm, fertilized ovum, blastula, morula, or any of the developmental stages,
as involving the life of a person. Working within a different historical and
methodological tradition, Professor White [18] observes that the law plays
a crucial role in the analysis of the concept of person and its relationship
to the ethical use of the fetus in biomedicine. Since the function of the law
is to prescribe and proscribe the behavior of persons toward others, it reflects
a community's commitment in different ways not only to the person who

carries the 'to-be-aborted entity', but also to the fetus as the 'person-to-be'. In her historical overview of the American law's attempt to define 'person', White can find no single concept of person 'in the whole sense' and is led to conclude that "(t)here is no single shortcut to deciding the answers to the increasingly difficult moral questions that the phenomenal growth of biomedical capability has thrust so urgently upon us" ([18], p. 130). While Biggers remains optimistic about the ability of biomedicine to provide background data for technical problem-solving, White underscores the challenges involved in fashioning public policy solutions. Despite these dissimilarities, Biggers and White share a common vantage point and task: they recognize the fragmented notions of modern ethical viewpoints [1], encourage clarification and synthesis of the evaluative considerations of the facts at the core of the abortion debate [2], and envision a future which involves fashioning common bases for cooperation [3].

In contrast with McCartney and Moraczewski, Biggers and White recognize the condition in which contemporary moral philosophy finds itself when confronted with any of the numerous moral dilemmas of the twentieth century. What marks the dilemma of modern men and women is not disagreement over diverging accounts of human ensoulment by a Creator, but rather the realization that they live in a Post-Christian, industrial society that spans from America to Japan. Further, there is the realization that we do not share a common moral understanding of the nature of the fetus, the morality of abortion, and the moral significance of sexuality. Since moral fragments are created within particular moral communities, and since nations such as America are not *one* community with regard to a number of moral issues, much cannot be decided as an element of national morality. The problem is then the extent to which any common moral consensus can be found. That is, the charge is rationally and generally to establish moral claims. Much to the contemporary philosopher's dismay, there is no way to unitarily accept this challenge. For example, where Engelhardt [2] holds that certain moral constraints can be discovered in the very notion of a pluralistic and peaceful community in which respect for the freedom of the members of such communities is essential (fetuses not being self-conscious, are not free), Professor Solomon [13] is convinced that Engelhardt's optimism is without grounding.

Consider in greater detail how Engelhardt and Solomon compare. According to Engelhardt, persons in the strict sense are self-conscious, rational, self-determining ([2], p. 184), "moral agents of the universe" ([2], p. 185). Since fetuses do not possess these characteristics, they cannot be considered persons in and of themselves and "therefore need not be extended the special protection we give to persons' ([2], p. 184). In terms of public policy making: if persons (e.g., women) are to be respected as the very condition for the possibility of a peaceable society, then a criterion of viability, namely, one "*not* based on the capacity of medical knowledge to render fetuses viable, but rather one based on the need to allow sufficient latitude for women to make their own decisions ... " ([2], p. 195) needs to be developed with regard to abortion. On this view, a rationally defensible view of the status of the fetus and of the morality of abortion is possible.

In contrast to Engelhardt, Solomon rejects the contention that a rationally defensible view of the status of the fetus or of the 'intrinsic worth' of persons can be established. Instead, he is convinced that "there is no answer (to the abortion dilemma), because there is no single principle or ontology that we can agree upon in this still (thankfully) heterogeneous and pluralistic society" ([13], p. 223). At best there can only be agreement on the level of the extrinsic worth or value that the fetus might have to members of a particular moral community. Yet, this agreement is open to change at any time and is not subject to rational assessment across communities with widely differing moral commitments. In this assertion, Solomon suggests that moral pluralism is none other than moral relativism or subjectivism.

However, despite the disagreement, one must note what is shared in Engelhardt and Solomon's approaches. Both are working with the recognition of the pluralism of beliefs or values that marks the contrast of modern societies. Both seek a rational framework in which rules and principles could constrain and guide all moral agents in light of the realization that concrete moral viewpoints can be framed only within particular historical contexts. Here in varying degrees they join C. L. Stevenson [14], Thomas Nagel [9], and Alastair MacIntyre [6] in the view that there is no single and univocal view of morality since concrete moral principles and values or beliefs are relative to individuals or communities.

In *After Virtue*, MacIntyre attempts to account for this state of moral relativism or pluralism in twentieth century moral philosophy. What we possess today, he affirms,

are fragments of a conceptual scheme, parts of which now lack those contexts from which their significance derived. We possess simulacra of morality, we continue to use many of the key expressions ... we have − very largely, if not entirely − lost our comprehension, both theoretical and practical, of morality ([6], p. 2).

With MacIntyre, Engelhardt and Solomon recognize the pluralism of normative principles and metaethical presumptions in contemporary society.

Since Solomon foresees no possible resolution to this untidy circumstance, he in part joins MacIntyre in his lament over the state of contemporary moral philosophy. In contrast, Engelhardt holds that a rational and peaceable solution to a state of widely divergent moral viewpoints may be obtained. His view is allied with Nagel's as expressed in 'The Fragmentation of Value' [9]. Both view the condition of moral pluralism as the result of a loss of the presumption that there will in the end be a single and univocal view of the good life that can and ought to be embraced. Engelhardt holds that answers can be negotiated or created relying on what one might term the very grammar of the ethical enterprise: commitment to the mutual respect of moral agents.

While this volume may not succeed in producing a final understanding of the status of the fetus and the morality of abortion, it can at least show what is not likely to be secured by general rational argument: namely, that the fetus is a person and that abortion is a serious moral wrong. After all, the burden of proof is on those who would wish to make such bold claims. Such claims are likely to be securable, if at all, only within particular communities already sharing a number of normative and metaethical assumptions. This, in itself, is conclusion enough with regard to the morality of proscribing abortion by law in societies constituted out of numerous communities with radically divergent opinions regarding the status of the fetus. But this point is part of a yet larger view. One may be witnessing the loss of what Engelhardt has called the monotheistic presumption in ethics: that there is one univocal moral viewpoint. When societies were marked by one orthodox interpretation of a monotheistically grounded ethics, there was the presumption that reason could establish one concrete moral viewpoint. It is clear that this is no longer the case. While MacIntyre laments the contemporary state of moral philosophy, Engelhardt celebrates this return to the polytheistic presumption that there are numerous communities each following their own gods, living together peaceably. This is a tradition closer to the presumptions of our pagan polytheistic forebears with regard to abortion and the purposes of sex. Having passed through and learned much from the Christian orthodoxy which constrained and instructed the West over the past millennium and a half, we are today confronted with the realization that there is no longer a reasonable presumption that one will be able to deliver a single, rational, and concrete view of moral life. Abortions will not be forbidden though many may hold them to be immoral. Sexual pleasures will be pursued by some as ends in themselves though many will hold that to be immoral. In short, the abortion debate as a controversy illustrating the untidiness of moral pluralism reflects an acceptance of the limitations of human reason and the obligation to respect the self-determination of competent individuals.

This returns us to the articles by Feen [3], McCartney [7], and Moraczewski [8] who sketch various approaches to this control of human reproduction through abortion and infanticide. Given the assessment that I forward of our condition of moral pluralism, their articles suggest our present approach in fact constitutes an historic compromise. On the one hand, the Greek approach allowed the avoidance of unwanted births and of defective children through abortion and infanticide. On the other hand, the Christian approach traditionally forbade both of these. With the collapse of the Christian world beginning in the West, and with the availability of not only effective contraception and safe abortion techniques but prenatal diagnosis as well, much of the need for infanticide, recognized in Greek customs and in formal practices generally has disappeared. Abortion and this current treatment of fetuses as non-personal, albeit human biological life, is a middle way between interests seeking respect for human life on the one hand, and the rights of women and the avoidance of unwanted births on the other. In short, the Feen article and the McCartney and Moraczewski articles seen against the backdrop of the other articles in this volume help us to recognize better the historical significance of *Roe v. Wade* [10] as a compromise between competing moral interests, given the recognition of new technological abilities, the pluralism of moral beliefs, and the rights of persons.

Center for Ethics, Medicine, and Public Issues
Baylor College of Medicine, Houston, Texas

NOTES

[1] Professors Feen [3] and Perkoff [11] provide a background substantiating the observation that morals are culture-laden, resulting in a clash between incompatible ethical valuations of fundamental disagreement.

[2] What is at stake in the abortion debate is not such facts as those of fetal physiological development, its biological relationship (or dependence) to its mother, or any other datum discoverable by methods used in the natural sciences, but rather the evaluation of these facts by members of society. This point finds emphasis in Professor Whitbeck's essay [17].

[3] Fashioning an answer is to be distinguished from discovering a correct truth. Walters' essay [16] is a core study of a collaborative investigation of individuals interested in formulating guidelines for ethical research involving fetuses. In other to attain this goal, peaceful harmonization of the divergent views of the participants on the status of the fetus and its ethical importance in the development of research practices is essential.

BIBLIOGRAPHY

1. Biggers, J. D.: 1983, 'Generation of the Human Life Cycle', in this volume, pp. 31–53.
2. Engelhardt, H. T., Jr.: 1983, 'Viability and the Use of the Fetus', in this volume, pp. 183–208.
3. Feen, R. H.: 1983, 'Abortion and Exposure in Ancient Greece: Assessing the Status of the Fetus and 'Newborn' from Classical Sources', in this volume, pp. 283–300.
4. Haeckel, E.: 1897, *The Evolution of Man*, D. Appleton, New York.
5. Haeckel, E.: 1866, *Generelle Morphologie der Organismen*, George Reimer, Berlin.
6. MacIntyre, A.: 1981, *After Virtue*, University of Notre Dame Press, Indiana.
7. McCartney, J. J.: 1983, 'Some Roman Catholic Concepts of Person and Their Implications for the Ontological Status of the Unborn', in this volume, pp. 313–323.
8. Moraczewski, A. S.: 1983, 'Human Personhood: A Study in Person-alized Biology', in this volume, pp. 301–311.
9. Nagel, T.: 1977, 'The Fragmentation of Value', in H. T. Engelhardt, Jr. and D. Callahan (eds.), *Knowledge, Value, and Belief*, the Hastings Center, New York, pp. 274–294.
10. *Roe v. Wade*, 410 U.S. 113 (1973).
11. Perkoff, G. T.: 1983, 'Toward a Normative Definition of Personhood', in this volume, pp. 159–166.
12. Shannon, T. A.: 1983, 'Abortion: A Challenge for Ethics and Public Policy', in this volume, pp. 3–14.
13. Solomon, R.: 1983, 'Reflections on the Meaning of (Fetal) Life', in this volume, pp. 209–226.
14. Stevenson, C. L.: 1963, *Facts and Values*, Yale University Press, New Haven, Connecticut, Chapter 3.
15. Teilhard de Chardin, P.: 1959, *The Future of Man*, trans. N. Denny, Harper Torchbooks, New York.
16. Walters, L.: 1983, 'The Fetus in Ethical and Public Policy Discussion from 1973 to the Present', in this volume, pp. 15–30.
17. Whitbeck, C.: 1983, 'The Moral Implications of Regarding Women as People: New Perspectives on Pregnancy and Personhood', in this volume, pp. 247–272.
18. White, P. D.: 1983, 'The Concept of Person, the Law, and the Use of the Fetus in Biomedicine', in this volume, pp. 119–157.

CONCLUDING REMARKS

Neither this section nor this volume comes to a single conclusion. That is not unexpected in a pluralist society where in addition to a general secular viewpoint there are the views of disparate religious and metaphysical communities. However, there is a convergence of views among the essays written from a secular perspective: there are no general strong arguments available to hold abortion to be a serious moral matter. To perceive abortion as a serious moral problem requires a set of very particular moral premises not generally supportable without special metaphysical or ethical assumptions. Similarly, one can understand within a particular religious or metaphysical viewpoint why oral intercourse should be considered a very serious moral offense [9], or why Kant, given his particular moral commitments, apart from his general philosophical arguments, would hold masturbation to be one of the most heinous of crimes [6]. But there are no general warrants for such positions [5]. One needs special religious or metaphysical views regarding the immorality or sinfulness of certain sexual acts to justify such condemnations. The problem of the morality of abortion would appear to have analogies to such moral issues. As a result, one would expect general societal policy to shift to the acceptance of abortion, as it becomes more widely appreciated that strong moral condemnation of abortion depends upon moral premises not generally available in a secular pluralist society. One finds, thus, that even in a nominally Catholic country such as Italy the use of abortion is accepted. There were, for example, 345.3 abortions for every 1000 live births in Italy in 1980 [12]. These changes, however, were not made without the usual societal agonies involved in reassessing the cardinal ethical presuppositions of public policy.

The continuing disputes regarding the morality of abortion are indices of a major conceptual shift that is taking place in our culture regarding the significance of sexuality, reproduction, the status of fetuses, and the rights of women. As the essays in this volume show, these current controversies have deep classical roots. They are a part of the ongoing endeavor of persons to understand the meaning of their development as humans. The availability of cheap and efficient means of procuring abortion with less risk to a woman than a full-term pregnancy forwards abortion as a reasonable second means

William B. Bondeson et al. *(eds.), Abortion and the Status of the Fetus*, 333–336.

of choice for controlling unwanted pregnancies. Indeed, current information suggests that the risk of dying during childbirth is ten times greater than that from abortion, up through the fifteenth week of pregnancy [4]. Further, the availability of genetic knowledge and the capacity to know in advance whether a particular fetus is severely deformed raises the issue of whether abortion would not be morally obligatory, or at least praiseworthy, under such circumstances. Indeed, one must wonder why a technique which so increases the freedom of women and which avoids such undesirable outcomes as unwanted or defective children could be held to be morally problematic.

The essays in this section should in part suggest why abortion is seen to be morally suspect, at least in the minds of many in our culture. The contributions of Feen, Moraczewski, and McCartney sketch the moral and particularly theological roots of much of our current debates. To understand the moral controversies engendered by abortion, one must, as these essays show, place them in a particular culture which views fetuses as persons, harbors suspicions regarding the manipulation of life, or considers the separation of the recreational and reproductive dimensions of sexuality to be improper. But beyond the backdrop of any particular culture, abortion is likely to be troubling because it alters major assumptions of most traditional societies. Men and women alike have traditionally been seen as instruments of social and communal goals. It has thus been natural to view them as reproductive units for the state or for society. There has in addition been an acceptance, at times stoical, of nature and its processes. The ready availability of safe and efficient means of abortion calls these assumptions into question.

Abortion is becoming a linchpin of modern culture. It marks one of the elements of viewing women as free participants in society. It requires them to be regarded no longer as producers of children for the community or for the state. It requires a further departure from what Robert Nozick has termed ownership of the people by the people [10]. By placing reproductive decisions in the hands of women, even to the point of deciding on the quality of the children they will bear, it offers a special liberation from state and communal reproductive policies. Individuals become arbiters of their own reproductive destinies. As such, abortion fulfills and completes the liberation offered through effective contraception, in that it provides not only a safeguard should contraception fail, but a means, with prenatal testing, for choosing the quality of reproductive outcomes. This offers not simply a social liberation but a liberation from the blind forces of nature.

It is in this sense, as has already been observed in this volume, that not only contraception and abortion are unnatural, but transplantation of organs and immunization as well. Modern medical technology liberates by setting the blind forces of nature under the control of medicine. It personalizes nature in the sense of fashioning nature in the image and likeness of the goals and aspirations of persons. Such powers introduce new responsibilities and require new virtues of prudence and circumspection. Further, they augment the human world by increasing the powers of persons to do that which is reasonable, compassionate, and loving. In this sense Joseph Fletcher is correct in holding that controlled reproduction is the most truly human reproduction, in that it can represent the responsible choices of free persons [7]. If, as many of the papers have argued in this volume, fetuses are not persons, and there is no serious moral evil involved in the destruction of mere human biological life, then the only true moral constraints upon the use of abortion are those obligations one fashions freely with others. Abortion then becomes a morally neutral instrument often uniquely appropriate for the realization of important moral goals.

Since such an understanding of abortion requires major shifts in traditional cultural attitudes, it can be accepted only with time. Even Japan, a predominantly non-Christian country with over thirty-five years' history of fairly easy access to abortion, still shows some signs of ambivalence [8]. In our own culture it should be quite clear that the conflicting views are even more bitterly and starkly drawn. They range from a reported kidnapping of a physician-owner of an abortion clinic by a group styled the Army of God [11], to continued condemnations of abortion by Pope John Paul II [2] and President Ronald Reagan [1]. The acceptance of divergent views of the significance of sexuality and reproduction, and tolerance of the free choices of individuals in these matters, has been hard fought. It has been nearly a decade and a half since the case of Norma McCorvey, a young divorcee gang-raped and lacking funds to go outside of Texas to secure an abortion began to move to the Supreme Court and make judicial history, as the case of *Roe v. Wade* [3]. The decade since *Roe v. Wade* has shown if anything the possibility of in fact living with divergent views regarding the morality of abortion and of allowing women the freedom of abortion on request.

Though such divergent views are likely to endure, a secular morality regarding abortion is in fact developing and is required as the possibility of a tolerant society. Even if particular religious or cultural groups see abortion as immoral, such will be, as essays in this volume argue, a difficult proposition to sustain on general secular premises alone. The very notion of a community peaceably spanning divergent moral viewpoints requires contribution to this major intellectual task: the fashioning of its own moral presuppositions [5].

This volume is offered as a moral language to span numerous moral communities with divergent viewpoints with regard to the propriety of abortion and the personal control of reproduction. This task is integral to the perennial endeavor of philosophy and the special undertaking of the philosophy of medicine.

BIBLIOGRAPHY

1. Anonymous: 1983, 'Reagan Endorses Anti-Abortion Bill', *Houston Chronicle* (January 23), 1–8.
2. Anonymous: 1983, 'What's News: World-Wide', *The Wall Street Journal* (January 19), 1.
3. Brasher, P.: 1983, ' "Jane Roe": Woman Behind Landmark Ruling on Abortion Says Battle Worth it', *Houston Chronicle* (January 22), 6–8.
4. Cates, W., Jr., *et al.*: 1982, 'Mortality from Abortion and Childbirth', *Journal of the American Medical Association* 248 (July 9), 192–196.
5. Engelhardt, H. T., Jr.: 1982, 'Bioethics in a Pluralist Society', *Perspectives in Biology and Medicine* 26 (Fall), 64–78.
6. Kant, I.: 1963, *Lectures on Ethics*, Harper Torchback, New York, p. 170.
7. Fletcher, J.: 1960, *Morals and Medicine*, Beacon Press, Boston, pp. 222–223.
8. Lehner, U.: 1983, 'Japanese Ceremonies Show Private Doubts Over Use of Abortion', *The Wall Street Journal* (January 6), 1, 11.
9. Noonan, J. T., Jr.: 1966, *Abortion*, Harvard University Press, Cambridge, Mass.
10. Nozick, R.: 1974, *Anarchy, State, and Utopia*, Basic Books, New York, pp. 289–290.
11. Peter, B.: 1982, 'Kidnapping Focuses Tensions and Fears on Abortion Clinic', *The Washington Post* (August 22), A2.
12. Tosi, S. L., M. E. Grandolfo, and A. Spinelli: 1983, 'Legal Abortion in Italy', *New England Journal of Medicine* 308 (January 6), 51–52.

NOTES ON CONTRIBUTORS

George J. Agich, Ph.D., is Associate Professor, Department of Medical Humanities, Department of Psychiatry, Southern Illinois University, School of Medicine, Springfield, Illinois.

John D. Biggers, Ph.D., is Professor of Physiology, Department of Physiology and Laboratory for Human Reproduction and Reproductive Biology, Harvard Medical School, Boston, Massachusetts.

H. Tristram Engelhardt, Jr., Ph.D., M.D., is Professor, Center for Ethics, Medicine, and Public Issues, Baylor College of Medicine, Houston, Texas.

Richard Harrow Feen, Ph.D., is currently writing a book on the evolving moral basis of Greek medicine. He was recently a post-doctoral student at Harvard Divinity School as well as a University Chapel Associate at Tufts University, Boston.

Mary Ann Gardell, B.S., M.A., Research Associate, Center for Ethics, Medicine, and Public Issues, Baylor College of Medicine, Houston, Texas.

Leonard Glantz, J.D., is Assistant Professor of Law and Medicine, Department of Socio-Medical Sciences and Community Medicine, Boston University Medical Center, Boston, Massachusetts.

Rev. James J. McCartney, OSA, Ph.D., is Dean of the College, Biscayne College, Miami, Florida.

Rev. Albert S. Moraczewski, O.P., Ph.D., is Vice President of Research, Pope John XXIII Medical-Moral Research and Education Center, St. Louis, Missouri.

Gerald T. Perkoff, M.D., is Curator's Professor and Associate Chairman, Department of Family and Community Medicine; Director, Robert Wood Johnson Family Practice Academic Fellowship Program; and Professor of Medicine, University of Missouri-Columbia, Columbia, Missouri.

Roland Puccetti, Ph.D., is Professor, Department of Philosophy, Dalhousie University, Halifax, Nova Scotia, Canada.

Nancy L. Schimmel, J.D., is an attorney at the Law Division of the First National Bank of Chicago, Illinois.

Thomas A. Shannon, Ph.D., is Associate Professor of Social Ethics, Worcester Polytechnic Institute, Worcester, Massachusetts.

337

Margery W. Shaw, M.D., J.D., is Director, School of Biomedical Sciences, The University of Texas Health Science Center at Houston, Houston, Texas.

Holly M. Smith, Ph.D., is Professor, Department of Philosophy, University of Illinois at Chicago Circle, College of Liberal Arts and Sciences, Chicago, Illinois.

Robert C. Solomon, Ph.D., is Professor, Department of Philosophy, The University of Texas at Austin, Austin, Texas.

Pierre Soupart, M.D., Ph.D., was Professor of Obstetrics and Gynecology, Vanderbilt University School of Medicine, Nashville, Tennessee. He died on July 10, 1981.

LeRoy Walters, Ph.D., is Director, Center for Bioethics, Kennedy Institute of Ethics, Georgetown University, Washington, D.C.

Caroline Whitbeck, Ph.D., is Associate Professor at the MGH Institute, Boston, Massachusetts, and Research Fellow, Center for Policy Alternatives, M.I.T., Cambridge, Massachusetts.

Patricia D. White, J.D., is Associate Professor of Law, Georgetown University Law Center, Washington, D.C.

INDEX